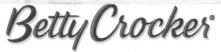
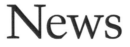

News

FOR IMMEDIATE RELEASE:
Contact: Claire Holzman / 201-748-5627 / cholzman@wiley.com

An inspiring special edition published in partnership with
Susan G. Komen for the Cure® and General Mills' Pink Together

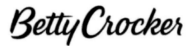

Living with Cancer Cookbook
Pink Together Edition

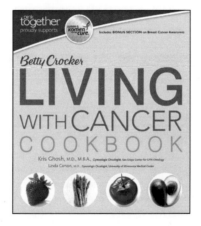

By Kris Ghosh, M.D., M.B.A and Linda Carson, M.D.

Plus a Message from Nancy G. Brinker
Founder & CEO of Susan G. Komen for the Cure®

Having a diagnosis of cancer rearranges your life and priorities. Many things change, including what used to be the simple tasks of cooking and eating. Nutrition is a critical factor in the fight against cancer, and patients searching for information on how to change their diet need look no further than **BETTY CROCKER LIVING WITH CANCER COOKBOOK PINK TOGETHER EDITION** (Wiley Paperback; September 26, 2011; $19.99)—a collection of more than 150 delicious recipes that provide the best in nutrition without sacrificing taste. Written with the expertise of two oncologists, along with a nutritionist, and presented in Betty Crocker's friendly and authoritative style, this book tackles the challenge of eating while undergoing treatment.

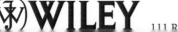

111 River Street • Hoboken, NJ 07030-5774

Partnering with Susan G. Komen for the Cure® and the General Mills' Pink Together initiative, this special edition also includes a 32-page section filled with additional nourishing recipes, thoughtful ideas, and inspiring stories from Pink Together Ambassadors. Pink Together selects five Survivor Ambassadors each year, and their stories and personal photographs will bring an uplifting note to this publication.

BETTY CROCKER LIVING WITH CANCER COOKBOOK PINK TOGETHER EDITION is designed for those undergoing cancer treatment as well as their care-takers. All recipes are geared for easy preparation for both patients—often tired from treatment—and non-cooks, such as a spouse or child who are helping out with the cooking.

Recipes are flagged throughout to show which ones can help mitigate the four most common side effects of cancer treatment: nausea, mouth sores, diarrhea, and constipation. Dr. Kris Ghosh also answers specific questions submitted by real patients on how to handle these side effects, with suggested recipes interspersed in a Q&A format.

Chapters like "Fatigue Fighting Snacks" and "Make-Ahead Meals" really speak to the needs of those going through treatment. Readers will also find a 7-day menu plan based on six small meals and snacks spread throughout the day.

With all-new design and photography, **BETTY CROCKER LIVING WITH CANCER COOKBOOK PINK TOGETHER EDITION** combines the nutritious recipes and health information that patients need with personal stories of survival that can inspire them to keep fighting and winning the battle against cancer.

ABOUT BETTY CROCKER
With more than 63 million cookbooks sold since 1950, Betty Crocker is the name readers trust for reliable, tasty, easy-to-prepare recipes and great ideas. For over 75 years, Betty Crocker has provided advice to millions of Americans through cookbooks, magazines, radio, and television.

ABOUT GENERAL MILLS and PINK TOGETHER
Launched in 2005, Pink Together is a national breast cancer awareness program that engages half a million breast cancer survivors and the many people supporting them in a unique online community. Susan G. Komen for the Cure® is proud to be the beneficiary of the Pink Together™ program. During the month of October, General Mills' iconic brands will turn the packaging pink in recognition of National Breast Cancer Awareness Month and Komen for the Cure®. General Mills' Pink Together program has contributed over $10 Million to Susan G Komen for the Cure®

Visit the website at www.pinktogether.com.

Living with Cancer Pink Together Cookbook
Betty Crocker Editors
Wiley Paperback | September 26, 2011 | $19.99 | ISBN: 978-1-1180-8314-7 | 288 pages

Withdrawn from
Troy Public Library

Betty Crocker®
LIVING
WITH CANCER

pink together edition

WILEY

John Wiley & Sons, Inc.

Nancy G. Brinker

Ambassador Nancy G. Brinker is the Founder and CEO of Susan G. Komen for the Cure®. She has served as Ambassador to Hungary and the United States Chief of Protocol and is currently the Goodwill Ambassador for Cancer Control for the United Nations World Health Organization. She has been the recipient of many prestigious awards, including the 2009 Presidential Medal of Freedom, the nation's highest civilian honor.

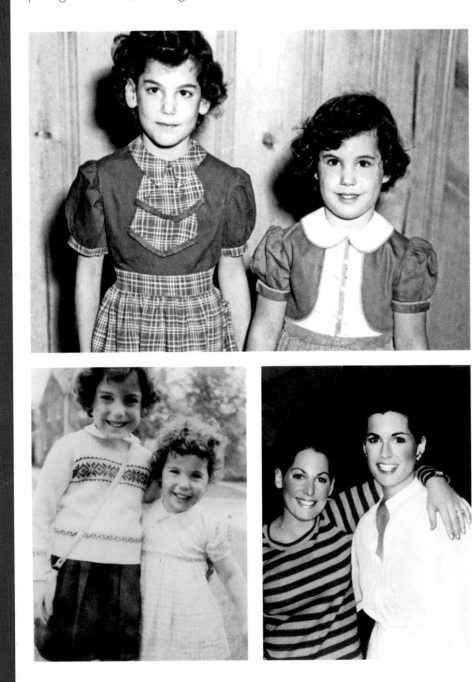

The Goodman sisters were always close, and a promise between them launched the global movement to end breast cancer. **Susan G. Komen,** who died of breast cancer at age 36, is on the left, and **Nancy G. Brinker,** who founded Susan G. Komen for the Cure® to rid the world of this disease, is on the right in all three photos.

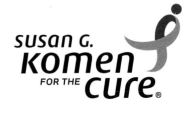

A Message from Ambassador Nancy G. Brinker

Founder and CEO of Susan G. Komen for the Cure®

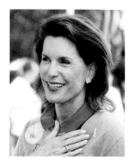

My sister Suzy was born in Peoria, Illinois, in the fall of 1943. She was three years old when I was born.

Suzy and I grew up watching our parents put faith into action. We learned the importance of volunteering and people coming together with a purpose. Suzy was the queen bee of the neighborhood—she was very sweet, but she had a mischievous streak. When Suzy was grounded, I was the hostage negotiator. When Suzy exceeded her curfew, I was the peace envoy. When Suzy died, my life's work was born.

Millions of people know the name Susan G. Komen as an icon for breast cancer awareness. But I wanted you to know the real Suzy—the Suzy I loved—the bright little girl, the homecoming queen in her dress with pink ribbons, the young woman who loved art and longed to see the world, the dedicated mother who fought for every last moment with her children.

This was a real woman—just like your sister, your daughter, your best friend.

When Suzy was diagnosed with breast cancer in her early thirties, we faced it with such limited information. There were no websites, no support groups, very limited treatment options.

From the beginning, Susan G. Komen for the Cure® has sought to empower women with knowledge, access to care and better treatment that comes from a wider understanding of this disease.

Just before Suzy died, she said, "Promise me, Nanny. Promise me you'll change it so other families won't have to go through this." I told her, "I promise. If it takes the rest of my life." I didn't realize at the time that it actually would.

It all began with a small group of committed women in my living room in Dallas, Texas, and has grown to a movement that reaches around the world. Our community affiliates—from Illinois to Italy—are peopled with remarkable volunteers. The Susan G. Komen Race for the Cure®, which started as one event with 800 runners, is now a global series with more than 1.6 million participants across five continents.

Komen Today

Susan G. Komen for the Cure® is the boldest community fueling the best science and making the biggest impact in the fight to end breast cancer. And we've gone global. Not because it's the trendy thing to do, but because it is the right thing to do.

We've touched people in more than 50 countries.

You can join us in the global movement to end breast cancer forever. There are many ways you can get involved in our fight—and I know there are many other efforts in your community that could benefit from your help. Never doubt your ability to make an impact. Never doubt your power to touch a life or change a society. We all have the capacity within us.

Our network redefined grassroots while our corporate partnerships redefined cause-related marketing—partners like our friends at General Mills, who have helped us invest millions in the cause. Together we changed the culture and science of breast cancer in America. Now we're reaching out to women around the world.

We aim to transform fear into understanding, ignorance into knowledge and tragedy into hope. Expand your knowledge at **komen.org.**

Nancy G. Brinker

Nancy G. Brinker, Founder and CEO, Susan G. Komen for the Cure®

My sister, Suzy, loved a good meal, and so I am delighted to share some of my favorite recipes in this cookbook as a tribute to her. I promised Suzy that I would do everything I could to end breast cancer; after her death from the disease in 1980, I made ending breast cancer my life's work. Three decades later, I still look back on so many special moments that I shared with Suzy, with our family and with our wonderful friends. More often than not, those special memories were shared over a meal. I hope that this collection of recipes inspires the same special moments, and special memories, in your life. Bon appétit.

Butternut Squash

From Ambassador Nancy G. Brinker, Founder and CEO of Susan G. Komen for the Cure®

Prep Time: 20 Minutes | **Start to Finish:** 1 Hour 10 Minutes | 4 servings

2	tablespoons organic agave sweetener
2	tablespoons olive oil
1	tablespoon brandy
¾	teaspoon sea salt
½	teaspoon freshly ground black pepper
1	butternut squash (1 to 1½ lbs), peeled, seeded

1 In medium bowl, mix all ingredients except squash. Cut squash into quarters lengthwise. Cut each quartered piece into ¼-inch-thick slices. Add squash to sweetener mixture; stir to coat. Let stand at room temperature 30 minutes to marinate.

2 Heat oven to 400°F. Spray 12x8-inch (2-quart) glass baking dish with cooking spray. Spread squash in dish with marinade.

3 Bake 15 to 20 minutes, stirring once halfway through bake time, until squash is tender.

1 Serving: Calories 150 (Calories from Fat 60); Total Fat 7g (Saturated Fat 1g, Trans Fat 0g); Cholesterol 0mg; Sodium 440mg; Potassium 360mg; Total Carbohydrate 21g (Dietary Fiber 2g); Protein 1g
% Daily Value: Vitamin A 280%; Vitamin C 15%; Calcium 6%; Iron 4%; Folic Acid 6%; Magnesium 10%
Exchanges: 1 Other Carbohydrate, 1 Vegetable, 1 ½ Fat **Carbohydrate Choices:** 1 ½

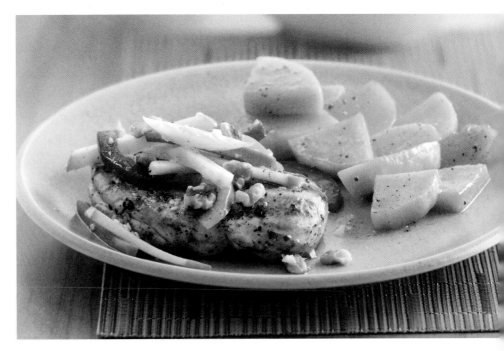

Grilled Chicken with Julienne Vegetable Salad

From Ambassador Nancy G. Brinker, Founder and CEO of Susan G. Komen for the Cure®

Prep Time: 35 Minutes | **Start to Finish:** 1 Hour 45 Minutes | 4 servings

SALAD

- 3 tablespoons olive oil
- 1 tablespoon champagne vinegar or white wine vinegar
- 1 teaspoon sesame seed
- ¼ teaspoon sea salt
- ⅛ teaspoon freshly ground black pepper
- 1 small clove garlic, finely chopped
- ½ small red bell pepper, julienne sliced
- ½ small yellow bell pepper, julienne sliced
- ½ carrot, julienne sliced
- ½ small bulb fennel, julienne sliced
- ½ Granny Smith apple, very thinly julienne sliced

CHICKEN

- 3 tablespoons olive oil
- 3 tablespoons lemon juice
- 1 teaspoon herbes de Provence
- ¾ teaspoon sea salt
- ½ teaspoon freshly ground black pepper
- 2 cloves garlic, finely chopped
- 4 boneless skinless chicken breasts
- ⅓ cup chopped walnuts

1. In medium bowl, mix 3 tablespoons oil, the vinegar, sesame seed, ¼ teaspoon sea salt, ⅛ teaspoon pepper and 1 clove garlic. Add remaining salad ingredients; toss to coat. Cover; refrigerate.

2. In 12x8-inch (2-quart) glass baking dish, mix all chicken ingredients except chicken and walnuts; blend well. Place chicken in marinade mixture; turn to coat. Cover; refrigerate about 1 hour to marinate.

3. Heat gas or charcoal grill. Remove chicken from marinade; reserve marinade. Place chicken on gas grill over medium heat or on charcoal grill 4 to 6 inches from medium coals. Cover grill; cook 10 to 15 minutes, turning once and brushing occasionally with reserved marinade, until juice of chicken is clear when center of thickest part is cut (at least 165°F). Discard any remaining marinade.

4. To serve, place chicken on serving plates. Top each with about ½ cup salad; sprinkle with walnuts. Reserve any remaining salad for a later use.

Broiling Directions: Set oven control to broil. Grease rack in broiler pan with shortening or cooking spray. Place chicken on rack in pan. Broil 4 to 6 inches from heat 10 to 15 minutes, turning once and brushing occasionally with reserved marinade, until juice of chicken is clear when center of thickest part is cut (at least 165°F). Discard any remaining marinade.

1 Serving: Calories 440 (Calories from Fat 280); Total Fat 31g (Saturated Fat 4.5g, Trans Fat 0g); Cholesterol 75mg; Sodium 670mg; Potassium 500mg; Total Carbohydrate 10g (Dietary Fiber 3g); Protein 29g **% Daily Value:** Vitamin A 35%; Vitamin C 35%; Calcium 6%; Iron 10%; Folic Acid 8%; Magnesium 15% **Exchanges:** ½ Starch, 1 Vegetable, 2 Very Lean Meat, 1 ½ Lean Meat, 5 Fat **Carbohydrate Choices:** ½

> **"This is one of my favorite healthy lunches."**
> **—Nancy G. Brinker**

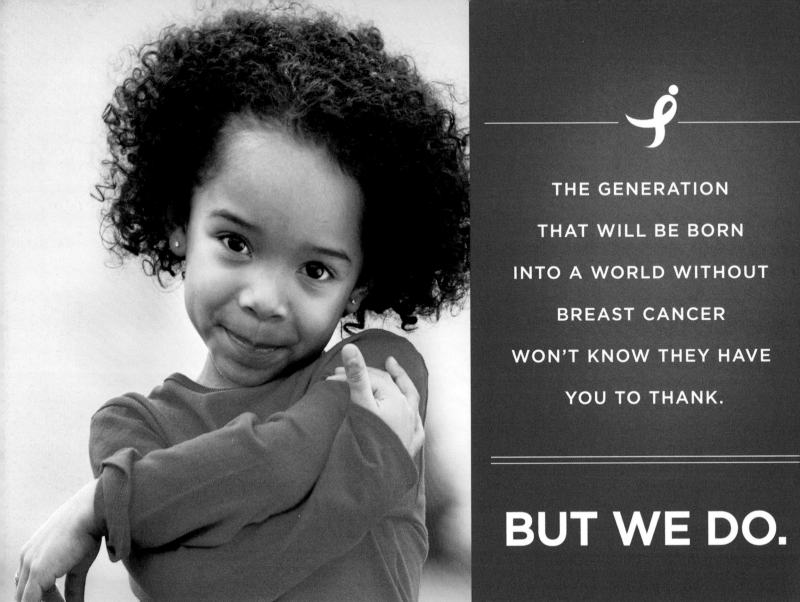

THE GENERATION THAT WILL BE BORN INTO A WORLD WITHOUT BREAST CANCER WON'T KNOW THEY HAVE YOU TO THANK.

BUT WE DO.

That day will be the legacy of the volunteers who give their time, the donors who fund access to treatment and screening, the advocates who give breast cancer a voice in the halls of power, the walkers and racers, the tweeters and bloggers and passionate wearers of pink, the researchers who unlock the answers and the grantors who fund their search, the corporate partners who share their profits, and the survivors who lend us inspiration. Thank you on behalf of those whose lives you save today.

And the ones who won't need saving tomorrow. **Join us at komen.org.**

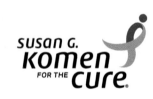

Best science. Boldest community. Biggest impact.
United in the fight against breast cancer.

© 2011 SUSAN G. KOMEN FOR THE CURE®
The Running Ribbon is a registered trademark
of Susan G. Komen for the Cure.

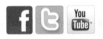

What You'll Find at pink**together**.

*P*ink Together is a national breast cancer awareness program that engages thousands of online community members. Everyone here understands the power of personal connections in the fight against breast cancer. It's a place where you can give strength, or borrow strength. It is where survivors, supporters, family and friends can send messages of hope and encouragement.

Pink Together began with the understanding that we can inspire one another by connecting and uniting people. We are proud to be a part of the *Betty Crocker Living with Cancer Cookbook* and hope that these recipes and stories nurture you throughout your journey.

Real People

You should not have to face breast cancer alone. That is why the **Pink Together Survivor Ambassadors** embody the spirit of our mission. Like many members of our online community, each one is a breast cancer survivor who is committed to sharing hope through their support, encouragement and inspiration.

Few things are more inspiring than the stories of people who triumph over challenges in their paths. The stories you'll find on Pink Together are filled with courage, determination and strength. Join our community at **pinktogether.com** and share your strength today.

Real Stories

As you read through the stories on Pink Together, you'll see how members of this special community inspire strength and hope. Receiving simple notes of encouragement from somebody who has read your story will remind you that you are not alone. At Pink Together, there is a whole community of support rooting for you.

Real Strength

You can meet and interact with women who understand what you are going through, because they've been there. We invite you to take a look!

Celebrating Hope

Since 2007, Pink Together has supported Susan G. Komen for the Cure®'s mission to save lives and end breast cancer forever. We would like to thank Ambassador Nancy G. Brinker, founder and CEO of Susan G Komen for the Cure®, for her contributions to this book. Special thanks go out to the Pink Together Survivor Ambassadors for their presence, involvement and willingness to share hope within their communities and ours.

Dedicated to M. B.

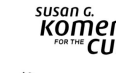

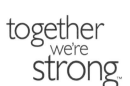

Introducing our Pink Together Survivor Ambassadors

The embodiment and spirit of **pinktogether.com**

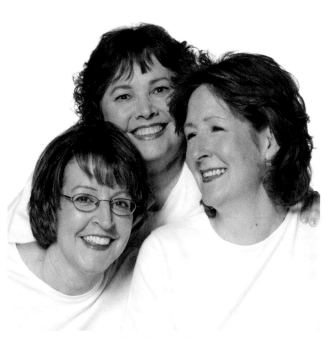

Sue, Fran, & Ann

Our founding **Pink Together Survivor Ambassadors** (pictured at left and below) are our friends and colleagues here at General Mills, most of whom have benefited from the work of Susan G. Komen for the Cure®. We hope you will be inspired by the stories and strength of all of the ambassadors. And of course, we hope that you find comfort in the special recipes that they have shared.

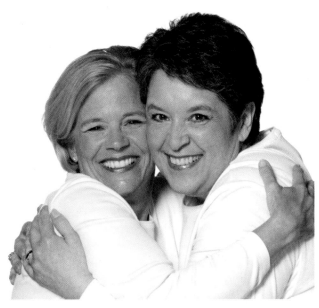

Betty & Linda

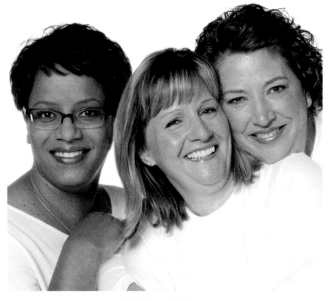

Val, Mary, & Mary

Cornish Pasties

From Betty, 2007 Pink Together
Survivor Ambassador

Prep Time: 1 Hour 15 minutes
Start to Finish: 2 Hours 20 Minutes

8 pasties

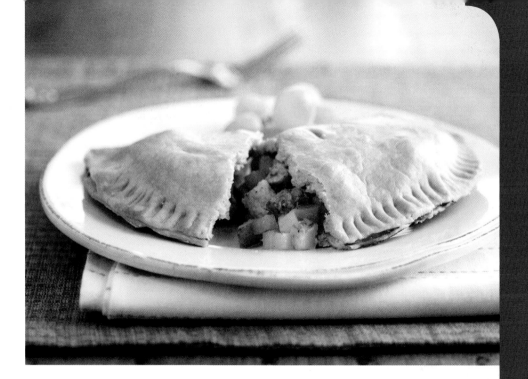

CRUST

4	cups all-purpose flour
1	teaspoon salt
1	cup shortening
¾	to 1 cup ice cold water

FILLING

½	lb boneless lean pork steak, finely chopped
½	lb boneless beef round steak, finely chopped
2	large baking potatoes (1 lb), unpeeled, finely chopped (3 cups)
½	rutabaga (about 6 oz), finely chopped (1 cup)
1	medium onion, chopped (½ cup)
1	teaspoon salt
½	teaspoon pepper
4	tablespoons butter, cut into 8 equal pieces

EGG WASH

1	egg
1	tablespoon milk

> 66 During my cancer treatment, a hot pasty was the comfort food that I enjoyed the most! 99
> —Betty

1. In medium bowl, stir together flour and salt. Using pastry blender (or pulling 2 table knives through ingredients in opposite directions), cut in shortening until particles are size of small peas. Slowly add cold water, tossing with fork and adding only enough water to hold dough together in ball. Cover bowl with plastic wrap; set aside. (If desired, wrap dough in plastic wrap; refrigerate up to 2 days. Allow dough to stand at room temperature 1 hour before rolling out.)

2. In large bowl, mix all filling ingredients except butter.

3. Heat oven to 400°F. Place sheet of parchment paper on cookie sheet, or spray cookie sheet with cooking spray. Divide dough into 8 balls; keep covered in bowl. On lightly floured surface, flatten 1 ball at a time slightly. Using floured rolling pin, roll flattened ball into 8-inch round. Repeat with remaining balls.

4. To make each pasty, place about ¾ cup filling onto one half of each dough round. Place 1 piece of butter on top of filling. Carefully lift other half of dough over filling to form crescent-shaped pasty. Seal edges with fork; cut small slits in top crust to vent. Place on cookie sheet.

5. In small bowl, beat egg and milk with whisk until blended. Brush tops of pasties with egg wash.

6. Bake 15 minutes. Reduce oven temperature to 350°F; bake 45 to 50 minutes longer or until golden brown.

1 Pasty: Calories 670 (Calories from Fat 330); Total Fat 37g (Saturated Fat 12g, Trans Fat 4.5g); Cholesterol 80mg; Sodium 670mg; Potassium 560mg; Total Carbohydrate 60g (Dietary Fiber 3g); Protein 23g **% Daily Value:** Vitamin A 4%; Vitamin C 8%; Calcium 4%; Iron 25%; Folic Acid 25%; Magnesium 10% **Exchanges:** 4 Starch, ½ Vegetable, 1 ½ Lean Meat, 6 Fat **Carbohydrate Choices:** 4

Caramel Chex® Mix

From Sue, 2007 Pink Together Survivor Ambassador

Prep Time: 15 Minutes | **Start to Finish:** 15 Minutes | 24 servings (½ cup each)

4½ cups Rice Chex® cereal

4½ cups Corn Chex® cereal

1 cup pecan halves

1 cup packed brown sugar

½ cup butter or margarine

¼ cup light corn syrup

½ teaspoon vanilla

1 In large microwavable bowl, mix cereals and pecan halves; set aside.

2 In 2-cup microwavable measuring cup, microwave remaining ingredients uncovered on High 1 to 2 minutes, stirring after 1 minute, until melted and smooth.

3 Pour mixture over cereal; gently stir until evenly coated. Microwave mixture uncovered on High 3 minutes, stirring every minute. Spread on waxed paper to cool. Store in tightly covered container.

1 Serving: Calories 150 (Calories from Fat 60); Total Fat 7g (Saturated Fat 2.5g, Trans Fat 0g); Cholesterol 10mg; Sodium 135mg; Potassium 50mg; Total Carbohydrate 21g (Dietary Fiber 0g); Protein 1g
% Daily Value: Vitamin A 6%; Vitamin C 0%; Calcium 4%; Iron 20%; Folic Acid 20%; Magnesium 0%
Exchanges: ½ Starch, 1 Other Carbohydrate, 1 ½ Fat **Carbohydrate Choices:** 1 ½

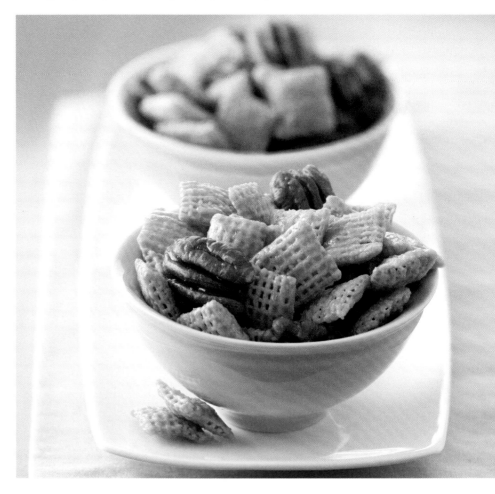

Jeanine

"I saw that there were 10-year and 15-year survivors. So it was hope that I can survive this a lot longer."

Jeanine and her husband proudly flaunt a permanent reminder of her triumph over breast cancer—matching pink ribbon tattoos. But Jeanine's initial reaction to her diagnosis was anything but triumphant. "I'm only 32." She remembers curling herself into a knot and crying, feeling as if her life was over. She admits to being fearful about the operations and the chemo, but what was most troubling was the thought of losing her hair.

Jeanine wants breast cancer patients to know that there is hope and there is life after breast cancer. "I went through chemo; I was sick. It was horrible." On those days when Jeanine felt she couldn't continue, the thought of her children spurred her on. "Who else would love them as much as me?" she thought.

On the days that Jeanine couldn't get out of bed, her close-knit family was a blessing. "Everyone took care of me because I couldn't take care of myself," she recalls. She became engaged during her treatment. "For him to go through that and say, 'You're still beautiful to me. I don't care if you don't have hair, you still look good to me and I want you to be my wife,' it was just amazing."

Truly grateful for her family's support, Jeanine also reached out to others online who could directly relate to her experience. "To have somebody on the web site say, 'Yeah, I know what you're talking about,'" at pinktogether.com, Jeanine found hope from survivors' stories. "I saw that there were 10-year and 15-year survivors. So it was hope that I can survive this a lot longer," she says. Being a survivor gives her daughter hope, too. "If she happens to get breast cancer, when she looks at me, she knows that she will be able to overcome it."

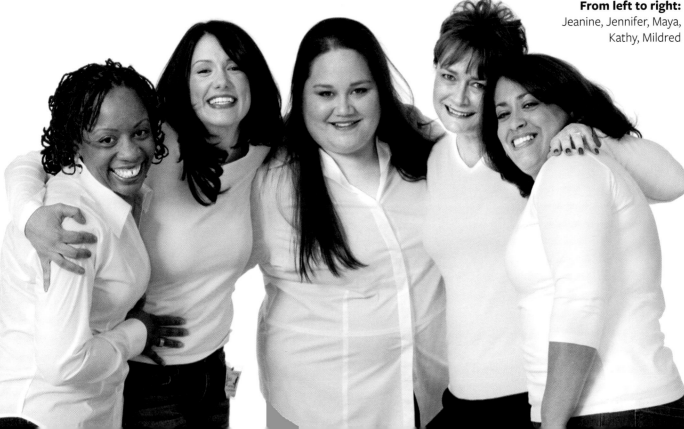

From left to right:
Jeanine, Jennifer, Maya, Kathy, Mildred

Kathy

> **I want people to feel hopeful, that they are not alone.**

Diagnosed for the first time in 1990, Kathy remembers, "There wasn't a lot of support available back then." "I chose to surround myself with positive, happy people because I was determined to beat this disease," she says. Kathy underwent a lumpectomy, followed by chemotherapy and radiation treatments, and remained cancer-free for twelve years.

Then in 2002, she was diagnosed with another type of breast cancer. I put on the survivor-mode hat and was determined to press on," Kathy says.

"I think the pinktogether.com web site is a phenomenal tool for people who are just diagnosed and looking for a place to go," she says. To provide hope for others, Kathy posted her story and invited people affected by breast cancer to visit the site. "I want people to feel hopeful, that they are not alone—that there are many survivors pulling for them."

Kathy has also become a resource for breast cancer patients and survivors by turning her own frustration into the inspiration for her business. A year after her bilateral mastectomy, Kathy was trying to find a mastectomy swimsuit in preparation for her son's wedding in Cancun. "This shouldn't be that difficult. I can't be the only woman who's having difficulty finding these things. Someday I'm going to have a facility where woman can go and find the things they need,'" says Kathy. After five years of envisioning her dream Kathy's shop, Absolute Dignity, first opened its doors.

At Absolute Dignity, women can find wigs, soft headwear, hats, lingerie and compression hosiery, including lymphedema sleeves, and of course, mastectomy swimwear. In addition, as a certified mastectomy fitter and a breast cancer survivor, Kathy is able to skillfully and compassionately assist women in a supportive and empowering way that provides her with great fulfillment.

I've never worked anywhere where you get hugged by every customer that walks out the door," Kathy says joyfully.

Maya

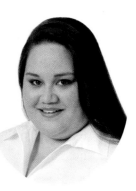

> **There is nothing like somebody who is in the same spot as you, who can say, 'It's gonna be okay.'**

At 27, Maya was diagnosed with breast cancer. Her reaction was to blame herself, questioning everything from the food she ate to her cell phone use. Then Maya focused on what she could do to beat the disease.

"People are generous and loving and supportive, but there is nothing like somebody who is in the same spot as you, who can say, 'It's okay, it's gonna be okay,'" she says. Providing this kind of support and compassion is one of the reasons Maya originally posted her messages on Pink Together. "I want people to see my story and learn about my situation and realize there's a way to heal. You have to fight. You fight and you win."

Maya admits that accepting support was difficult initially. Accustomed to solving problems on her own, Maya quickly realized this was one situation she couldn't remedy by herself. "Ask for what you need from others," says Maya. Let them in. It actually enriches their lives as much as it does yours."

Maya also advises those going through breast cancer treatment to be assertive and informed. Being a survivor has completely changed the way she deals with others. "It's restructured my place on the planet. I've been given the chance to stop this from happening to anybody else. I have a purpose."

Grandma Eva's Gingersnaps

From Maya, 2008 Pink Together Survivor Ambassador

Prep Time: 1 Hour 25 Minutes | **Start to Finish:** 2 Hours 25 Minutes | 4½ dozen cookies

2	cups all-purpose flour
1½	teaspoons baking soda
1½	teaspoons grated gingerroot
½	teaspoon salt
2	teaspoons ground cinnamon
½	teaspoon freshly ground black pepper
¼	teaspoon ground nutmeg
¼	teaspoon ground cloves or cardamom
¾	cup butter, softened
⅔	cup sugar
¼	cup molasses
½	teaspoon vanilla
1	egg
¼	cup sugar

1 In medium bowl, stir together flour, baking soda, gingerroot, salt, cinnamon, pepper, nutmeg and cloves.

2 In large bowl, beat butter with electric mixer on medium speed until light and fluffy. Add ⅔ cup sugar; beat until well blended. Beat in molasses, vanilla and egg. On low speed, beat in flour mixture until combined. Cover dough; refrigerate 1 to 2 hours for easier handling.

3 Heat oven to 350°F. Shape dough into 1-inch balls. Roll in ¼ cup sugar; place about 3 inches apart on ungreased cookie sheets.

4 Bake 9 to 12 minutes or until golden brown. Cool 2 minutes; remove from cookie sheets to cooling racks.

1 Cookie: Calories 60 (Calories from Fat 25); Total Fat 2.5g (Saturated Fat 1.5g, Trans Fat 0g); Cholesterol 10mg; Sodium 75mg; Potassium 30mg; Total Carbohydrate 8g (Dietary Fiber 0g); Protein 0g
% Daily Value: Vitamin A 0%; Vitamin C 0%; Calcium 0%; Iron 0%; Folic Acid 0%; Magnesium 0%
Exchanges: ½ Starch, ½ Fat **Carbohydrate Choices:** ½

66 A recipe that soothed my heart as I fought breast cancer was my great-grandmother's gingersnaps. 99 —Maya

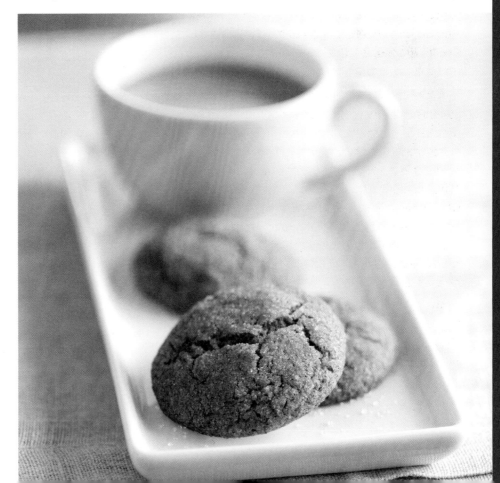

Jennifer

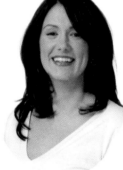

> **❝You can borrow hope by reaching out to someone.❞**

Jennifer was in Las Vegas for a friend's wedding when she scratched her chest and noticed a small lump. After returning home, a mammogram and ultrasound detected an aggressive form of breast cancer.

"Had it been six months later, I probably wouldn't be here," she says. Jennifer was diagnosed with early-onset breast cancer at age 28. "It was quite frightening for me because my grandmother passed at age 50 and her daughter, my aunt, passed away at 30," Jennifer recalls. In addition, Jennifer's mother was diagnosed with breast cancer at age 47.

Finding hope and a sense of connection is what Jennifer wants people visiting pinktogether.com to experience. "There's a lot of isolation with breast cancer," she says. "You get to read people's stories and you immediately feel a sense of community."

Jennifer encourages breast cancer patients to seek support from others, especially during difficult times. "Speaking with them, seeing that they've made it. You're simultaneously borrowing their hope without even realizing it."

"We get so caught up in things that, in the end, really don't matter. Having cancer gives you a clear perspective of what does matter."

Jennifer's life also was touched deeply by her friend Christine, who was taken by breast cancer at age 32. During a heart-to-heart conversation, Christine expressed her fear.

"If I leave this earth and I haven't helped someone, my life didn't mean as much as I wanted it to," Christine confided to Jennifer. "I got the chance to tell Christine, 'You've changed my life and helped me. I wouldn't have gotten through it without you.'"

Christine replied, "Thanks, that's all I needed to hear."

Mildred

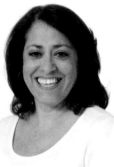

> **❝Don't be afraid to seek out support from other women. Know that hope is out there.❞**

Mildred has a mission to help women understand that there is much to be done in the fight against breast cancer. "We need to come together because we will not be finished until we find a cure," says Mildred.

Mildred recalls feeling numb upon being diagnosed with breast cancer at age 37. After the initial shock, Mildred's concerns were for her three small children. She remembers thinking, "Who is going to take care of them? Who is going to raise them?"

Mildred immediately began to educate herself. "Part of me was afraid to seek help. I thought I was the sole person going through this," she admits.

"Chemo was one of my main challenges. There were times when I gave up hope. I remember my husband pointing at my three children and saying, 'Don't do it for me. Do it for yourself and most importantly, do it for your three kids.' All of the side effects you have with it: How your body changes. Within a month or two, I looked like I was eighty." Today, Mildred vibrantly embodies her victory over breast cancer.

Mildred believes the stories at pinktogether.com can be an uplifting resource for people whose lives are affected by breast cancer. "I want them to see that there is hope out there. That we can go on. We're not alone," she says.

"Please have a mammogram. Getting checked, that's the key. The faster we can find breast cancer, if there is any. The faster we can get a cure."

Surviving breast cancer has given Mildred a new purpose in inspiring and helping others, and a new perspective on life. "Now I see things totally different. My attitude is different. Any little thing, a flower, it's wonderful. I want a butterfly garden. I love butterflies. They're beautiful. To me it's hope."

Mildred's Tres Leches Cake

From Mildred, 2008 Pink Together Survivor Ambassador

Prep Time: 15 Minutes | **Start to Finish:** 1 Hour 45 Minutes | 15 servings

1 box white cake mix with pudding

Water, vegetable oil and egg whites called for on cake mix box

1 can (14 oz) coconut milk (not cream of coconut)

1 can (12 oz) evaporated milk

1 can (14 oz) sweetened condensed milk

1 container (8 oz) frozen whipped topping, thawed

1 cup flaked or shredded coconut

½ cup chopped maraschino cherries, drained

1 Heat oven to 350°F. Make and bake cake mix in 13x9-inch pan as directed on box, using water, oil and egg whites. Cool in pan 10 minutes.

2 Meanwhile, in medium bowl, mix 3 cans of milk; set aside.

3 Using long-tined fork, poke holes in cake every ½ inch, wiping fork occasionally to reduce sticking. Slowly pour milk mixture over top of cake. Refrigerate at least 1 hour or until milk mixture is absorbed into cake.

4 Spread whipped topping over cake; sprinkle with coconut. Top with cherries.

1 Serving: Calories 420 (Calories from Fat 180); Total Fat 20g (Saturated Fat 13g, Trans Fat 0g); Cholesterol 15mg; Sodium 330mg; Potassium 290mg; Total Carbohydrate 55g (Dietary Fiber 1g); Protein 7g
% Daily Value: Vitamin A 2%; Vitamin C 0%; Calcium 20%; Iron 6%; Folic Acid 2%; Magnesium 6%
Exchanges: 2 Starch, 1 ½ Other Carbohydrate, 4 Fat **Carbohydrate Choices:** 3 ½

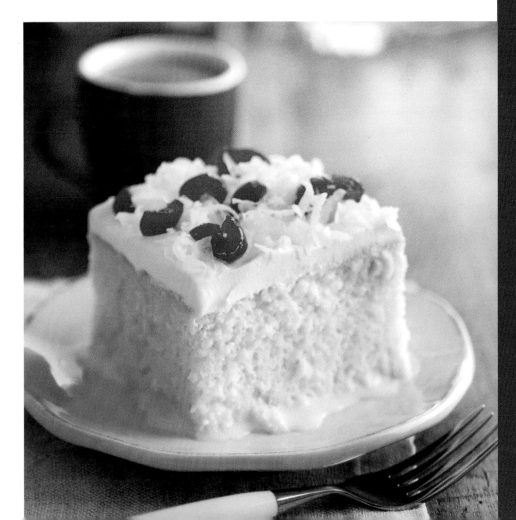

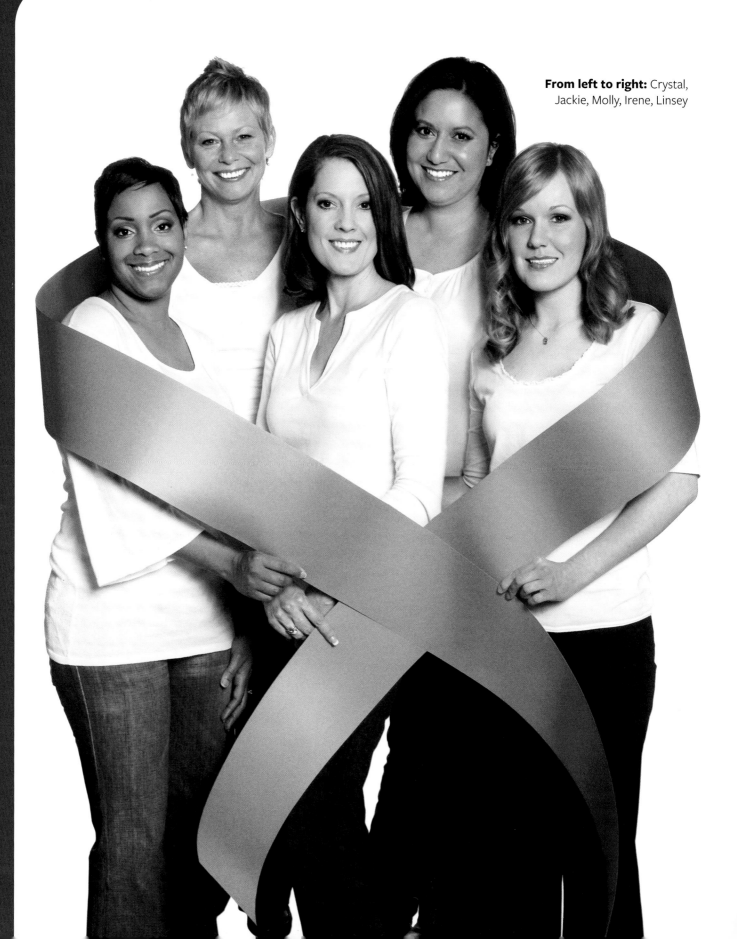

From left to right: Crystal, Jackie, Molly, Irene, Linsey

Crystal

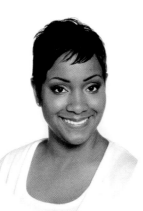

66 Just a simple note of support can help people believe there is life after breast cancer. 99

On New Year's Eve, 2003, Crystal was on top of the world. The New Year brought both a wedding proposal and a great new job as a sales manager. Crystal had been active during Breast Cancer Awareness Month since her mother had been diagnosed with breast cancer three years earlier.

That October, Crystal's doctor scheduled a mammogram and after that everything happened very quickly. Crystal went from exam to mammogram to biopsy to mastectomy within three weeks. "My mom was on a flight the next day and was there to walk me through the entire time."

"My son was not handling this well at all." Trying to comfort her son and plan a wedding and battle breast cancer was overwhelming for Crystal. "I walked out on faith and quit my job. I now work in the nonprofit sector and it has been more than rewarding. I have found a new passion in my life, helping others!" She hopes to continue this outreach by showing everyone that there is life after breast cancer.

Irene

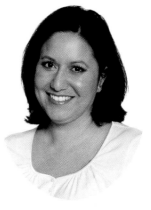

66 Making a personal connection with other women at pinktogether.com really opened up a door of hope for me. 99

Irene began her journey with breast cancer at the age of 34. Nine months earlier, Irene's younger sister was diagnosed with breast cancer at the young age of 30. Cancer runs in Irene's family and this caused Irene and her sister to be very careful about doing breast exams each month.

After her mastectomy, Irene and her sister were a constant support to each other. They even went wig shopping together. "Never did we imagine that in our lifetime we would be bald and breast-less at the same time!"

Irene also discovered a community of support on pinktogether.com. "It was nice to connect with other women, especially at a time when I felt so alone." Irene wants to spread the word that early detection saves lives.

Jackie

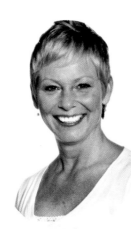

❝It is heartwarming to see so many women reaching out to each other at pinktogether.com.❞

Jackie may call herself a "biker chick" but she's also a loving wife and mother with a great sense of humor. Jackie is also a two-time breast cancer survivor whose life has been touched by cancer many times over. Her daughter survived a battle with cancer at a very young age and her mother was diagnosed with breast cancer at the age of 40.

"Having this history of cancer in her family caused Jackie to be extremely vigilant with her own health. She began having regular mammograms when she was just 35. And at 40, she discovered a lump in her breast, the same age her mother was diagnosed. After a lumpectomy and months of radiation treatment, Jackie was ready to be done with cancer forever. Just a few years later, during a routine checkup, Jackie's doctor unexpectedly found precancerous cells in the same breast as her previous cancer.

After the bilateral mastectomy, her doctor discovered an 8-cm area of Invasive Lobular Carcinoma in that breast. "My surgeon said I literally saved my own life making that decision." Jackie was very fortunate to have the support of her mother and her daughter and is glad to have a place like Pink Together, where she can inspire the same hope and strength in others that her daughter and mother inspired in her.

Linsey

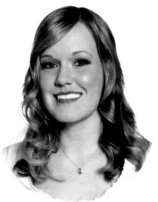

❝Pinktogether.com let me know someone was rooting for me.❞

Linsey has the kind of smile that lights up a room.

At the age of 23, Linsey was forced to make a decision to have a mastectomy of her left breast. Less than a year later, after a precautionary mastectomy of her right breast, her odds of ever having cancer again went down to three percent. It was a struggle for Linsey to deal with something so serious at a time when others her age were studying and hanging out with their friends.

That struggle was made even more difficult by the fact that there were no other young people she could turn to. "What does it mean to be 23 with breast cancer?" Until she found Pink Together, Linsey felt like she was alone in her fight, but now she has found a community of young women who understand what it means to be a breast cancer survivor.

"I never fully understood that I was at risk, and for a while I ignored the lump I felt in my breast because I assumed it was nothing." Linsey hopes her story will inspire young women across the country to become more active in the fight against breast cancer.

Meatball Sandwiches

From Linsey, 2009 Pink Together Survivor Ambassador

Prep Time: 35 Minutes | **Start to Finish:** 2 Hours 30 Minutes | 10 sandwiches

SAUCE

- ½ lb bulk Italian pork sausage
- 1 medium onion, chopped (½ cup)
- 1 small green bell pepper, chopped (about ½ cup)
- 2 cans (8 oz each) tomato sauce
- 1 can (14.5 oz) stewed tomatoes, undrained
- 1 can (12 oz) tomato paste
- 2 teaspoons packed brown sugar
- 1 teaspoon garlic powder
- ½ teaspoon dried oregano leaves
- ½ teaspoon dried basil leaves

MEATBALLS

- 2 eggs, slightly beaten
- 3 tablespoons milk
- 2 lbs lean (at least 80%) ground beef
- ½ cup unseasoned dry bread crumbs
- 1 teaspoon dried basil leaves
- ¾ teaspoon salt
- ½ teaspoon rubbed sage
- ⅛ teaspoon dried oregano leaves
- ⅛ teaspoon pepper

ROLLS AND CHEESE

- 10 hoagie or deli-style rolls
- 1 package (8 oz) sliced mozzarella cheese, slices cut in half diagonally

1 In 3-quart saucepan or Dutch oven, cook sausage, onion and bell pepper over medium-high heat, stirring occasionally, until sausage is brown; drain. Stir in remaining sauce ingredients. Heat to boiling. Reduce heat to low; cover and simmer 30 minutes.

2 Meanwhile, heat oven to 400°F. In large bowl, mix meatball ingredients until well blended. Shape into 40 (1½-inch) meatballs. Place meatballs in ungreased 15x10x1-inch pan.

3 Bake 20 to 25 minutes or until meatballs are thoroughly cooked and no longer pink in center. Add to sauce; cover and simmer about 1 hour.

4 Place 4 meatballs on bottom half of each bun. Top each with 2 cheese halves; cover with top of half of bun.

1 Sandwich: Calories 650 (Calories from Fat 230); Total Fat 25g (Saturated Fat 10g, Trans Fat 1.5g); Cholesterol 120mg; Sodium 1770mg; Potassium 1060mg; Total Carbohydrate 67g (Dietary Fiber 5g); Protein 38g **% Daily Value:** Vitamin A 25%; Vitamin C 20%; Calcium 35%; Iron 40%; Folic Acid 35%; Magnesium 20% **Exchanges:** 3 Starch, 1 Other Carbohydrate, 2 Vegetable, 2 Lean Meat, 1 ½ High-Fat Meat, 1 Fat **Carbohydrate Choices:** 4 ½

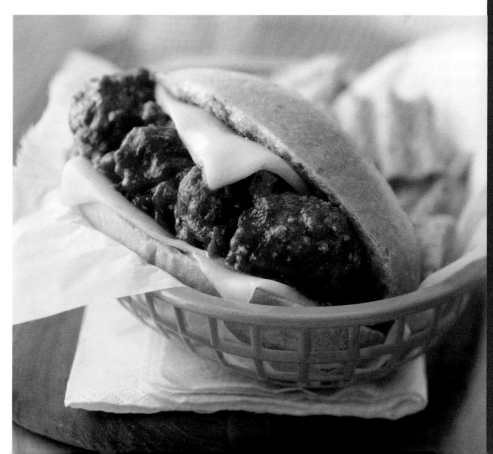

Molly

"It's in your heart. You want to help and Pink Together lets you do that."

Molly's joy for life comes out in everything she does, especially when she's onstage with her first love, her music. Molly shares this passion with her two closest friends, her older twin sisters. During her battle with breast cancer Molly was even brave enough to perform bald while she was undergoing chemotherapy.

Diagnosed at the age of 33, Molly was devastated. Despite her initial shock, Molly quickly discovered an inner strength that helped her overcome her fears. With her husband and sisters by her side, Molly was able to keep an incredibly positive outlook during her battle with breast cancer. After an initial lumpectomy and four rounds of chemotherapy and radiation, Molly thought she was done with the disease forever.

Then during an annual mammogram, Molly's second diagnosis was a new primary breast cancer, not a recurrence. This time around Molly required a double mastectomy. Throughout it all, she never let the disease control her life.

As a Pink Together Survivor Ambassador, she hopes to show others that despite the diagnoses you are still in charge of who you are and how you live your life. "I can imagine a world without breast cancer."

Clockwise: Jackie, Irene, Crystal, Molly, Linsey

Pepperoni and Sausage Bread

From Molly, 2009 Pink Together Survivor Ambassador

Prep Time: 20 Minutes | **Start to Finish:** 3 Hours 50 Minutes | 4 servings

1 loaf (1 lb) frozen white bread dough

1 egg, beaten

1.5 oz sliced pepperoni (about 22 slices)

½ lb bulk Italian pork sausage, cooked, drained

4 slices mozzarella cheese, halved, or 1 cup shredded mozzarella cheese (4 oz)

Bell peppers, olives or any other desired ingredients, if desired

1 cup marinara sauce

1 Heat oven to 350°F. Thaw and raise bread dough as directed on package.

2 On lightly floured surface, roll out dough to 14x10-inch rectangle. Brush dough with half of the beaten egg. Top with pepperoni, cooked sausage, cheese and other desired ingredients.

3 Roll up jelly-roll fashion, pinching edges to seal. Brush top with remaining egg. On ungreased large cookie sheet, place roll seam side down, curving into crescent shape if desired.

4 Bake 25 to 30 minutes or until golden brown. Serve with marinara sauce.

1 Serving: Calories 670 (Calories from Fat 260); Total Fat 29g (Saturated Fat 11g, Trans Fat 1g); Cholesterol 105mg; Sodium 1930mg; Potassium 520mg; Total Carbohydrate 73g (Dietary Fiber 3g); Protein 29g **% Daily Value:** Vitamin A 10%; Vitamin C 4%; Calcium 40%; Iron 35%; Folic Acid 35%; Magnesium 15% **Exchanges:** 3 Starch, 2 Other Carbohydrate, 1 ½ Medium-Fat Meat, 1 High-Fat Meat, 2 ½ Fat **Carbohydrate Choices:** 5

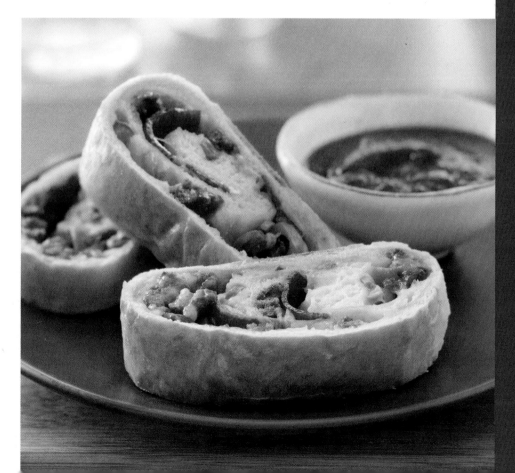

Ebony

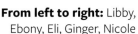

> **"Pink Together, my family and friends help me get through it all."**

Ebony is a strong, vivacious woman with an instinctive affinity for the spotlight. In August of 2007, Ebony relocated to Dallas to begin her dream job as co-host of the nationally syndicated Rickey Smiley Morning Show. One month later, she felt something strange in her breast. She thought it was nothing and was ready to dismiss it until her family convinced her to have it checked out. After a series of tests the unimaginable news was delivered that it was, in fact, breast cancer.

Ebony considered keeping her diagnosis to herself, but quickly realized that she needed the support of her friends and family. So she decided to face her new life head on, which meant sharing her diagnosis with her listeners around the country.

After sharing her story with her listeners, Ebony felt a surge of purpose and began looking for a way to help others whose lives had been touched by breast cancer. Ebony became a National Ambassador for the Susan G. Komen for the Cure® Circle of Promise, a program that promotes awareness of breast cancer in the African-American community.

"Everybody has different cancers in their life, whatever it is—as long as you take it and address it head on you can start moving in a positive direction."

From left to right: Libby, Ebony, Eli, Ginger, Nicole

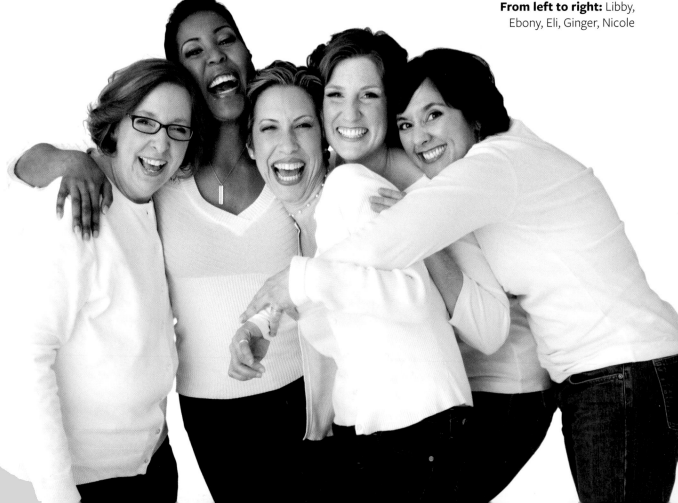

Hoppin' John

From Ebony, 2010 Pink Together Survivor Ambassador

Prep Time: 35 Minutes | **Start to Finish:** 35 Minutes | 6 servings (1 cup each)

1 tablespoon canola or olive oil

1 cup finely chopped cooked ham

½ cup mixture of finely chopped onions, red, green and yellow peppers

¼ cup cooked bacon pieces (from 3-oz jar)

1 tablespoon finely chopped garlic

1 cup chopped andouille sausage

2 cans (15.8 oz each) southern style black-eyed peas, drained

1 can (10 oz) mild diced tomatoes with green chiles, undrained

1 box (10 oz) frozen chopped collard greens, thawed and drained

Hot cooked rice, if desired

1 In 12-inch skillet, heat oil over medium heat. Add ham, onion-pepper mixture, bacon and garlic; cook 5 minutes, stirring occasionally, until onion is tender.

2 Stir in remaining ingredients except rice. Reduce heat to low; cover and cook 20 minutes, stirring occasionally. Serve over rice.

1 Serving: Calories 320 (Calories from Fat 110); Total Fat 13g (Saturated Fat 3.5g, Trans Fat 0g); Cholesterol 40mg; Sodium 1070mg; Potassium 630mg; Total Carbohydrate 30g (Dietary Fiber 7g); Protein 22g **% Daily Value:** Vitamin A 100%; Vitamin C 25%; Calcium 15%; Iron 25%; Folic Acid 70%; Magnesium 20% **Exchanges:** 1 Starch, 1/2 Other Carbohydrate, 1 1/2 Vegetable, 1 Very Lean Meat, 1 1/2 Lean Meat, 1 1/2 Fat **Carbohydrate Choices:** 2

Variation For an extra kick, use spicy sausage and hot diced tomatoes with green chiles.

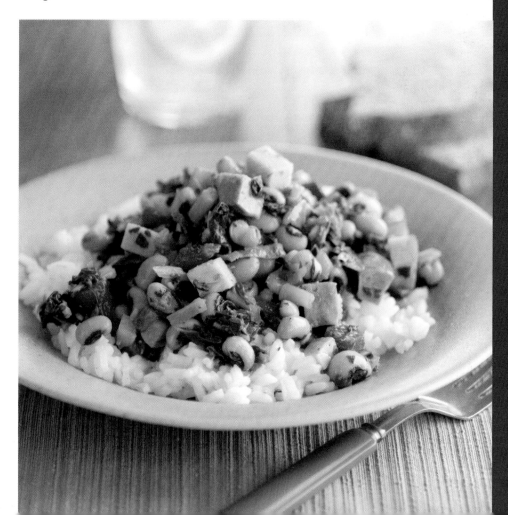

Nicole

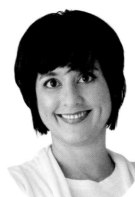

66It's important to know that you can fight and that you can win.99

Nicole's smile and her joy for life are overwhelmingly infectious. She has refused to let breast cancer temper her enthusiasm or her positive outlook on life. Nicole was just 34 years old when she felt a lump in her breast.

A mammogram confirmed her worst fears: Nicole was diagnosed with an especially aggressive form of breast cancer called triple negative breast cancer, which is resistant to most therapies. Nicole underwent chemotherapy, radiation and eventually a mastectomy.

Nicole turned to running to help her cope with the stresses of her treatments. "When I was going through chemo I tried to stay in shape because if I was going to lose my hair, I wasn't also going to lose my ability to run." After her recovery Nicole made it her mission to get the word out to young Latina women that early detection saves lives. This activism led her to take a job with Susan G. Komen for the Cure®, where she continues to support women whose lives have been touched by breast cancer.

Many Latina women are reluctant to talk about breast cancer. Nicole encourages them to get mammograms and become educated about the benefits of early detection and treatment. She's also helping Latina women overcome the difficulties caused by their language barrier when they communicate with doctors and insurance companies. "Stay strong, stay positive . . . don't be afraid to reach out to the women who have already walked in your shoes."

Eli

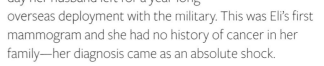

66Pink Together lets me say thank you and extend my hand to others.99

Eli exudes a strength and wisdom you can't help but admire. Eli received the news that she had breast cancer the day her husband left for a year-long overseas deployment with the military. This was Eli's first mammogram and she had no history of cancer in her family—her diagnosis came as an absolute shock.

With her husband overseas, Eli's son became her star supporter during this difficult time. His positive attitude helped ease Eli's journey through her treatment and recovery. "Without him it would have been a very difficult journey for me." After two surgeries, chemotherapy and radiation, Eli has now been cancer-free for more than two years.

She has started a program called Amando Lavida, which brings volunteers together to provide emotional support and translation services for Latina women who have been diagnosed with breast cancer. She's also working on outreach efforts to ensure Latina women in the area are educated about breast cancer prevention, detection and treatment. "Through my journey, I have come across some of the most fabulous people—the love, courage and hope they have given me is priceless. I am blessed to be able to extend my hand and make a difference."

Lentil Soup

From Eli, 2010 Pink Together Survivor Ambassador

Prep Time: 20 Minutes | **Start to Finish:** 45 Minutes | 8 servings (1 cup each)

2 tablespoons olive oil

1 large onion, chopped (1 cup)

1 medium carrot, finely chopped (½ cup)

1 stalk celery, chopped (⅓ cup)

2 medium green onions or scallions, chopped

3 cloves garlic, finely chopped

1 sheet kombu or wakame seaweed (from 10-oz package), if desired

2 cups (12 oz) dried lentils, sorted, rinsed

1 small butternut squash, peeled, seeded and cubed (2 cups)

1 tablespoon chopped fresh or 1 teaspoon dried oregano leaves

1 tablespoon tamari sauce

¾ teaspoon sea salt

2 sprigs fresh or 1 teaspoon dried thyme leaves

1 dried bay leaf

6 cups water or vegetable broth

1 In 3-quart saucepan or Dutch oven, heat oil over medium heat. Add onion, carrot, celery, green onions and garlic; cook about 5 minutes, stirring occasionally, until onions are tender. Soak seaweed in 2 cups water about 5 minutes or until softened; drain.

2 Stir remaining ingredients and drained seaweed into onion mixture. Heat to boiling. Reduce heat; cover and simmer 20 to 25 minutes or until lentils are tender. Remove and discard bay leaf and thyme sprigs before serving.

1 Serving: Calories 200 (Calories from Fat 35); Total Fat 4g (Saturated Fat 0.5g, Trans Fat 0g); Cholesterol 0mg; Sodium 350mg; Potassium 600mg; Total Carbohydrate 30g (Dietary Fiber 8g); Protein 11g
% Daily Value: Vitamin A 90%; Vitamin C 8%; Calcium 6%; Iron 25%; Folic Acid 60%; Magnesium 15%
Exchanges: 1 ½ Starch, 2 Vegetable, ½ Very Lean Meat, ½ Fat **Carbohydrate Choices:** 2

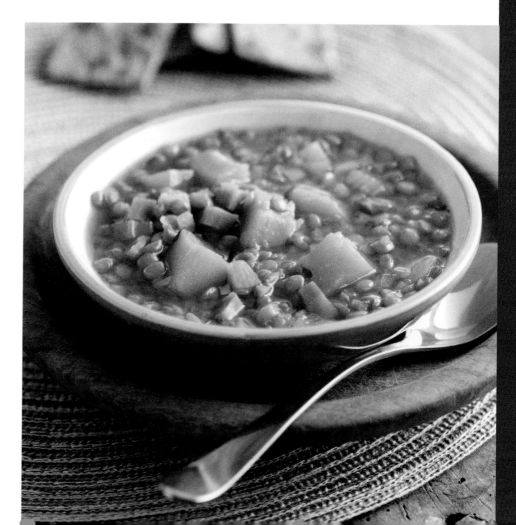

Ginger

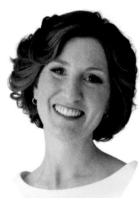

66Stories provide great hope and support for the newly diagnosed.99

Ginger has an amazing ability to find ways to turn any challenge into an opportunity. This positive attitude is doubly amazing given that Ginger was five months pregnant at the time of her diagnosis.

Ginger was forced to make one of the scariest decisions any young mother will ever face: begin treatments immediately and risk the health of her unborn baby or delay treatments and risk her own health. With her loving husband by her side, Ginger made the difficult decision to start treatments after she gave birth.

"Now I have this beautiful little boy who's running around telling me how much he loves me."

During chemotherapy treatments, Ginger noticed how sad and melancholy the people around her were and made it her mission to bring smiles to these survivors by collecting gifts from local businesses and giving them out as "prizes" to the people in the chemotherapy room whenever she went in for treatment. "I'd just give out prizes . . . awards for just being alive, for being a fighter, for taking our chemo medicine and for living one more day."

Ginger is a cancer survivor determined to bring joy to the lives of those who have been touched by breast cancer. "What I want to get across is that good things can come from bad experiences if we are willing to open our hearts to others and share the goodness inside."

Today, Ginger's HappyChemo.com is her way of continuing to do good together.

Libby

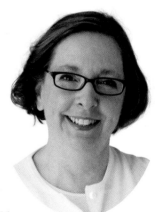

66My life has changed from going through cancer, mostly by enjoying every day.99

Libby is a devoted mother of two and a two-time breast cancer survivor who unwaveringly refused to let cancer derail her life—or the lives of her family.

At the age of 38 her diagnosis came as a complete shock. Fortunately, her cancer was stage one and required only outpatient surgery.

Nine years later another mammogram detected a new mass in her breast. This time, a harder course of treatment was required. Through both of her battles with breast cancer, Libby focused on keeping her life and her family as normal as possible.

"The treatments got progressively harder and I didn't feel well, but I always thought this could be so much worse. I'm a pretty 'glass is half full' person, so keeping a positive outlook was pretty easy." Today, Libby is a two-time breast cancer survivor who believes in the power of early detection.

Chris's Taco Chili

From Libby, 2010 Pink Together Survivor Ambassador

Prep Time: 35 Minutes | **Start to Finish:** 35 Minutes | 6 servings (1½ cups each)

1 lb lean ground turkey

1 can (29 oz) tomato puree

1 can (15.25 oz) whole kernel sweet corn, drained

1 can (15 oz) black beans, drained, rinsed

1 can (14.5 oz) diced tomatoes (any variety), undrained

1 can (4.5 oz) diced green chiles, undrained

1 package (1 oz) taco seasoning mix

Crushed red pepper flakes, if desired

Tortilla chips, if desired

1 In 3-quart saucepan or Dutch oven, cook turkey over medium-high heat 5 to 7 minutes, stirring occasionally, until no longer pink; drain. Return to saucepan.

2 Stir in tomato puree, corn, beans, diced tomatoes, chiles and taco seasoning mix. Add crushed red pepper flakes, ½ teaspoon at a time, to desired taste. Heat to boiling over medium heat. Reduce heat to low; simmer uncovered 20 minutes, stirring occasionally. Serve with tortilla chips.

1 Serving: Calories 320 (Calories from Fat 45); Total Fat 5g (Saturated Fat 1.5g, Trans Fat 0g); Cholesterol 50mg; Sodium 1650mg; Potassium 1020mg; Total Carbohydrate 43g (Dietary Fiber 10g); Protein 24g
% Daily Value: Vitamin A 25%; Vitamin C 25%; Calcium 8%; Iron 30%; Folic Acid 30%; Magnesium 20% **Exchanges:** 1 ½ Starch, ½ Other Carbohydrate, 2 ½ Vegetable, ½ Very Lean Meat, 1 ½ Lean Meat
Carbohydrate Choices: 3

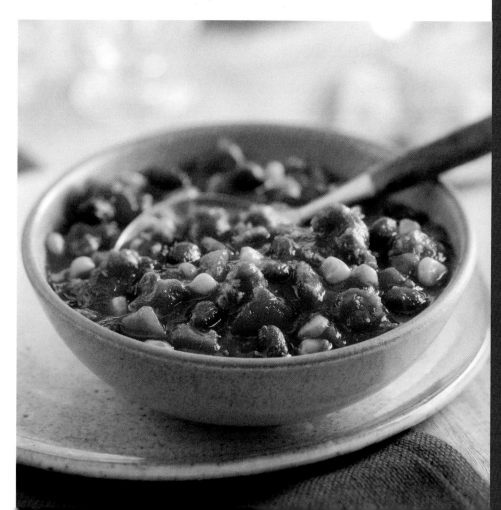

❝ This super-simple chili recipe from my friend Chris was my go-to dish during chemo. It was quick to make, and the bold flavors overpowered the metallic taste in my mouth after treatment.❞ —Libby

2011 marks the five-year partnership of Pink Together and Susan G. Komen for the Cure®. During that time, we have donated over $10 Million in support of Community Outreach and Research initiatives.

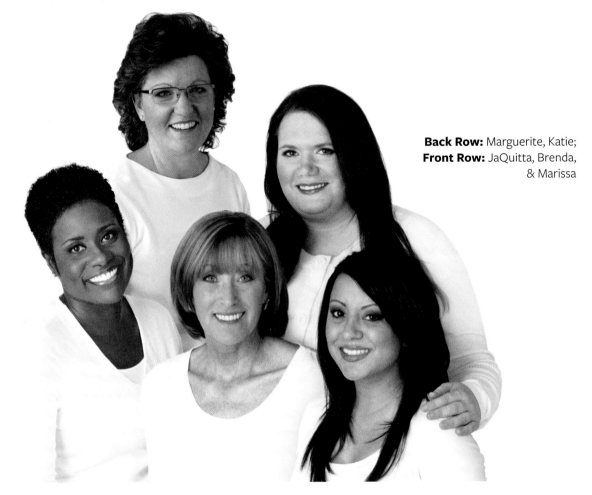

Back Row: Marguerite, Katie;
Front Row: JaQuitta, Brenda, & Marissa

Marissa

"We are here. We are alive. We can beat it."

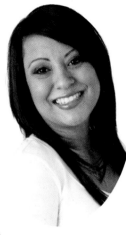

Marissa is a funny, vibrant young woman with so much strength that even though she was diagnosed at the young age of 24, cancer never stood a chance.

When Marissa was diagnosed with breast cancer she was in such a state of shock that she didn't really understand what was happening to her for several days. Once the reality set in though, she knew exactly what kind of a fight she was in for. Cancer has been an unfortunately all too common occurrence in Marissa's family for many generations. Marissa has lost cousins to breast cancer and a great aunt to ovarian cancer. She also watched her grandmother battle and defeat ovarian cancer 16 years earlier. Inspired by her Grandmother's recovery Marissa vowed to not let cancer get the best of her either.

"The thing I remember grandma always telling me was, 'Look at me, I'm here.'"

With the love and support of her family and grandmother, who had raised her since the 3rd grade, Marissa undertook a bilateral mastectomy in May of 2009. Marissa was the youngest patient many of her doctors had ever treated and she felt very alone. Then she discovered all the stories on pinktogether.com and learned that she is far from being the only young survivor out there.

Though her journey has been long and painful, Marissa feels that being faced with breast cancer at such a young age has opened her heart and mind to life in a way she never would have viewed it otherwise. While other girls her age were finishing college and starting careers, Marissa was fighting a battle for her life and learning the true value of family and what it means to be alive.

"I have so much more living to do, my life has just begun. I have fought and conquered this battle! Other young survivors can too!"

JaQuitta

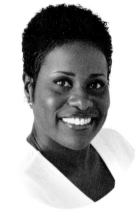

"Pink Together is a sisterhood—a team of champions in the fight against breast cancer."

JaQuitta is a strong, self-confident woman who never backs down from a challenge. So when breast cancer entered her life, she did the only thing she knew how to do: She faced it head on with a fierce determination until she had kicked the disease to the curb.

JaQuitta's breast cancer journey began on Thursday July 19, 2007. She discovered her tumor by doing a breast self-exam, as she had been doing since her 20s because she knew she was "supposed to". A young, healthy woman who ate right, exercised and had no family history of cancer, JaQuitta never imagined she would discover anything. But she did.

JaQuitta's tumor was diagnosed as infiltrating ductal carcinoma, about 2 point 3 centimeters between a stage 2 and 3, which meant surgery, chemo and radiation--even though there was no cancer detected in the lymph nodes.

"The hardest part about the cancer was the diagnosis--hearing the words, trying to understand what I was hearing other than, blah-blah-blah cancer, and blah-blah-blah specialist."

In the beginning JaQuitta felt overwhelmed all the time, but she soon realized she had to get it together. So she set out to find out more about breast cancer, options, treatment, empowerment, and recovery and to find doctors who she felt comfortable with.

She also came to understand how important it is to be open to accepting support. As a TV Anchor-Reporter in Atlanta, she decided to make her diagnosis and her journey public She didn't want people feeling sorry for her. She wanted to show people first hand that a person can take the challenge of cancer head on.

As a breast cancer survivor JaQuitta is grateful for the lessons she has learned about how to be strong and how to slow down and appreciate the little things. And, she's grateful to have discovered a community of women who understand how breast cancer changes everything in your life.

"Pink Together for me means unity. It's a sisterhood. The unity of it comes from knowing that another woman understands all the stuff that you have to go through. If you wanna cry, you can. If you wanna laugh, you can. There is no judgement there."

Katie

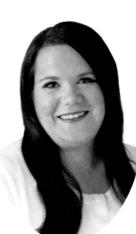

❝Pink Together is a place to find strength, hope and courage.❞

Katie is a small town girl with a big personality. She is bubbly and delightful and she can talk a mile a minute. She is also a fiercely independent, strong willed woman who refused to let breast cancer dampen her high sprits or her joy for life.

At the young age of 36, Katie discovered she had breast cancer in an unusual way. Working at a clinic that was offering free breast exams, she decided to have one done so she would have a baseline when she started regular breast cancer screenings in a few years. Katie had no family history of breast cancer and had never experienced pain in her breasts so she expected to simply have the mammogram and be done with it.

Not wanting to miss a great deal of time from work, she scheduled an appointment on a Friday at 7:20 am, before her shift started. A few minutes later her doctor returned and immediately wanted to do an ultrasound. Then before she knew it, they prepped her for a biopsy followed by some shocking news: the cells would likely be cancerous and even if they weren't, she'd have to have the mass removed. It was only 8 am, but Katie went to work with ice packs to keep the pain from the biopsy in check.

The call came on Sunday evening: Katie had early stage invasive ductile breast cancer. Katie's first instinct was to talk about her diagnosis with her co-workers, her friends and her family, which helped her work through the rollercoaster of emotions she was experience right after her diagnosis.

Fortunately for Katie her mass was caught at a very early stage, which meant her doctors were able to offer her a number of options for treatment. Katie chose to take a hands-on, intellectual approach to her diagnosis. She wanted her treatment decision to be her own so she did an incredible amount of research and chose to have a partial mastectomy.

"I know that many women don't have the choice and I was blessed to have a choice. I did a lot of my own research and had many conversations with my newly assembled healthcare team."

Katie's cancer was discovered early enough that it could be completely removed through surgery, and after a round of radiation treatments Katie has been happily cancer free for nearly 2 years. Through her diagnosis and her treatments, Katie found a new strength—a strength that she is now using to help other young women understand the risks of breast cancer and the importance of early detection.

"I knew that if it happened to me, it could happen to anybody. That is why I wanted to share my story on pinktogether.com. No two cancer experiences are the same, but I've been there and want to let other women know that early detection can mean that cancer isn't necessarily the end. I hope I can provide support and encouragement to my fellow survivors!"

Marguerite

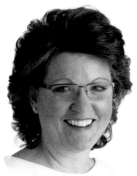

> **"Pink Together can help others walk the road that I walked."**

Marguerite is thoughtful, warm and friendly, but most of all she is a problem solver. And that is exactly how she approached her cancer diagnosis: as a problem to be solved.

Marguerite's family has been touched many times over by the devastating effects of breast cancer; her great-grandmother, grandmother, mother and aunt were all diagnosed. Marguerite always thought that breast cancer would be something she'd have to deal with given her family history, yet she was blindsided when she was diagnosed at the age of 44.

Because of her family history, Marguerite had been diligent about getting regular mammograms and this was not the first one that had caused a red flag, so she wasn't too worried. That changed when she was given the news that it was cancer. At first, the doctors thought the cancer was contained in the duct, but a second surgery found that the cancer had invaded the breast tissue.

Marguerite soon learned that surgery was just the beginning and really the easiest part of her journey. The information and choices that were thrown at her were overwhelming. Chemo, no chemo. Radiation, no radiation. Drugs, no drugs. Survival statistics and probabilities of reoccurrence all started to run together.

"When you're first diagnosed as a cancer patient you just want to know everything, and you want to know what other people have done."

Before Marguerite made any decisions on treatment she went through genetic testing to see if she was carrying the breast cancer gene. Fortunately she was not, so after very carefully weighing all her options she decided to bypass chemotherapy and instead underwent 6-1/2 weeks of daily radiation therapy. Marguerite also started seeing a holistic practitioner and worked to improve her diet. She will happily celebrate her 5-year anniversary of being cancer-free this year by using the things she learned through her treatment to help other women through their treatments.

"I want to share my story in hopes that it might help someone else who will walk the road that I walked. Pinktogether.com helps me do that."

Brenda

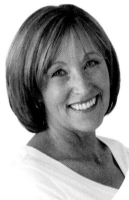

> **" The longer you are a survivor, the stronger you become. "**

Brenda is soft spoken and contemplative by nature, but underneath her quiet exterior lays a fierce strength and determination. She is a fighter with a heart of gold. A woman who always puts the needs of her loved ones first and worries about herself second.

When Brenda was first diagnosed with breast cancer she was understandably angry at the world. Brenda had no family history of cancer, and her head was reeling with the diagnosis. Then, just two weeks later, her world turned upside down again: Her mother was diagnosed with breast cancer, too. This dual diagnosis came as a complete shock to everyone and doctors could find no genetic link between Brenda's cancer and her mother's. The doctors said they considered the odds of mother and daughter both going through a breast cancer diagnosis under such unique circumstances to be extremely rare. It was devastating for Brenda and her entire family. It also gave Brenda a newfound reason to fight. Despite her own battle, Brenda picked up and moved several thousand miles away to be by her mother's side.

"It was an experience I would never forget with us going though the breast cancer together. We had bonded a lot over the years but never on this level. She was my strength and I was hers and it brought us even closer together."

Sadly, Brenda's mother eventually lost her battle with breast cancer which led Brenda to strengthen her resolve to fight even harder. She is now celebrating six-years as a survivor and she is more determined than ever to not let breast cancer rule her life. Through her time with her mother, Brenda also realized how much she could offer other women who are going through a breast cancer diagnosis. She is now on a mission to help as many women as she can.

"I realize now that there is so much more I can be doing to help. That is one of the great things about pinktogether.com. I'm able to reach out to other women, to be there for support for them, to help them. That's the whole point, to get the word out there and to be supportive."

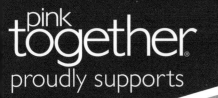

pink together® proudly supports

susan G. komen FOR THE cure®

Includes BONUS SECTION on Breast Cancer Awareness

Betty Crocker®
LIVING
WITH CANCER
COOKBOOK

Kris Ghosh, M.D., M.B.A. *Gynecologic Oncologist*, San Diego Center for GYN Oncology

Linda Carson, M.D. *Gynecologic Oncologist*, University of Minnesota Medical Center

Elyse Cohen, M.S., L.N. Bell Institute of Health and Nutrition

General Mills

Editorial Director: Jeff Nowak

Publishing Manager: Christine Gray

Editors: Diane Carlson
Cheri Olerud
Kathy Saatzer
Karen Schiemo
Grace Wells

Recipe Development and Testing:
Betty Crocker Kitchens

Photography: General Mills Photography
Studios and Image Library

Photographers: Andy Swarbrick
Maja Sahlberg

Food Stylists: Carol Grones
Susan Brosious

John Wiley & Sons, Inc.

Publisher: Natalie Chapman

Executive Editor: Anne Ficklen

Editorial Assistant: Heather Dabah

Senior Production Editor:
Jacqueline Beach

Cover Design: Suzanne Sunwoo

Art Director and Interior Design:
Tai Blanche

Interior Layout: Nick Anderson

Manufacturing Manager: Kevin Watt

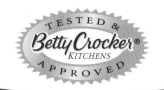

The Betty Crocker Kitchens seal guarantees success in your kitchen. Every recipe has been tested in America's Most Trusted Kitchens™ to meet our high standards of reliability, easy preparation and great taste.

Find more great ideas at
BettyCrocker.com

This book is printed on acid-free paper. ∞

Copyright © 2011 by General Mills, Minneapolis, Minnesota. All rights reserved.

Published by John Wiley & Sons, Inc., Hoboken, New Jersey

Published simultaneously in Canada

No part of this publication may be reproduced, stored in a retrieval system, or transmitted in any form or by any means, electronic, mechanical, photocopying, recording, scanning, or otherwise, except as permitted under Section 107 or 108 of the 1976 United States Copyright Act, without either the prior written permission of the Publisher, or authorization through payment of the appropriate per-copy fee to the Copyright Clearance Center, Inc., 222 Rosewood Drive, Danvers, MA 01923, (978) 750-8400, fax (978) 750-4470, or on the web at www. copyright.com. Requests to the Publisher for permission should be addressed to the Permissions Department, John Wiley & Sons, Inc., 111 River Street, Hoboken, NJ 07030, (201) 748-6011, fax (201) 748-6008, or online at http://www.wiley.com/go/permissions.

Trademarks: Wiley and the Wiley Publishing logo are trademarks or registered trademarks of John Wiley & Sons and/or its affiliates. All other trademarks referred to herein are trademarks of General Mills. John Wiley & Sons, Inc., is not associated with any product or vendor mentioned in this book.

Limit of Liability/Disclaimer of Warranty: While the publisher and author have used their best efforts in preparing this book, they make no representations or warranties with respect to the accuracy or completeness of the contents of this book and specifically disclaim any implied warranties of merchantability or fitness for a particular purpose. No warranty may be created or extended by sales representatives or written sales materials. The advice and strategies contained herein may not be suitable for your situation. You should consult with a professional where appropriate. Neither the publisher nor author shall be liable for any loss of profit or any other commercial damages, including but not limited to special, incidental, consequential, or other damages.

For general information on our other products and services or for technical support, please contact our Customer Care Department within the United States at (800) 762-2974, outside the United States at (317) 572-3993 or fax (317) 572-4002.

Wiley also publishes its books in a variety of electronic formats. Some content that appears in print may not be available in electronic books. For more information about Wiley products, visit our web site at www.wiley.com.

Library of Congress Cataloging-in-Publication Data

Crocker, Betty.
    Betty Crocker living with cancer cookbook / Betty Crocker. — Pink together ed.
        p. cm.
    Includes index.
    Summary: "Designed for those undergoing cancer treatment as well as their family and/or caretakers who are looking to enjoy delicious and nutritious meals"— Provided by publisher.
        ISBN 978-1-118-08314-7 (pbk.)
    1. Cancer—Diet therapy—Recipes. 2. Cancer—Treatment—Complications—Diet therapy—Recipes. 3. Cancer—Nutritional aspects. I. Title. II. Title: Living with cancer cookbook.
    RC271.D52C76 2011
    641.5′631—dc23
                            2011028231

Manufactured in the United States of America

10 9 8 7 6 5 4 3 2 1

A special thanks to the following individuals who provided tasty recipes and insightful quotes:
Theresa H., Pat Y., Randie N., Susan S., Marie E., Anne R., Catherine H., Lois K., Marilyn T., Patty N., Mary W., Joan K., Ellen T., MaryElaine W., Kathy S., Joyce K., Carol N. and Judy O.

Since its launch in 2002, the *Betty Crocker Living with Cancer Cookbook* has helped many survivors with their battle against cancer. A collaboration between the trusted kitchens of Betty Crocker, cancer doctors, nutrition experts and real cancer survivors, this book offers guidance for a time when the simple tasks of eating and cooking are a challenge. Awarded an International Association of Culinary Professionals award in 2003, this guide has received worldwide support and praise among many leaders in nutrition and cancer care.

New technology and new medications are helping us continue to win battles in our fight. However, our patients' struggles and priorities remain the same, including how to gain control of their lives and perform the simple tasks of cooking and eating. As some of our newer therapies offer new challenges, we find that, for our patients, combating the side effects of treatment and maintaining some sense of normalcy and quality of life remain the foundation for success.

Inspired by the questions posed by our patients and their families, we offer some direction to the nutritional hurdles that cancer patients confront daily. Nutritional health is still the most important indicator for the way our patients handle their treatment and their survival. This book offers general nutritional guidelines for our patients undergoing surgery, radiation or chemotherapy. These recipes have been tried by many patients and their families over the past decade, and offer tasty recipes that are simple to prepare and help target specific side effects.

Nutrition and quality of life go hand in hand, and are the focus of cancer care. Everyone who contributed to this book will be remembered for their wisdom and guidance and for paving the way for survival for many to come.

Betty Crocker has been the name that people count on for healthy cooking, easy recipes and great taste. The *Betty Crocker Living with Cancer Cookbook* was the first of many books targeting this specific dietary need. We continue to hope that the *Betty Crocker Living with Cancer Cookbook* will bring back the joy of eating to you and those you love!

Kris Ghosh, M.D., M.B.A.   **Linda Carson, M.D.**

Key to Common Side Effects

The four most common symptoms in cancer treatment are nausea, mouth sores, diarrhea and constipation. Eating the right foods can help these symptoms, and to make it easier to find foods that work for you, we have marked recipes that are especially good for these symptoms. Remember, any of the recipes in this book will help you during cancer treatment—your personal preference is always the best indicator of what recipe is best for you.

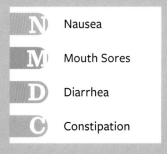

N	Nausea
M	Mouth Sores
D	Diarrhea
C	Constipation

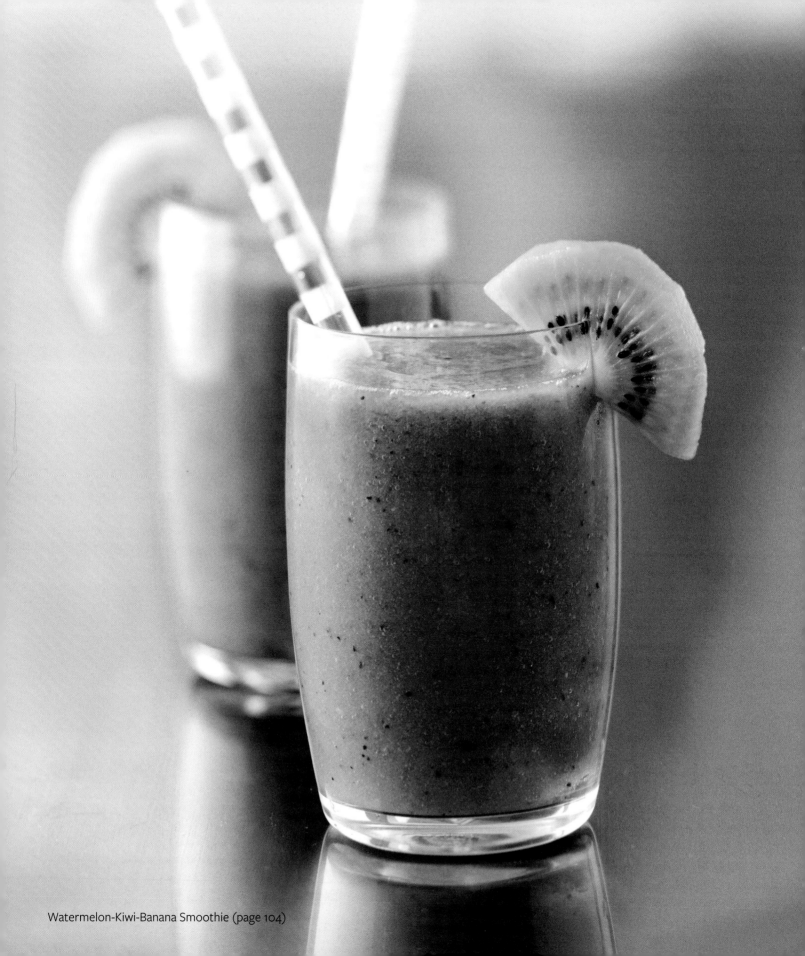

Watermelon-Kiwi-Banana Smoothie (page 104)

CONTENTS

Bring Back the Joy of Eating   6

1   Coping with Side Effects   26

2   Energy-Boosting Breakfasts   50

3   Fatigue-Fighting Snacks   78

4   20-Minute Main Dishes   110

5   Make-Ahead Meals   140

6   Family-Pleasing Main Dishes   170

7   Comforting Side Dishes   202

8   Treat-Yourself Desserts   220

Easy Menus During Treatment   236

Recipes to Use After Treatment   245

Nutrition and Medical Glossary   247

Additional Resources   248

Metric Conversion Guide   249

Recipe Testing and Calculating Nutrition Information   250

Index   251

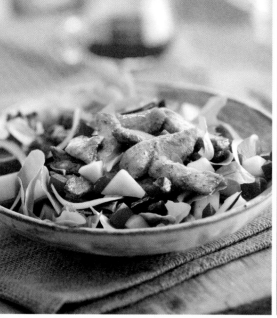
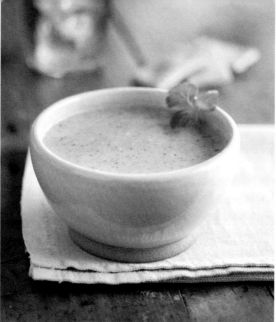
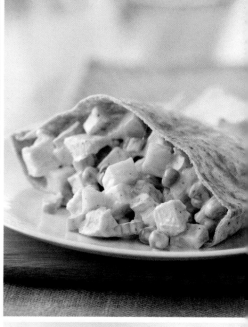
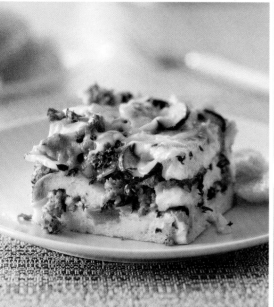
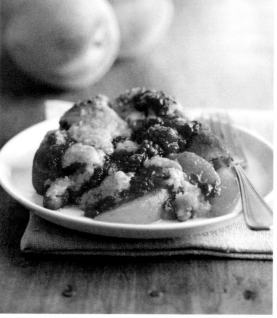
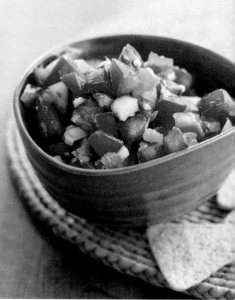
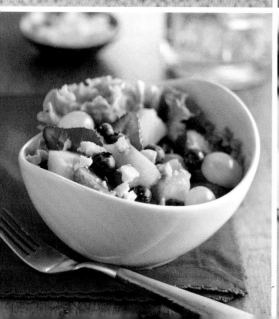
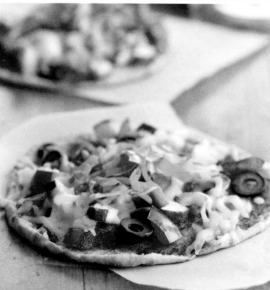
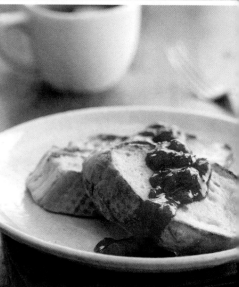

Bring Back the Joy of Eating

Although your life is changing and you are extremely frightened, a diagnosis of cancer does not have to take over your life. You may feel that way at first, but that feeling need not stay. Some cancer survivors have told us they prefer to focus on the future and their life after cancer because doing so offers hope.

One way to regain control in your life is to plan what to cook and eat every day. Nutrition and eating well are absolutely essential to your recovery and quality of life.

Included in this book are secrets of survival from cancer patients. These individuals share the small hints and the big ideas that worked for them as they navigated their cancer diagnosis and treatment. They offer bits of advice and wisdom they found to be helpful in their personal struggles to thrive and that brought back the joy of eating for them.

Be Prepared for a Roller Coaster Ride

If you've recently learned that you—or a loved one—has cancer, you may wonder how you, your friends and family can possibly cope. Living with cancer and its treatment can be compared to a roller coaster ride: from day to day, you never know what to expect; the ups, downs and side curves are unknowns. Not knowing the outcome is also very scary.

Understandably, you are experiencing many thoughts, emotions and feelings that are overwhelming. It's normal to feel a lack of control over your life. Take the time you need to accept your or your loved one's diagnosis. Talk to your doctor, dietitian, nurse, counselor, member of the clergy, family and friends. Seek out information to learn everything you can about the disease, treatment and side effects, and learn what you can do for yourself.

As different as each person's DNA, cancer affects people in different ways. Your—or your loved one's—experience with cancer is an individual challenge, a personal roller coaster ride. As you are presented with options, you must decide what is right for you. The plan that's effective for one individual may not work well for another. And rather than follow a road map that may have been developed for someone else, it's best to create your own plan. Trial and error, your own energy level and listening to your body are the best guides to determine what works for you. If you are supporting someone during this time, try to help by gathering information, or taking notes when you meet with doctors, providing child care during medical visits, and discussing possible options for treatment.

In this section, the focus is on the nutritional needs of individuals with cancer and ways to help you meet these needs. Information on eating out, grocery shopping and special diets is also included. In addition to discussing a traditional medical perspective, some of the alternative or complementary therapies are also addressed.

In Chapter 1, you'll find a helpful Coping with Side Effects guide that includes expert medical advice on ten common side effects, a recipe to help each particular side effect and a list of the top recipes in the book that are helpful for the four most bothersome side effects. Following that are seven chapters of recipes to use in planning your meals and mini-meals, including foods that your whole family can help you prepare and enjoy, or that you can prepare to help your loved one with cancer.

Though primarily written for the newly diagnosed cancer patient, this cookbook is also for families and friends and those survivors who remain in treatment for an extended period of time. Because the needs of each cancer patient are unique, we invite you to use this cookbook as a guide. You may adopt the information and recipes that meet your needs and skim over the remainder. We hope this book will bring back the joy of eating for you and those you love.

What Is Cancer All About, Anyway?

In the beginning, understanding the basics about cancer and treatment and what you can expect is important. Here are the answers to some frequently asked questions:

What is cancer?

Cancer is a family of diseases with a wide variety of symptoms. It is often described as an abnormal growth of cells—any cells—in some part of the body. Some cancers produce tumors or growths while others are blood-borne, like leukemia. Cancer affects women, men, children and the elderly. The foods we eat, our genetic makeup and the environment we've been exposed to all impact the risk of developing cancer. A diet high in animal fat has been linked to cancer. Thus, a well-balanced, lower-fat diet is an important part of cancer prevention. In addition, scientific research estimates that almost one-third of cancer cases are related to diet—and numbers are increasing.

How is cancer treated?

Treatment of most cancers requires several approaches. Depending on the type and stage of cancer, treatment may include surgery, radiation, chemotherapy or biological therapies. The success of any treatment is related to the overall health of the survivor.

Complementary therapies including meditation, herbal remedies and acupuncture as well as nutritional therapies have been used with conventional treatments. Always consult your healthcare team when starting a new therapy. Eating a well-balanced diet rich in vitamins and minerals is often a best practice during cancer treatment. In addition, a positive attitude, a sense of humor, courage and having a strong support system of friends and family can have a tremendous impact on your healing and happiness.

Why me?

Though it is very common to pose the question "Why me?" (as almost every newly diagnosed cancer patient does), there is no exact answer. Individually, each patient must seek out answers to his or her own personal satisfaction. Asking the question "Why me?" is a normal response to grief about cancer, and it is the beginning of healing.

According to experts, grief has six stages. As we work through our grief, we move through these stages. And as the word "stage" implies, we may be in more than one grief stage at a time or we may move in and out of these stages in different orders, depending upon how we work through our grief. Eventually, as we heal, we reach acceptance, which allows us to move forward with our lives.

Here's a quick overview of the grief stages as they may relate to cancer:

- **Shock and Denial.** To protect us, our brains use shock, numbness and denial to cope with the traumas we experience, whether the traumas are physical or emotional. And for many, a cancer diagnosis is trauma. During this stage, denying the diagnosis of cancer is common. You may feel as though the diagnosis is a bad dream from which you will awaken and realize isn't true. You may go about your daily routine in a very surreal or disconnected way.

- **Bargaining.** When physical or emotional pain becomes unbearable, engaging in some form of negotiation is typical. Consciously or unconsciously, you may try to negotiate with a higher power, your spouse, your friend, your doctor or whomever you see as being able to help cure cancer and rectify the potential outcome. Bargaining is really an attempt to postpone your grief.

- **Anger.** You may become angry about cancer—angry with yourself, family members, doctors and even the world. You may play out your anger as hurt, frustration, fear, helplessness or guilt. The reasons and targets of anger are as unique as the individuals dealing with them. You may even surprise yourself with your rage. To help you cope, ask others to listen to how angry you feel about cancer.

- **Guilt.** You may blame yourself or others and often may feel helplessly guilty about a cancer diagnosis. You may say to yourself or others, "If only I had or hadn't done this." Or you may think, "What could I have done to prevent cancer?" Unfortunately, there may be nothing you can do or could have done to prevent or change a cancer diagnosis.

- **Depression.** A sense of helplessness and the reality of a cancer diagnosis sinks in deeply and you feel depressed. Symptoms of depression often include loss of appetite, feelings of worthlessness, an inability to enjoy anything, insomnia or difficulty concentrating and making decisions. If depression is lasting a long time, you may want to speak about how you feel with a caring friend, or go to a mental health professional if you feel that's the care you need.

- **Acceptance.** One day, you notice that the sun is shining and you have more good days than bad. You have hope, and you can begin to enjoy life again. At first, acceptance can be so subtle that you may not even recognize it. With time, you realize that there is life with cancer and, hopefully, life after cancer.

As you work through the stages of grief, recognizing and talking about your feelings is healthy, regardless of which stage you're in. Talking to others about how you feel is key to healing. And as you heal and accept cancer, you can begin to move on.

What resources are available to help me?

Continue to rely on your doctor as your first resource throughout your treatment. Other professionals who may be able to assist you are oncology nurses, dietitians and counselors. It takes an entire integrated team to provide good care. And you may find talking with other cancer survivors to be useful. If speaking with a cancer survivor would be helpful for you, ask your doctor for the names of survivors with the same type of cancer you have who have agreed to share their experiences.

On the internet, there are many blogs, support groups and resources. Just remember that everyone's journey is special and unique, and that not everything you hear or read will be relevant to you. If you find comments that are helpful, you may also want to share comments about your journey with newly diagnosed patients.

A cancer support group comprised of others who are going through experiences similar to your own can be an important source of support and strength. Ask your doctor to provide you with a contact or information about where and when local support groups meet. Organizations such as the American Cancer Society have an endless number of resources to share, from answering questions on hot lines to providing wigs and clothing for survivors to wear, to a website full of useful and helpful information. See page 248 for additional resources.

How quickly can life return to normal?

Depending on the type and stage of cancer you have and the kind of treatment you are undergoing, the time it takes can vary considerably. Then again, realizing that you may have to accept a "new normal" may be crucial to your self-esteem and your survival. Talking to your doctor and to other cancer survivors will give you some perspective, but realize that each type of cancer, each survivor and each situation is unique.

What can I expect from treatment day to day?

According to one cancer survivor, "Expect the unexpected." The common side effects of chemotherapy include fatigue, nausea, vomiting and diarrhea. As you undergo treatment, you will most likely experience days when you feel quite ill, days when you feel a bit better and days when you feel almost like your normal self. Tracking your own side-effect patterns relative to your treatments will give you some sense of what to expect, but realize, too, that your course may change. And there is a small percentage of patients who are fortunate enough to have little or no side effects at all.

Focus on and enjoy the days you feel well. On those days when you feel ill, remember that you will feel better again and your energy will return. As another survivor said, "This, too, shall pass."

Take Control of Your Life

Most cancer survivors say the best way to deal with your own recovery is to take charge. That means taking control of your life, control over your cancer and control over treatment options and potential side effects. So much about survival depends upon your outlook. Choose to educate yourself and learn as much as you can in order to make wise choices that are right for you.

Although each course is individual, survivors say there are six universal themes that are key to coping with and living with cancer.

1. Eat nutritious foods.

The link between diet and health continues to grow stronger with each new study published. In fact, the American Cancer Society estimates that more than 35 percent of new cancer diagnoses are related to diet. With obesity becoming an epidemic crisis, cancer rates are increasing among those who are overweight.

In addition to affecting physical health, food plays a major role in your mental health and well-being. The food you eat affects your energy level and how well you sleep and think. In your cancer battle, you may find that as your energy level drops, food will bring it back up. One survivor said, "During cancer treatment, eating was a tool to ward off both physical and mental fatigue."

Cancer patients have increased nutritional needs. And sound nutrition has a tremendously positive impact on healing. During treatment, your body has a greater need for calcium, iron, magnesium and potassium. This increased need is based on two reasons: (1) Your body is fighting the disease, which requires more energy and more nutrients than usual, and (2) your treatment kills cells, both cancerous and healthy cells, thereby disrupting the nutrient balance in your body.

Food can help you regain strength and vitality, but how do you know what to eat and how much? Eating can make you feel worse, so how do you know which foods to avoid? Fortunately, eating well does not have to mean preparing complicated foods or gourmet recipes. The simpler and easier the recipes are to prepare, the better—and the more likely you are to have the energy to eat.

One cancer survivor feels that eating well is the most important factor in her own healing: "Eating is a time of enjoyment and socialization. It goes beyond food. It is a ritual that brings people together for support, communication and pleasure. It is a way for us to feel 'normal' with family and friends."

2. Remain positive and hopeful.

"Keep a positive attitude, because it will help you physically and mentally," says another survivor. Though being "up" all the time is not possible, finding at least one thing to be thankful for each day can lift your spirits and give you courage. With a little practice, you will find more and more things you can appreciate.

To achieve the hopeful part, you can try to face your worst fears. Being able to identify what it is that you fear most may be helpful. Do you fear death? Leaving others behind to live out their lives while you are gone? Perhaps you fear life—if there's pain and discomfort. Whatever your fears are, trying to face them and coming to terms with them is very helpful for healing.

Once you've worked through your fears, it is possible to have hope and to go on living. Although imagining this seems difficult at first, some survivors say they think about having cancer as being presented with a gift, a unique ability to grow, to build inner strength and to make positive changes in their lives.

3. Use prayer, meditation and relaxation techniques.

Studies among patients in hospitals have indicated that there is a strong connection between healing and prayer. Having faith in a higher being, one who can help guide you through difficult times, is beneficial to many survivors. Spiritual connections, whether through prayer or meditation, can provide comfort, stress relief and focus for many people. For these reasons, prayer and meditation can be extremely beneficial to those who are sick. Even knowing that others are thinking about you in their prayers can provide relief. You are not alone. If you aren't comfortable with the concept of a higher being, practice relaxation techniques and realize that you are connected with all parts of the universe—the trees, waterfalls, the birds—those things that give you comfort.

4. Remember to laugh.

Laughter is like internal jogging. It promotes better blood circulation, can help lower blood pressure, relieves pain and stimulates the release of certain hormones that can have a calming effect. Laughing and smiling are contagious and can have a profound, positive effect on healing. One survivor said, "People must think cancer patients don't have a sense of humor. My family doesn't say anything funny to me anymore." Laughing at yourself or telling a joke can help ease tension, especially for family or friends who may not know what to say during this particularly difficult time. Letting others know you want to laugh and need to laugh may help ease their discomfort as well as yours.

5. Stay connected to others.

Isolating yourself from others during this difficult time may be tempting, but don't! Staying in touch with family and friends is very helpful to cancer survivors. Everyone needs support, and who better to provide support than people who know you and care about you? Cancer survivors offer advice to other survivors and their families: "Surround yourself with those you love!" "Just keep talking and sharing." "Join a support group!" "You don't need to do this completely on your own."

6. Take care of yourself.

"This is one time when it's okay to be selfish. Concentrate on yourself and getting well." "Don't be afraid to ask for help!" Advice from survivors includes tips on letting others help. Many cancer survivors find that asking for assistance isn't as hard as they think it might be. Anticipating the asking seems to be the hardest part, especially for those of us who pride ourselves on self-sufficiency. You may be surprised to find that friends and family are willing to help in any way they can; they just need guidance on where to put their efforts.

Find ways to be especially good to yourself, and include as many of the following options as you can each day and each week:

- Exercise daily. Thirty minutes of walking or light exercise is recommended each day to improve appetite and strength and to reduce fatigue. Try doing light housework, walking around the house or climbing the stairs. Because some days you will feel more energetic than others, be sure to exercise whenever you feel up to it. Many survivors have found that even a few minutes of exercise or activity stimulates their appetite. Your own energy level and how you feel are your best gauges to the frequency and amount of exercise that's right for you.

- Enjoy nature. Take a walk through the woods, picnic outside or stop to listen to the birds. Immersing yourself in nature will refresh and nourish you. Nature can be very healing for body, mind and soul. If you can't go outside, relax by an open window and breathe in the fresh air, or gaze at nearby trees, faraway cloud formations or a fresh snowfall. Listen to the sounds of flowing water, even if it means simply running a bath!

- Celebrate! Celebrate simple accomplishments, such as reaching treatment hurdles or survival milestones. Take time to set the table and use the good china, just for fun. Put flowers or a plant on the table to represent life. Ask a friend to drop off some colorful balloons to create a party atmosphere. Plan a backward dinner where the whole family is silly and eats dessert first, then the main meal.

- Express yourself. Express your feelings, thoughts, hopes and frustrations in a journal. Write, type on the computer, tweet or record your thoughts by whatever means works best for you. You may be surprised by what's going on in your head and heart. Being able to share your feelings releases tension and aids healing.

- Try something new. Some survivors find that trying something new is rejuvenating. It's one way to lessen fears and boost spirits. Try a new food, a new body stretch or even a new adventure. Experience life to keep yourself feeling alive. One survivor who describes herself as "not too athletic" took up yoga for the first time and found she really enjoyed the stretching and breathing. Yoga helped her tune into her body in a new, healthy way.

- Rest. No matter what time the clock says, if you're tired, take a nap. Sleep is your body's way of shutting down to recharge, to regain energy and start anew. Try to sleep well at night by slowing down before bedtime and limiting caffeine late in the day. And if you need to snooze during the day, allow yourself this wonderfully healing renewal.

- Use relaxation techniques. Find a comfy spot and listen to calming music or try deep breathing to relax. Use meditation—even for a short time—by repeating a simple word or sound to focus your energy and center yourself. Visualize being in pleasant surroundings enveloped in healing light and warmth. Stretch out on the bed or floor and let the tension ease out of your body. If you're feeling up to it, have a gentle massage, or take a yoga class.

FOODS RICH IN ESSENTIAL NUTRIENTS

Potassium	Calcium	Iron	Magnesium
Tomatoes	Milk	Ready-to-eat cereals (fortified with iron)	Green leafy vegetables
Bananas	Yogurt	Hot cereals (fortified with iron)	Nuts
Oranges	Orange juice (fortified with calcium)	Spinach	Soybeans
Fruit juices	Tofu	Red meats (beef, pork)	Peanut butter
Vegetable juices	Salmon (with bones)	Peas	Ready-to-eat cereals (fortified with iron)
	Sardines	Nuts	Hot cereals (fortified with iron)
	Spinach	Green leafy vegetables	Bananas
	Broccoli		Fish
	Cheese		

Eat Well and Enjoy Food

Eating well means keeping your body healthy through the foods you eat. Making nutritious food selections, enjoying eating and maintaining a healthy body fit together. It takes some planning, but the payoff is well worth the effort.

You may have questions about which foods to eat now that you've been diagnosed with cancer. You may wish to consider these factors when making your food selections:

- Choose foods you like. Eating will be easier if you're eating foods you like, even if it means eating for breakfast what you'd normally eat for dinner. If the food is appealing to you, enjoy it.
- Select foods with healing nutrients. Potassium, calcium, iron and magnesium are nutrients beneficial for your body, especially during healing. For easy planning, the recipes in this cookbook list how much of each of these nutrients they contain.
- Ask your doctor. For your particular type of cancer or treatment, there may be some dos and don'ts for success that others may have learned from past experiences. Check with your doctor to be sure you're on the right track.

The Importance of Sound Nutrition

Planning meals and eating can be real challenges when you aren't feeling well, and sound nutrition has perhaps never been more important to your life than right now—your very survival may depend on it. Keep these important nutrition basics in mind as you plan and eat your meals.

Balance Is Key

Eating a balanced diet including a variety of foods each day helps ensure that you get the fuel and all the vitamins and minerals your body needs. The fuel, or energy your body requires, comes from calories. And calories come from balanced sources of carbohydrates, protein and fat.

Carbohydrates provide quick energy and are your body's favorite fuel source. That's why the bulk of your calories (about 55 to 60 percent) is made up of carbohydrates. Foods such as bread, cereal, pasta, rice and potatoes are all examples of carbohydrates, along with simple sugars, honey and fruits. Easy to eat, these foods provide calories that can help sustain you through treatment and healing.

Radiation (Radiotherapy) Remedies

Radiation is recommended for some types of cancers. If you'll be undergoing radiation treatments, you'll want to know these facts:

1. Fatigue is the most common side effect from radiotherapy and can last for months after treatment.

2. Other side effects from radiotherapy depend upon where the radiation is directed. If you have radiation in the stomach area, a common side effect is nausea. If you have radiation to the pelvis, you may experience diarrhea or pain with urination.

3. A low-residue/low-fiber diet is recommended during abdominal and/or pelvic radiation. Avoid popcorn—it may cause diarrhea or bowel obstruction if eaten soon after abdominal/pelvic treatments. Ask your doctor for a list of low-residue and low-fiber foods. Also refer to pages 19 to 20 for a list of these foods, and look through this cookbook for recipes that are flagged as "low fiber" and "low residue."

4. Eat foods that contain high concentrations of iron, and eat these foods with an orange or another food high in vitamin C so the iron in the food can be more easily absorbed. Many of the recipes in this cookbook are flagged as being high in iron. Also, ask your doctor if you need iron supplements to keep your iron stores high; preventing anemia can help the radiation work better.

Protein helps build new cells. It makes hormones and enzymes that keep your body functioning and makes antibodies to fight off infection. Protein comes primarily from animal foods, such as meats, fish, poultry and dairy sources, along with some plant foods such as dry beans, vegetables, rice and pasta. As your body fights the cancerous cells, it needs plenty of protein to keep going.

Fat helps to build new cells, shuttle vitamins through your body and make certain hormones that regulate your blood pressure, along with other vital functions. Fats come from oils, butter, margarine, nuts and sweets (such as chocolate and ice cream). Experts recommend that no more than 35 percent of calories should come from fat. But as you progress through your treatment, you may find you need a bit of extra fat to maintain your weight. When adding fat, try to stay away from fried or greasy foods because they may be difficult to digest.

Vitamins help release energy from the fuel sources of carbohydrate, protein and fat. Your vision, hair and skin, as well as the strength of your bones, all depend upon the vitamins that come from the foods you eat. The more variety you have in your diet, the more likely you are to get all the vitamins your body needs.

Minerals help your body with many functions under the surface. Of particular importance during cancer treatment, certain minerals may be needed in greater than normal amounts. Iron, for example, a mineral that carries much-needed oxygen to your body cells, is in great demand. Calcium (key to strong bones and teeth) and potassium (important for proper nerve and muscle function) are also required in greater amounts than usual by cancer survivors.

Surgery and chemotherapy deplete the body of many essential vitamins and minerals. The Foods Rich in Essential Nutrients chart on page 13 shows food sources that can help provide some of these important minerals. Check with your doctor or dietitian to be sure your diet is supplying sufficient quantities of nutrients or to see if you require supplements. It's best not to take vitamin and mineral supplements on your own, without the supervision of your doctor or dietitian.

Enjoy Cooking, Shopping and Eating

With this emphasis on the increased need for certain nutrients, what needs to change in your diet, if anything, isn't always clear. Less clear is how to handle family meals and what you do with grocery shopping when battling cancer. Read on to learn more hints to help you and your family cope.

Should I make changes to my eating routine?

Much of the answer to this question depends upon your current eating habits, the particular kind of cancer you have, the treatment you are undergoing, any side effects you experience and the foods your body will tolerate. It is best to discuss any potential dietary changes with your dietitian and doctor.

There will be times when you won't be hungry, so eat whenever you can, even if it's only a small portion. If you crave a specific food, go ahead and eat it. If a regular-sized meal looks unmanageable, try eating several smaller meals or snacks throughout the day. Avoid eating just before bedtime because lying down after eating may cause nausea. A short brisk walk after dinner may help digest your food.

How do I cook for my family?

If cooking for your family has always been part of your daily life and you enjoy it, by all means continue. Simply plan what to eat, allowing for any dietary limitations. Then apply the sound nutrition advice from the previous pages and follow the simple tips below to ensure success:

- Plan menus together. Though patience and planning are needed to choose meals that satisfy everyone, family members want to feel they are doing something to help. And greater success is achieved when tasks are shared among the family.

- Save your strength. Overcoming fatigue can be a challenge. Focus on the tasks you enjoy and those that are manageable for your level of energy. Take advantage

of offers to help from friends and family members by allowing them to assist in food preparation and cooking, especially when you're feeling tired.

- Season foods to your tastes. Separate a serving or two after cooking each dish. Then season, spice or salt the smaller serving to your tastes! By adding extra flavor this way, one recipe can appeal to all members of the family.

- Enjoy eating. Just talking with and enjoying your family or friends in a pleasant environment can lead to successful eating. You don't have to be elaborate. Set the table, adjust the lights, play soft music, light candles or light a fire. Then sit back, eat and enjoy each other's company.

- Give up the cleanup. When the meal is over, let family or friends clear the table and clean the kitchen. That way, everyone plays a vital role and is contributing to the workload. Use your time to catch up on a little rest.

How do I go grocery shopping?

Shopping when you have cancer can be difficult, particularly when you don't feel well, you're overcome by fatigue or food sights and smells nauseate you. Take advantage of grocery stores and Web sites that offer home delivery. Or have family and friends pick up several items for you while they are doing their own shopping.

If you must go to the grocery store yourself, try these tips to make the most of your shopping trips:

- Shop in the morning or at times when you feel less fatigued.

- Make a detailed grocery list so you aren't tempted to binge shop. Visit smaller grocery stores and park close to the building.

- Visit only those aisles of the store that are necessary. Do the rest in a separate trip.

- Purchase prepared foods to ease food preparation. Bagged salads, baby-cut carrots, deli items and meat that's boned and trimmed of fat can make things easier for you at home.

Make MyPlate Your Plate

MyPlate is a simple visual approach to building a healthy plate at meal times and making healthier food choices every day. It is built on the 2010 *Dietary Guidelines for Americans*.

My Plate emphasizes eating a variety of nutritious foods from five major food groups (fruits, vegetables, grains, proteins and dairy) within a place setting—and includes awareness of eating these foods in the right proportions too.

The importance of nutrition is coupled with daily exercise for overall health. When you are feeling up to it and having a good day, try to go for a walk or swim or whatever keeps you moving. Following the 2010 *Dietary Guidelines* and MyPlate can indeed help in your healing. The points below can help you plan healthy meals for yourself and your family today... and for the future.

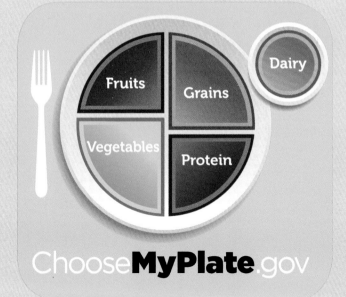

Choose**MyPlate**.gov

- **Enjoy your food, but eat less.**
Eating smaller amounts now when you aren't feeling your best may be the norm, but as you recover, you'll want to remember not to overdo it. Even when you eat small portions, include foods loaded with nutrients that aid recovery and replenish your increased needs for calcium, iron, potassium and magnesium. Be sure to eat lean protein foods (beef and pork loin, poultry breast, fish and shellfish, dry beans, eggs and nuts) for iron and magnesium.

- **Fill half your plate with colorful fruits and vegetables.** Eat a bounty of plant foods in a variety of forms for plenty of vitamins A and C, folic acid and potassium—all nutrients necessary for a healthy body. If eating fruits and vegetables is difficult, try sipping juices or eating applesauce or pureed fruits from the blender.

- **Switch to fat-free or low-fat (1%) milk and milk products.**

Fat-free milk, lower fat cheeses and light yogurt offer bone-building calcium and vitamin D benefits without extra fat. Seek out nutrition information to be sure you know what you're getting—at least 10 to 20% Daily Value of calcium and vitamin D or more per serving.

- **Consume at least half your grains as whole grains.** Read labels and replace refined grains with whole wheat breads and tortillas, whole grain oats, barley, and whole grain cereals. These foods are good sources of B vitamins, iron. They also contain fiber to keep foods moving through the digestive tract. Look for the words "whole" at the top of the ingredient list.

- **Compare foods and recipes to help reduce sodium.** As you continue to feel better, you'll want to examine labels on canned and packaged foods such as soups, breads and frozen meals—choosing foods

with lower numbers. Read nutrition information on recipes too.

- **Drink water to keep calories down.** Experts generally recommend drinking plenty of water for healthy individuals. And that holds true for cancer survivors, too. Beverages such as milk, juices and herbal teas also count, but remember to quench your thirst with plain water as well. Add a spritz of lemon or lime, if it agrees with you.

- **Balance calories to help manage your weight.** Right now this may not be top of mind—as you eat to keep your weight up. But as eating and activity return to normal, it is important to remember that calories consumed must equal calories expended by activity to keep weight stable. Avoid oversized portions when eating out or bring half home. If you're trying to lose weight, tip the scales in your favor by eating less and exercising more.

- Buy convenience foods that stay fresh for a long time. Pastas, rice mixes, canned tuna and soups keep on the shelf for a long time.
- Shop at farmers' markets whenever you can. Open air promotes less nausea than closed-in grocery stores.
- And when you do have assistance in the grocery store, try these suggestions:
- Buy large quantities of foods to decrease the number of shopping trips.
- Purchase lots of produce. Fresh fruits and veggies are heavy to carry, but they are loaded with vitamins A and C, folic acid and other important nutrients.
- Minimize extra walking by asking family members to come along with you. They can run back for items you missed.
- Delegate carrying the grocery bags and putting the food away to an able-bodied family member or friend.

How can I stock my kitchen and pantry?

When you return home from grocery shopping, store your foods where they stay fresh the longest. To minimize smells and flavor changes, throw out questionable food items right away and keep packaged fresh foods only to their expiration date. Because food flavors and smells often become stronger over time, you may want to turn over this freshness duty to another household member, especially if you're experiencing nausea.

To make cooking for the family easier for you:

- Keep your kitchen well stocked.
- Organize your refrigerator and freezer so you and others can find foods easily.
- Ask family and friends to prepare meals.
- Use simple recipes that can be prepared quickly and easily. Many easy recipes are contained in this cookbook.
- Enlist help from others to rinse and cut fresh fruits and vegetables for easier eating.
- Prepare only foods that you and your family enjoy.

- Break up food preparation tasks, and rest when you can. Start some of the preparation early in the day when you have more energy.
- Use timesaving kitchen appliances such as a slow cooker, rice cooker, food processor and microwave oven that keep food odors contained.
- Cherish leftovers. Cook more food than you need for your immediate meal, and refrigerate or freeze unused portions for another time.
- Plan and prepare foods ahead of treatment times. If food preparation is difficult for you during chemotherapy, for example, rely on foods that have been cooked ahead of time and frozen, or ask friends or family to help out. Some of the recipes in this cookbook can be made ahead and refrigerated or frozen.
- Keep foods covered and sealed and take out the trash at the end of each meal to reduce lingering food odors.

How can I eat out?

Eating out is a great alternative to cooking. It can offer even more food choices than eating at home and eliminates the preparation and cleanup.

To ease your concerns, ask these important questions at the restaurant or phone ahead:

How is the food prepared?

- Limit fat and, therefore, the amount of fried or greasy foods you eat. High-fat choices can induce nausea and are difficult to digest. The best choices include broiled and grilled meals, because the flavor of the food is preserved without adding extra fat.

What ingredients are used in a particular dish?

- Explain what you cannot eat, because a dish may contain hidden ingredients such as onions, garlic, or spices that could cause discomfort. Knowing ahead of time about problem menu items and avoiding them is better than sending dishes back to the kitchen.

How hot or spicy are the foods?

- Some cancer patients can tolerate highly spiced foods and even prefer them, and others desire mild foods.

After-Surgery Suggestions

Read on for the most important things to do after cancer surgery:

1. Ask your doctor to explain the surgery that was performed. Did surgery involve the removal of tissue or organs? Were part of your intestines or colon removed, and will that affect the foods you can or cannot eat?

2. Ask if you need to be on a special diet and about any foods you may or may not be permitted to eat. Find out how long the dietary restrictions will last, either short term or long term.

3. Ask if you need specific vitamins or mineral supplements. Some nutrients must be supplemented after intestinal surgery, and others may help healing.

4. Eat six small meals per day. Small meals, rather than three large meals, are more easily tolerated after surgery. Try to eat half the normal serving size you ate before surgery. See Easy Menus, page 236.

5. Regular bowel movements are important after surgery to help get your system moving again. Talk to your doctor if you have not had a bowel movement within a 24-hour period after surgery.

6. Protein foods are needed for restoring strength and building new cells. In the first few weeks after surgery, eat plenty of protein-rich foods (found on page 14) and lower fat foods (to avoid cramping and bloating).

7. Vitamin C, calcium, iron, magnesium and potassium are essential healing vitamins and minerals. Make sure that you eat foods that contain these nutrients. For a list of good food sources, turn to page 13.

8. Start walking or doing light activity or simple exercises as soon as you feel up to it. Movement will help restore your appetite and the regularity your healing body needs. Before starting exercise, consult your doctor regarding any restrictions.

9. Remain properly hydrated post-surgery. Sip beverages—particularly water—throughout the day.

Spice level, sweetness and saltiness can often be tailored to your taste. Just let your server know what you need.

Can I order a small portion?

- Try to order à la carte items or lunch-size portions if possible. Select different kinds of foods and flavors when available. New food adventures often lead to greater success in finding foods that you enjoy.

Am I familiar with this restaurant or cuisine?

- Choose restaurants you know, if that eases your concerns. Or try new ones that sound appealing to you. Either way, request seating that's far away from the kitchen to avoid cooking smells that may cause nausea.

Is outdoor seating an option?

- Choose outside or patio dining whenever you can, weather permitting. Nature is known to be beneficial in the healing process, so be sure to indulge. Fresh air can help settle your stomach, and pleasant surroundings can enhance your overall eating experience.

Can I have the recipe?

- When you find a restaurant dish that appeals to you, request the recipe. Then try it at home and share the new food with family and friends. If others enjoy it, too, add it to your meal planning.

Will I be rushed through the meal?

- Getting ready and dining out does require some extra effort. If eating has been taking longer because of discomfort and you're concerned about feeling rushed, call ahead to be sure you can have a leisurely meal. Request a table that isn't on a tight reservation schedule so you can take your time eating and enjoy yourself.

Can I order dessert first?

- Yes, indeed! You're dealing with enough stresses related to cancer right now, and you certainly deserve a break. When eating out, choose to dine at a restaurant with a sense of humor and fun. If it's a stuffy place, you may want to select another restaurant that's more comfortable for you. And remember, dessert can offer many calories per bite, so indulge!

Special Diets

Depending on the type of cancer you have and your treatment plan, you may need to follow a special diet at different times during treatment. Check with your doctor or dietitian to clarify any eating restrictions or questions you may have. And follow the advice you've been given to ease discomfort and aid in your healing.

Some dietary restrictions involve terms such as fiber and residue. Fiber and residue may not be food descriptions you thought much about before your cancer diagnosis. To help aid your understanding, let's define the two words. Sometimes used interchangeably, the terms fiber and residue do have different meanings.

Fiber describes the type of carbohydrate in a food that isn't broken down before passing through to your stool. Sometimes people refer to fiber as providing roughage or bulk. For a diet to be high in fiber, it must contain foods that supply substantial amounts of fiber, totaling at least 25 to 35 grams daily. Check the Nutrition Facts on packaged food products or check the recipe nutrition information for the fiber content of foods you eat.

Residue is the material left in the colon after digestion. It includes intestinal cells and breakdown products including fiber from the foods you eat. Increasing the amount of fiber you eat will increase residue and, therefore, the amount of stool you produce.

High-fiber foods are also high-residue foods. And low-residue foods are low in fiber. However, some low-fiber foods contain residue, too. For example, milk is low in fiber but high in residue. The components in milk have a considerable effect on stool production, even though milk contains no fiber.

Information about residue is not listed on Nutrition Facts labels, nor is it usually included in recipe nutrition information. However, any recipe in this cookbook that is low residue is listed that way. Check out the information below to find foods that fit your individual dietary needs.

Foods for Special Diets

Low Residue

Some survivors, particularly those who have had stomach or colon cancer, find that a low-residue diet works well for them. If your doctor or dietitian has recommended following a low-residue diet, follow the suggestions listed below.

These foods are allowed on a low-residue diet:

- Beef and pork
- Chicken and turkey
- Fish and seafood
- Eggs
- Milk, no more than 1 to 2 cups per day
- Potatoes
- Cooked spinach, asparagus, beets, eggplant, green beans and rutabaga
- Canned tomato paste and jarred tomato sauce (no seeds, no onions)
- Avocado (limit to 1 serving per day)
- Cooked or canned applesauce, fruit cocktail and pears
- Nectarines, peaches, cantaloupe and honeydew (limit fresh to 1 serving per day)
- Fruit and vegetable juices and purees
- Pasta (white) and couscous
- White bread and crackers
- White-flour pancakes
- Cooked oatmeal, cornmeal, farina, hot wheat cereal, and cream of rice cereal
- Egg and rice noodles
- Plain cakes and cookies
- Graham crackers
- Saltine crackers
- Broth and bouillon
- Butter
- Gelatin
- Italian fruit ice

Avoid these foods if eating a low-residue diet:

- No whole grains, coarse wheat and bran
- No seeds, nuts, dried fruits and fruit skins
- No coconut, popcorn and marmalade
- No apples, berries, citrus, pears and plums
- No watermelon, pumpkin and prunes
- No rice
- No peas, carrots, tomatoes and squash
- No broccoli, cabbage, cauliflower and rhubarb
- No dairy products

High Residue

If you don't have any restrictions on the amount of residue in your diet, you may eat a high-residue diet and also include the foods listed under "low residue" above.

Low Fiber

If you have been advised to follow a low-fiber diet, eat only foods containing less than 1 gram of fiber per serving. The amount of fiber in each recipe is included in this book. And you can read the Nutrition Facts labels to determine the fiber content of packaged food products.

Low-fiber foods include white bread, clear broth, clear liquids (tea, carbonated beverages), saltine crackers, fish, eggs, chicken, beef and flavored gelatin to name a few.

High Fiber

To follow a high-fiber diet, the more fiber you eat, the better. Experts recommend at least 25 grams of fiber daily. To get enough fiber each day, be sure to include:

- 10-ounce equivalents or more of whole-grain breads, cereals, bran, rice, pasta and other products made with whole grains
- 4 to 6 cups of vegetables and fruits, especially those with edible skins, seeds and hulls
- 2- to 3-ounce equivalents or more of legumes (dried peas and beans) and nuts for protein

Liquid Diet

A liquid diet is often prescribed for hospital patients immediately following surgery because it is soothing and easy to digest. It can also be helpful for times when you may be experiencing bouts of nausea, vomiting or diarrhea or when you're having difficulty chewing.

A clear liquid diet is comprised mainly of liquids and provides only about 500 calories per day. For this reason, a liquid diet is a short-term regimen only. Clear liquids do not provide enough calories and nutrients to maintain good health or to aid in long-term healing.

A clear liquid diet includes the following items only:

- Tea, clear beverages and carbonated beverages
- Clear fruit juices (such as apple and grape)
- Broth
- Flavored gelatin
- No milk or milk beverages
- No fruit juices with pulp
- Sports drinks and certain energy drinks

Sometimes cancer survivors may require a liquid diet, but it need not be only clear liquids. Check with your doctor or dietitian to see if a liquid diet with the addition of nutritional beverages, blended smoothies or shakes may be appropriate for you to increase calories and nutrients.

Neutropenic Diet

Cancer treatment can affect your immune system. Cancer survivors undergoing either bone marrow transplant or chemotherapy may be at risk for infection when their white blood cell count is below 500 cells per cubic millimeter of blood. If your white blood cell count is too low and you've been placed on a neutropenic diet, omit the following foods from your diet to reduce risk of infection:

- No raw or undercooked meat, chicken, pork, fish or shellfish.
- No raw eggs (no Caesar salad, homemade ice cream, cookie dough or cake batter). Use pasteurized egg products as a substitute.

- No unpasteurized or raw milk products.

- No honey, nuts or fruit or vegetable juices.

- No raw vegetables or fruits (except peeled, washed, thick-skinned fruits such as cantaloupe, honeydew melon, watermelon, oranges and bananas).

- No outdated products (out-of-code, past sell-by or use-by dates) or moldy products.

- No aged cheeses (such as Brie, blue, sharp Cheddar, Stilton, feta, Mexican hot cheese and Camembert).

Mind-Body-Spirit Connection to Healing

In conventional medicine, the mind-body connection is not the focus of the treatment. We rely instead on things outside of us, such as medications and surgery, to cure ailments. This is typical of cancer treatment practices today. Complementary, or alternative, medicine or therapies place more emphasis on using the inside, our thoughts and emotions, as an integral part of healing and overall wellness.

Complementary Therapies

Listed below are treatment options that could be tried in addition to your current treatment options. In the United States, more than 25 percent of all cancer patients will try at least one alternative therapy during the course of their treatment. Some claims of complementary therapies are poorly documented or unproven, but others are supported by years of scientific research.Alternative Medicine, established in 1991 gave rise to the National Center for Complementary and Alternative Medicine (NCCAM) in 1998. NCCAM collects research data on complementary practices and helps to establish safety guidelines and effectiveness of these therapies.

Connecting the brain, the physical body and good health as tools for wellness is easier in many complementary therapies. Many of the therapies listed here began thousands of years ago, in cultures spanning the globe, from Europe to China and India to Egypt. The treatments use herbs, needles or body manipulation as a means to heal ailments. Before you venture out to try them, read on for details about what

Chemotherapy Considerations

Chemotherapy, the most common type of cancer treatment, affects no two people the same way. Much of what happens depends on how you respond to the treatment, the particular drug or drugs you are taking, the dosage and the type and stage of the cancer. Consider these suggestions to help make your experience with chemotherapy one that works in the best way for you:

1. Ask your doctor what kind of drugs you are receiving. Ask about potential side effects and interactions that may occur and make changes as needed.

2. Raise questions about how the drug is administered and about any potential side effects so you are prepared for how you may feel and the changes your body may experience during and after treatment.

3. Whenever you have nausea, take the nausea medication provided because it generally will help you feel well enough to eat. If the medication isn't helpful, call your doctor right away and discuss alternate medication.

4. Your body is already tired just from having cancer, and chemotherapy adds to that feeling of fatigue. To help ease the tiredness, rest often and try to do some activity every day. More ideas about handling fatigue are provided on page 28.

5. Expect the common side effects of chemotherapy: decreased appetite, mouth sores, dry mouth, changes in the taste of foods and constipation.

6. If you are not having a bowel movement daily, ask your doctor about drinking more fluid, eating more fiber (25 to 35 grams) or taking a stool softener or laxative.

7. Vitamin and mineral stores in the body become depleted while you undergo chemotherapy. Ask your doctor if you need to take any nutrient supplements (especially iron, which can help reduce fatigue) or switch from the supplements you regularly take.

8. Neutropenia occurs when the white blood cell count drops to a dangerously low level—about 7 to 14 days after receiving chemotherapy—when you are at higher risk for infections and should avoid certain foods (listed on page 20 and 21).

they are and how they work; explore research and resources available from NCCAM. If you have questions about blending these therapies with your current medications or cancer treatment plan, be sure to check with your doctor.

Acupuncture

Part of traditional Chinese medicine, acupuncture is an ancient art and science of healing. The word acupuncture comes from two Latin words: acus, meaning "needles," and punctura, meaning "pricking." Like its definition, Chinese acupuncture involves the insertion of needles into specific points on your body.

Based on the belief that energy flows between body organs along channels, or meridians, healing occurs when the flow of energy in the entire body is balanced. The energy is called chi, or qi (pronounced CHEE). Chi changes with your mental, physical and spiritual well-being and is made up of two opposing forces called yin (the shady side of the mountain) and yang (the sunny side).

Worldwide scientific evidence exists to support that acupuncture is a successful treatment for headaches, lower back pain, angina, dementia and arthritis and for relief of other ailments or imbalances.

Aromatherapy

Aromatherapy, or scent therapy, was developed by ancient Egyptians and is the use of "essential oils" to increase relaxation, improve mood and enhance circulation. Essential oils are the concentrated forms of natural oils extracted from petals, leaves, roots, resin, bark, rinds, stalks, stems and seeds of various plants.

After they're extracted, essential oils are applied externally, inhaled or used in compresses or lotions. They are also used in soaps, candles, perfumes, potpourri, bath salts, massage oils, antiseptic solutions, sprays and shampoos.

Ayurveda

One of the oldest forms of medical practice, Ayurveda (pronounced I-YUR-VAYDA) originated in ancient India. It is based on the concept that energy, called prana, keeps the mind and body alive. Each of us is made up of five elements: air, water, earth, fire and space. These five elements are organized into three constitutional states called doshas, which govern our physical, mental and emotional processes. These doshas are vata, representing space and air; pitta, for fire and water; and kapha, encompassing water and earth. Each of us is a combination of all three doshas, but usually one of them dominates.

Ayurvedic practitioners observe, ask questions about your lifestyle, spirituality and physical health, touch you, and take pulses at different places to determine the diagnosis and assess the status of your doshas, depending upon which elements are out of balance. You are then further categorized based on the dietary changes needed to rebalance your doshas.

Most Ayurvedic remedies are diet-based, using foods, herbs and spices to regain balance by strengthening or weakening the doshas. In addition, other remedies and behavioral changes, such as minerals, gems, yoga postures and breathing, meditation, detoxification processes or hydrotherapy and massages, may be advised to reestablish the elements.

Bodywork

Bodywork is a catchall term for many different techniques that treat ailments and promote relaxation through proper movement, posture, exercise, massage and other body manipulations. Shiatsu and massage are two types of bodywork practiced more commonly in the United States.

Shiatsu, a traditional healing method from Japan, uses a form of acupressure, or finger pressure, on specific body sites to increase circulation and improve energy flow. The technique involves locating acupoints, sites on your body specific to certain tissues. Pressure is applied to these points for two to ten minutes until a pulse is felt. Then the pressure is released slowly. Acupressure techniques can be used in physical therapy and in various types of bodywork and massage.

Massage is the manipulation of soft tissues to relieve sore muscles and promote relaxation. It is used to reduce tension, improve circulation, aid in healing injured soft tissues, control pain and promote overall well-being.

Massage can stretch tissue, increase your range of motion and reduce certain kinds of swelling.

Herbal Medicine

Herbs come from plants, mainly the leaves, stems, flowers, twigs, roots, seeds, bark, fruit and saps of a variety of different plants. We typically think of herbs as substances that impart flavor to our foods, but some of these herbs also have medicine-like qualities.

In fact, many modern medicines are derived from plants discovered long ago to have medicinal properties. Though herbs can be predecessors to modern medicines, they are not regulated by the Food and Drug Administration (FDA), so use caution when obtaining them. You can buy herbal remedies in the form of capsules, tablets, powders and concentrated liquids (called tinctures or extracts), and they can be prepared using fresh or dried ingredients and can be steeped or infused, as in making a tea.

For your own safety, experts suggest you purchase prepared herbal medicines from reliable sources, because those grown or concocted yourself may be inconsistent or contain natural variations that can be toxic. Trained professionals in the fields of botany, Ayurvedic medicine, naturopathy and traditional Chinese medicine can be helpful in selecting the herbs, form and potency that are appropriate for you.

Herbal medicines are usually milder and may act more slowly than conventional medicines. Certain herbs, such as borage, chaparral, coltsfoot, comfrey, ma huang (ephedra), germanium and yohimbe should not be used because they are potentially harmful, causing liver disease, rises in blood pressure and kidney damage. Check with your doctor to be sure that the herbs you take don't interact with your medications or treatment regimens.

Meditation

Quiet forms of contemplation, mindfulness or meditation have been recognized worldwide for their effectiveness at establishing a sense of peacefulness, inner calm and relaxation. Developed in Eastern cultures, most techniques require closing your eyes and focusing on a single thought, word, image or sound and allowing other thoughts to float away. Traditionally used as a spiritual exercise, meditation has been helpful for people with chronic pain, panic attacks, high blood pressure and respiratory problems such as asthma and emphysema because meditation slows the heart rate and regulates breathing.

Naturopathy

Naturopathy originates from the traditions of early European health spas. Emphasizing preventive care, naturopathy takes advantage of your body's own natural healing powers. It avoids many of the traditions of conventional medicine and teaches healthful lifestyle habits. Naturopathic treatments vary by practitioner and encompass many elements, such as massage, physical activity, herbal remedies, natural foods, acupuncture and hydrotherapy (water treatments).

Yoga

Yoga is an ancient practice and philosophy first developed and practiced in India. The word yoga is derived from the ancient Sanskrit word yuj, meaning "union." Yoga is based on balancing the mind, body and spirit by using exercises, ethical beliefs and dietary restrictions.

Many different types of yoga are practiced worldwide. Western versions of yoga typically practiced in the United States include both body positions and movements, called postures, and breathing exercises, in addition to dietary practices. The postures, called asanas, are used to stretch and strengthen muscles; the breathing exercises, called pranayama, help with relaxation and stress relief. Yoga experts advise that you start slowly with basic breathing techniques and simple postures before moving on to the more advanced exercises.

Summing It Up

As you can see, the wide variety of complementary medicines and therapies from different parts of the world focus on different principles. All are available to you as you make the connection between your mind and body and wellness. Be sure to check with your doctor if you have any questions about your conventional medication or treatment plan or about one of these complementary therapies.

Beyond Treatment

Congratulations! You've made it through your treatment and have started to move on with your life. Cancer survivors have told us that treatment effects, particularly fatigue, may last for a period of time after treatment is complete. To minimize fatigue and continue your healing, you may wish to incorporate some basic principles about food and lifestyle that may help as you continue on your healing path.

Basics for a Healthy Lifestyle

The 2010 Dietary Guidelines for Americans and MyPlate, published by the U.S. Departments of Agriculture and Health and Human Services, can help you take action for good health and develop a healthy lifestyle. Some of the basic messages of a healthy lifestyle include being active each day, eating plant foods and making sensible food choices overall.

At first, following these suggestions may be difficult for some cancer survivors. If so, survivors may be better served by starting with a focus on eating plant foods and making sensible choices, and then including activity when they are feeling better.

Be Active Daily

As you probably know, obesity is linked to many diseases. Carrying extra weight may place you at greater risk for developing high blood pressure, heart disease, certain types of cancer, diabetes, stroke, arthritis and difficult breathing. Choosing a lifestyle that helps you increase your level of activity and strive for a healthy body weight may be helpful for maintaining good health in the long run.

Experts recommend monitoring body weight regularly by stepping on the scale every few weeks. Work with your doctor or dietitian to determine your Body Mass Index (BMI), a measure that links your height and weight to potential health risks. If you find you weigh more than you would like to, there is no better time than after treatment to take off excess weight. (During treatment is not a good time to try to lose weight, because your body is concentrating on fighting cancer cells.) But it's best to lose the weight gradually. Aim to lose about 10 percent of your weight in about six months—or about one-half to two pounds per week. Losing weight and maintaining a healthy weight should become part of your everyday lifestyle.

Being physically active on a daily basis can help you take off and keep off weight, strengthen and tone muscles and increase your flexibility. Aim for at least 60 minutes of physical activity daily or more if you are trying to lose weight. You don't have to do it all at the same time. Keep track of the times you go up and down the steps, walk through the parking lot and lift things, such as groceries. All these activities count and add up to your total activity for the day.

Eat Plant Foods

MyPlate on page 16 is a wonderful visual guide to remind you of the variety and proportions of foods you need daily. Use plant foods such as fruits, vegetables and whole grains, legumes, nuts and seeds as the mainstay of your diet. These foods supply much of the carbohydrate energy you need, along with many of the vitamins and minerals.

Plant foods should make up three-quarters of your plate and should be the focus of your eating. Scientific research has shown that whole grains (such as whole wheat and whole-grain oats), legumes (dried beans and peas), cruciferous vegetables (those in the cabbage family such as broccoli, kale and Brussels sprouts) contain fiber, vitamins, minerals and other natural components that may help prevent disease. Dark green vegetables (including spinach and broccoli) and orange-yellow fruits and vegetables (such as carrots, winter squash, sweet potatoes, cantaloupe and oranges) are rich in antioxidants (vitamins A and C) and folic acid, which are also important for maintaining a healthy body.

To these plant foods, add small amounts of lean cuts of meat, poultry, fish, eggs and low-fat dairy foods to balance out your diet. Variety is vital to a balanced diet that supplies the nutrients needed for health. Keeping the portions to a reasonable size is key to helping maintain a healthy body weight.

Make Sensible Choices

Fats supply energy. Too much fat supplies more energy than we need. Besides adding to weight gain, some fats, particularly saturated fats from animal sources, can increase risk of coronary heart disease by raising blood cholesterol levels. Unsaturated fats (monounsaturated and polyunsaturated fats), mainly from plant foods, do not raise blood cholesterol. Experts recommend you choose unsaturated fats over saturated fats.

Reading the Nutrition Facts label on food packages and recipe nutrition information can help you choose foods that are lower in fat and saturated fat. Experts recommend eating no more than 35 percent of calories from fat. To figure that out, keep track by adding up all the grams of fat you ate for the day and multiplying the total by 9 calories per gram to give you FAT CALORIES. Then divide the FAT CALORIES by the total number of calories you ate for the day. Multiply by 100 to get the number to a final percent. The final number should be less than 35 percent.

Choose beverages and foods that supply healthy nutrients as well as calories. Again, read the Nutrition Facts to help you select sensible food choices for life. To decrease added sugars and solid fats (called SoFAS) and the calories they contribute, limit fried foods, soft drinks, candy, cakes, cookies, desserts and ice cream.

Select foods and prepare foods with less salt whenever possible. Scientific research shows that we may be able to reduce our risk of developing high blood pressure by consuming foods that are lower in salt and sodium. In the body, sodium helps to control fluid balance and blood pressure. For some individuals, high levels of sodium in the diet can be associated with higher blood pressure. No one knows for sure who will develop high blood pressure, but limiting salt and sodium is recommended for all healthy individuals. Look for low-sodium canned soups, tomatoes and vegetables, choose reduced sodium soy sauce, remove salt shakers from the table and go easy on cheese, salty snacks, pickles, olives, mustard and ketchup to decrease the sodium in your diet.

Alcoholic beverages are harmful when consumed in large quantities because they can impair judgment and lead to dependency and other health problems. If you drink alcoholic beverages, do so in moderation. More than one drink per day for women or two drinks per day for men can increase risk of auto accidents, high blood pressure, stroke, violence, suicide, birth defects and cancer. Heavy drinkers also run the risk of malnutrition because they often substitute alcoholic drinks for nutritious foods.

Onward and Upward

Being active, focusing on eating healthy plant-based foods and making sensible choices are keys to establishing a healthy lifestyle. From time to time, though, thoughts of cancer returning to your body are bound to be on your mind. Risk of cancer recurrence is highest in the first five years after treatment, so staying in tune with your body and following up with your doctor regularly are important. Even with the sound nutrition and healthy lifestyle practices offered here and throughout this book, no single food or practice can be a guarantee against cancer recurrence.

To feel your best, remember to eat a well-balanced, low-fat diet and drink plenty of water. Be sure to get some exercise every day and continue to do the activities you enjoy. Spend time with people you love and care about. Listen to your body and get plenty of rest, especially when you feel tired. Taking care of yourself is the very best thing to do right now—and for the future as well.

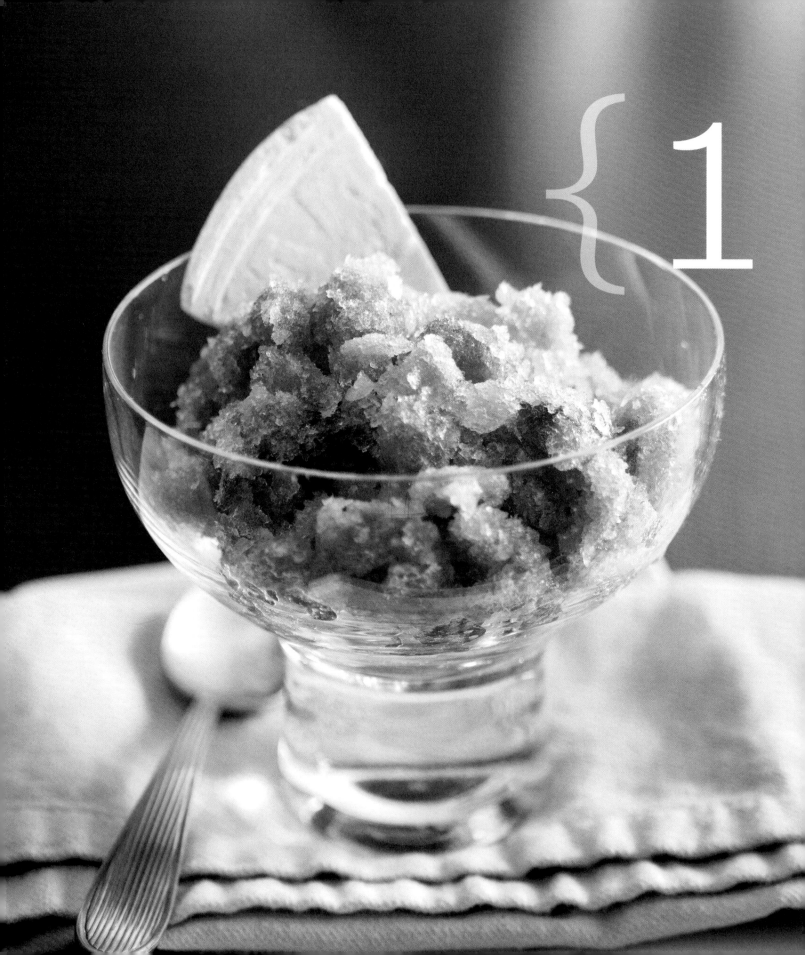

{1

Coping with Side Effects }

29   Berry-Banana Smoothie

31   Spicy Citrus Chicken

33   Refreshing Lemon-Lime Drink

35   Cranberry-Herbal Tea Granita

37   Hot Fruit Compote

39   Milk and Rice "Soup"

41   Creamy Seafood Risotto

43   Crunchy Fruit Snack Mix

45   Lentil-Rice Casserole

47   Roasted Garlic Mashed Potatoes

{Q & A}

Why am I too tired to eat anything?

Dr. Ghosh: Being tired is the most common complaint of cancer and treatment. The reasons for fatigue can include the cancer itself, stress, diarrhea, infections, radiation and anemia. Fatigue can make meal preparation exhausting, and when you're finished with preparation, you may not even feel like eating.

Make it easy on yourself during the times when you are most fatigued by taking a break from cooking. For easy meals and snacks, keep plenty of timesaving foods on hand.

Here are some tips to overcome fatigue:

- Prepare simple meals or snacks, and use timesaving convenience foods whenever possible.
- Take iron or vitamin supplements.
- Nap during the day and get quality sleep at night.
- Invigorate yourself by going for a walk or a swim.

These foods require little or no food preparation and are recommended during times of greatest fatigue:

- Fresh fruits and vegetables
- Potatoes, especially refrigerated and mixes
- Eggs
- Canned fruits, vegetables, soups, tuna, legumes, chili and beans
- Cereals and grains (bread, bagels, pasta, rice, oatmeal)
- Snacks (chips, crackers, popcorn, pretzels)
- Bakery items (muffins, pastries, cookies)
- Dairy foods (cheese, yogurt, milk)
- Beverages (fruit juices, cider, milk, sports drinks, nutritional beverages, lemonade, herbal teas, bottled water)

Berry-Banana Smoothie

Prep Time: 10 Minutes | **Start to Finish:** 10 Minutes | 2 servings (about 1 cup each)

1 cup vanilla, plain, strawberry or raspberry fat-free yogurt

½ cup Cheerios® or another round oat cereal

2 tablespoons ground flaxseed or flaxseed meal

½ cup fresh strawberry halves or raspberries, or frozen whole strawberries

½ cup fat-free (skim) milk

1 to 2 tablespoons sugar

½ banana

1 Place all ingredients in blender. Cover; blend on high speed 10 seconds. Stop blender; scrape down sides. Cover; blend about 20 seconds longer or until smooth.

2 Pour mixture into glasses. Serve immediately.

❝Yogurt and fortified cereal team up to make this protein-loaded, high-iron smoothie enjoyable any time you need an extra energy boost."—**Dr. Ghosh**

High in calcium, vitamin C and folic acid; good source of fiber

1 Serving: Calories 270 (Calories from Fat 30); Total Fat 3.5g (Saturated Fat 0.5g, Trans Fat 0g); Cholesterol 0mg; Sodium 170mg; Potassium 590mg; Total Carbohydrate 50g (Dietary Fiber 4g); Protein 10g
% Daily Value: Vitamin A 6%; Vitamin C 45%; Calcium 30%; Iron 15%; Folic Acid 25%; Magnesium 20%
Exchanges: 2 Fruit, 1 Skim Milk, 1 Fat **Carbohydrate Choices:** 3

{Q & A}

Why does food have a metallic taste?

Dr. Ghosh: Unfortunately, chemotherapy, radiation treatments and even medications can change the flavor of foods and beverages in your mouth. Chemotherapy commonly causes a bitter, metallic taste especially when eating high-protein foods like meats. Dry mouth may also lead to changes in taste.

To improve the taste of your food, try these hints:

- Rev up your taste buds by eating strong-flavored or spicy foods. Spice and strong flavors hide "off" tastes, too.

- Smell your food before eating to entice your appetite. Taste and smell are so closely linked that much of what you taste is actually what you smell. And foods that smell good will generally taste good to you, too.

- Dazzle your taste buds by eating either hot food or cold food. Skip the just-warm food because it may taste blah.

- Refrain from using flatware that contains silver. Opt for stainless steel or plastic utensils instead.

- Rinse your mouth frequently.

- Brush your teeth often.

- Drink cool liquids.

- Suck on sour hard candy.

Spicy Citrus Chicken

Prep Time: 15 Minutes | **Start to Finish:** 4 Hours | 6 servings

6 boneless skinless chicken breasts (about 1 ¾ lb)

½ cup unsweetened grape juice or red wine

1 tablespoon grated orange peel

½ cup orange juice

1 tablespoon grated lemon peel

½ cup lemon juice

2 tablespoons chopped fresh cilantro

1 ½ teaspoons chopped fresh or ½ teaspoon dried oregano leaves

1 teaspoon ground cumin

½ teaspoon salt

¼ teaspoon crushed red pepper flakes

2 medium green onions, chopped (2 tablespoons)

Orange slices, if desired

1 Place chicken in shallow glass or plastic dish. In small bowl, mix remaining ingredients except orange slices; pour over chicken. Cover; refrigerate at least 3 hours but no longer than 24 hours.

2 Heat oven to 375°F. Spray rack in shallow roasting pan with cooking spray. Remove chicken from marinade; place on rack in pan. Reserve marinade.

3 Bake uncovered 35 to 45 minutes, brushing with marinade every 15 minutes, until juice of chicken is clear when center of thickest part is cut (at least 165°F). Discard any remaining marinade. Serve chicken with orange slices.

❝The citrus flavors along with herbs and spices in this recipe may help you to disguise a metallic taste in your mouth."—Dr. Ghosh

Low fiber

1 Serving: Calories 190 (Calories from Fat 40); Total Fat 4.5g (Saturated Fat 1.5g, Trans Fat 0g); Cholesterol 80mg; Sodium 270mg; Potassium 340mg; Total Carbohydrate 7g (Dietary Fiber 0g); Protein 30g **% Daily Value:** Vitamin A 2%; Vitamin C 20%; Calcium 4%; Iron 8%; Folic Acid 4%; Magnesium 8% **Exchanges:** ½ Fruit, 4 Very Lean Meat, 1/2 Fat **Carbohydrate Choices:** ½

{Q & A}

Why do I feel nauseated all the time?

Dr. Ghosh: Nausea and vomiting are often associated with cancer—from chemotherapy, after surgery, from medications and radiation therapy. Sometimes even strong smells can cause nausea or vomiting. Medications that fight nausea work well for most people but may cause symptoms of dry mouth, sleepiness and light-headedness.

Here are some helpful hints to relieve nausea:

- Use a kitchen fan or open the windows when cooking.

- Keep pans covered to reduce cooking odors. Eat small, frequent meals slowly.

- Serve food cold because cold foods have less of an aroma.

- Avoid spicy, greasy or rich foods.

- Choose dry, salty foods such as dry toast, crackers and pretzels.

- Choose sugar-sweetened beverages over sugar-free drinks, because sugar slows digestion and doesn't tend to cause nausea.

- Drink chilled beverages because they go down easier.

- Consume foods separate from beverages by at least an hour, if you are not troubled by dry mouth.

- Sit up or stay up for at least 90 minutes after eating.

- Specific foods that may help include clear liquids, carbonated drinks, yogurt, sherbet, angel food cake, hot wheat cereal, rice, oatmeal, boiled potatoes, noodles, canned peaches or other soft fruits and vegetables.

Refreshing Lemon-Lime Drink

Prep Time: 5 Minutes | **Start to Finish:** 5 Minutes | 8 servings (½ cup each)

1 can (12 oz) frozen limeade or lemonade concentrate, thawed

1 cup chilled lime- or lemon-flavored sports drink

1 can (12 oz) lemon-lime carbonated beverage, chilled

1 In large pitcher, mix limeade concentrate and sports drink.

2 Just before serving, add carbonated beverage.

66 This cool drink, which contains a combination of beverages to replenish needed nutrients, may help ease feelings of nausea."
—Dr. Ghosh

Low fiber

1 Serving: Calories 130 (Calories from Fat 0); Total Fat 0g (Saturated Fat 0g, Trans Fat 0g); Cholesterol 0mg; Sodium 15mg; Potassium 25mg; Total Carbohydrate 33g (Dietary Fiber 0g); Protein 0g **% Daily Value:** Vitamin A 0%; Vitamin C 10%; Calcium 0%; Iron 0%; Folic Acid 0%; Magnesium 0% **Exchanges:** ½ Starch, 1 ½ Other Carbohydrate **Carbohydrate Choices:** 2

{Q & A}

Why is my mouth always dry?

Dr. Ghosh: Dry mouth can be the result of chemotherapy, certain medications or radiation treatment. Neglecting symptoms of dry mouth can lead to developing painful mouth sores, dental problems and changes in taste sensation.

To improve dry mouth:

- Drink at least eight to ten glasses of fluid each day.

- Avoid citrus fruits and dry foods.

- Rinse your mouth every few hours.

- Suck on hard candy, especially sour candy.

- Keep your lips moist.

- Try very sour or very sweet foods and beverages, such as lemonade or cranberry juice; these foods will cause more saliva to flow. (If you have a tender mouth or sore throat, though, sweet or sour foods can make that worse.)

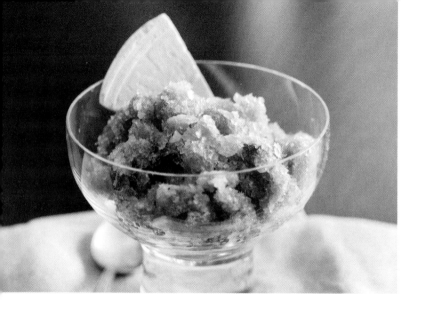

Cranberry-Herbal Tea Granita

Prep Time: 15 Minutes | **Start to Finish:** 5 Hours 35 Minutes | 8 servings

5 whole cloves

1 slice orange

2 cups water

½ cup sugar

1 stick cinnamon

3 tea bags red zesty herbal tea flavored with hibiscus, rose hips and lemongrass

1 ½ cups cranberry juice cocktail

1 ½ cups pineapple juice

Fresh fruit, if desired

Thin almond wafer cookies, if desired

1 Insert cloves into peel of orange slice. In 2-quart saucepan, heat water, sugar, cinnamon stick and orange slice to boiling, stirring occasionally. Remove from heat; add tea bags. Cover; let steep 5 minutes.

2 Remove tea bags, cinnamon stick and orange slice. Stir cranberry and pineapple juices into tea. Pour into 2-quart nonmetal bowl or 8-inch square (2-quart) glass baking dish. Cover; freeze about 2 hours or until partially frozen.

3 Stir granita with fork or whisk. Cover; freeze 3 hours longer, stirring every 30 minutes and breaking up any large chunks.

4 Remove granita from freezer 20 minutes before serving. Spoon into stemmed glasses. Garnish with fruit and cookies.

66 Try this zesty cranberry ice to wet your whistle and lessen symptoms of dry mouth."—Dr. Ghosh

High in vitamin C; low fiber

1 Serving: Calories 100 (Calories from Fat 0); Total Fat 0g (Saturated Fat 0g, Trans Fat 0g); Cholesterol 0mg; Sodium 0mg; Potassium 80mg; Total Carbohydrate 26g (Dietary Fiber 0g); Protein 0g
% Daily Value: Vitamin A 0%; Vitamin C 15%; Calcium 0%; Iron 0%; Folic Acid 2%; Magnesium 2%
Exchanges: 1 ½ Other Carbohydrate **Carbohydrate Choices:** 2

{Q & A}

Why am I constipated?

Dr. Ghosh: Constipation can be an unwanted side effect from chemotherapy, certain medications, not drinking enough fluid or lack of exercise or activity. It is crucial to relieve constipation, because not treating it can lead to nausea, vomiting and severe stomach pain.

To avoid or relieve constipation:

- Eat plenty of fiber, at least 25 to 35 grams per day. High-fiber choices include whole-grain cereals and breads, fruits (fresh, frozen, dried or canned), vegetables (fresh, frozen or cooked) and legumes (dried peas and beans).

- Drink eight to ten glasses of water daily.

- Exercise.

- Drink a hot beverage about half an hour before your usual bowel movement time.

Stool softeners and laxatives are available and sometimes necessary, but it's important to try foods, beverages and exercise first. Save the stool softeners and laxatives to use as a last resort, and take them only with the approval of your doctor.

Hot Fruit Compote

Prep Time: 15 Minutes │ **Start to Finish:** 1 Hour │ 10 servings

1 can (29 oz) pear halves
in heavy syrup

1 can (29 oz) peach halves
in heavy syrup

1 can (20 oz) pineapple
chunks in juice

½ cup dried apricots

½ cup dried prunes

½ cup dried cherries or raisins

2 tablespoons packed
brown sugar

¼ cup brandy, if desired

½ teaspoon ground cinnamon

¼ teaspoon ground nutmeg

½ cup slivered almonds,
if desired

1 Heat oven to 375°F. Drain canned fruits, reserving syrup and juice. In small bowl, mix syrup and juice; set aside.

2 Cut pears and peaches into bite-size pieces. In 3-quart casserole or 13x9-inch (3-quart) glass baking dish, layer canned and dried fruits.

3 In small bowl, mix brown sugar and brandy; pour over fruit. (If not using brandy, sprinkle brown sugar over fruit.) Pour syrup-juice mixture over fruit just until fruit is covered; discard any remaining mixture. Sprinkle cinnamon, nutmeg and almonds over fruit.

4 Bake uncovered about 45 minutes or until bubbly. Serve warm or cool.

❝Try this high-fiber recipe, along with a glass of water, to help ease constipation. You can make this the day before and simply warm it before serving. It's delicious hot or cold.❞—**Dr. Ghosh**

High in vitamin A; good source of fiber and potassium

1 Serving: Calories 250 (Calories from Fat 0); Total Fat 0g (Saturated Fat 0g, Trans Fat 0g); Cholesterol 0mg; Sodium 10mg; Potassium 390mg; Total Carbohydrate 60g (Dietary Fiber 4g); Protein 1g
% Daily Value: Vitamin A 15%; Vitamin C 8%; Calcium 4%; Iron 6%; Folic Acid 2%; Magnesium 6%
Exchanges: 2 Fruit, 2 Other Carbohydrate **Carbohydrate Choices:** 4

{Q & A}

Why do I have diarrhea?

Dr. Ghosh: Radiation and chemotherapy are common causes of diarrhea. And diarrhea causes an excess loss of fluids and nutrients.

There are medications available to treat diarrhea, but here are some things to try on your own:

- Try sports drinks, broths or Pedialyte® to replenish lost fluid and electrolytes. Avoid tea, coffee and prune juice.

- Take a vitamin and mineral supplement that includes vitamins A, B12, E and K, as well as folic acid.

- Eat frequent, small meals that are low in fat and high in carbohydrates and protein.

- Avoid milk and milk-based foods because the sugar in milk can stimulate diarrhea.

- Eat applesauce.

- As diarrhea ends, add these foods to your diet: rice, noodles, potatoes, white bread, yogurt, cottage cheese, hot wheat cereal, eggs, creamy peanut butter, canned peeled fruit, well-cooked vegetables, skinless chicken or turkey, lean beef and fish.

- Slowly add small amounts of fiber from fruits and grains.

Milk and Rice "Soup"

Prep Time: 10 Minutes | **Start to Finish:** 35 Minutes | 4 servings

1 cup uncooked regular
long-grain rice

2 cups water

2 bananas

2 ½ cups fat-free (skim) milk

2 tablespoons sugar

1 In 2-quart saucepan, heat rice and water to boiling. Reduce heat to low; cover and simmer about 15 minutes or until water is absorbed and rice is tender. Let stand about 10 minutes or until cool enough to eat, or refrigerate.

2 In medium bowl, completely mash bananas. Stir in cooked rice, milk and sugar. Serve immediately. Cover and refrigerate any remaining soup.

❝This soup is great for breakfast or just about any time. I normally recommend avoiding milk for diarrhea, but in this recipe the milk is added to bananas and rice, which makes it an effective remedy for diarrhea."—Dr. Ghosh

High in calcium and folic acid; good source of potassium

1 Serving: Calories 310 (Calories from Fat 5); Total Fat 0.5g (Saturated Fat 0g, Trans Fat 0g); Cholesterol 0mg; Sodium 70mg; Potassium 500mg; Total Carbohydrate 67g (Dietary Fiber 2g); Protein 9g
% Daily Value: Vitamin A 8%; Vitamin C 4%; Calcium 20%; Iron 10%; Folic Acid 15%; Magnesium 15%
Exchanges: 1 ½ Starch, ½ Fruit, 2 Other Carbohydrate, ½ Skim Milk **Carbohydrate Choices:** 4 ½

{Q & A}

How can I eat with mouth sores?

Dr. Ghosh: Mouth sores can be a troublesome side effect of chemotherapy or radiation therapy and usually occur a few days after treatment. The inside of the mouth can become raw and ulcerated, making eating and swallowing difficult. If pain from mouth sores becomes unbearable, discuss with your doctor because there are medications that may help. You may also try oral topical pain medications such as Orabase®. Rinse your mouth after meals and at bedtime with 8 ounces warm water mixed with 1 teaspoon salt; brush teeth with a soft toothbrush at least twice a day.

Be sure to discuss your mouth sores with your doctor and try the following suggestions:

- Omit hard, rough-textured or irritating foods.

- Drink nutritional energy beverages, such as Carnation® Instant Breakfast Essentials™ drink, Boost®, or Ensure®.

- Avoid spicy or peppery foods.

- Avoid citrus foods such as tomatoes, oranges, grapefruit and lemons because of their high acid content.

- Eat small, high-calorie, high-protein meals frequently.

- Eat only room-temperature foods, not hot or cold foods.

- Pour liquids over foods to soften them (milk over toast, for example).

- Use buttermilk as a mouthwash to soothe irritations.

- Eat soft, easy-to-swallow foods: shakes; bananas; applesauce; watermelon and other soft fruits; yogurt; cottage cheese; mashed potatoes; pasta; noodles; custard; puddings; gelatins; scrambled eggs; oatmeal or other cooked cereals; mashed sweet potatoes, peas or carrots; pureed meats.

- Use a straw to drink liquids.

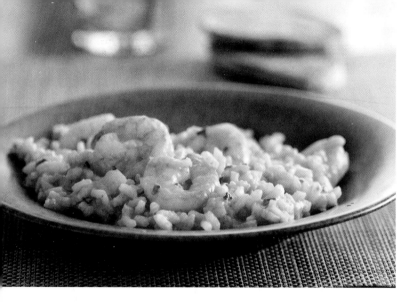

Creamy Seafood Risotto

Prep Time: 30 Minutes | **Start to Finish:** 30 Minutes | 6 servings

2   tablespoons olive or
     vegetable oil

8   oz uncooked medium shrimp
     (thawed if frozen), peeled,
     deveined

1   can (14.5 oz) whole tomatoes,
     undrained

¼   cup whole milk

¼   cup butter or margarine

1   small onion, chopped (¼ cup)

2   cups uncooked Arborio rice

1   cup dry white wine, water or
     chicken broth

¼   teaspoon salt

¼   teaspoon ground red pepper
     (cayenne), if desired

4   cups chicken broth

2   tablespoons chopped fresh
     arugula or spinach

½   cup grated Parmesan cheese

1   In 12-inch skillet, heat oil over medium heat. Add shrimp; cook 2 to 3 minutes, stirring frequently, until shrimp are pink and firm.

2   In food processor or blender, place shrimp, tomatoes and milk. Cover; process about 1 minute or until smooth. (If you are up to chewing the shrimp, leave them whole and blend just the tomatoes and milk together in food processor.)

3   In 3-quart saucepan, melt butter over medium heat. Add onion; cook about 5 minutes, stirring occasionally, until tender. Stir in rice. Cook about 5 minutes, stirring frequently, until edges of rice kernels are translucent. Stir in wine, salt and red pepper. Heat to boiling. Reduce heat; simmer uncovered 10 minutes, stirring occasionally.

4   Stir in broth. Cook over low heat 12 to 14 minutes, stirring occasionally, until liquid is absorbed.

5   Stir in shrimp-tomato mixture and arugula. Cook 3 minutes. Stir in cheese. Serve immediately.

66 Try this soft, easy-on-your-mouth risotto. It's an Italian staple and is a great source of many nutrients, like iron, folic acid and potassium."—Dr. Ghosh

High in iron and folic acid

1 Serving: Calories 450 (Calories from Fat 160); Total Fat 18g (Saturated Fat 8g, Trans Fat 0g); Cholesterol 80mg; Sodium 1440mg; Potassium 370mg; Total Carbohydrate 52g (Dietary Fiber 2g); Protein 18g **% Daily Value:** Vitamin A 8%; Vitamin C 6%; Calcium 15%; Iron 30%; Folic Acid 4%; Magnesium 6% **Exchanges:** 3 Starch, 1 Vegetable, ½ Very Lean Meat, ½ Lean Meat, 3 Fat **Carbohydrate Choices:** 3 ½

{Q & A}

How come I'm not hungry?

Dr. Ghosh: Loss of appetite during cancer treatment is due to many factors that include your type of treatment or level of stress. Treat appetite loss by managing your symptoms (pain, nausea or diarrhea) and discussing anything that's bothering you with your doctor, nurse, dietitian, member of the clergy, trusted friend or family member or mental health professional. Also, keep track of the foods, people, things or places that stimulate your appetite.

Your doctor can prescribe medications that can improve appetite, but try these suggestions to overcome lack of hunger first:

- Eat small, frequent meals.

- Choose foods high in protein and calories, such as shakes, custards and nutritional beverages (Boost® or Carnation® Instant Breakfast Essentials™ drinks).

- If you crave a particular food, eat it.

- Eat whenever you're hungry, no matter what time of day.

- Drink plenty of liquids; eight to ten glasses daily are recommended.

- Make meals and your eating environment attractive by playing soft music and dimming the lights.

- Keep easy snacks on hand to enjoy often, even at bedtime. It's important to eat whenever you feel up to it. Good choices are cheese and crackers, pudding, yogurt, fruit, raisins, muffins and other breads, cereal, nuts and popcorn.

Crunchy Fruit Snack Mix

Prep Time: 15 Minutes | **Start to Finish:** 1 Hour | 10 servings (about ¾ cup each)

4 cups Total® Raisin Bran cereal

⅓ cup sliced almonds

1 bag (8 oz) dried mixed fruit (1 ½ cups), cut into ½-inch pieces

¼ cup packed brown sugar

2 tablespoons butter or margarine

2 teaspoons ground cinnamon

1 teaspoon ground ginger

1 Heat oven to 300°F. In large bowl, place cereal, almonds and fruit; set aside.

2 In 1-quart saucepan, heat brown sugar and butter over low heat, stirring occasionally, until butter is melted. Stir in cinnamon and ginger. Pour over cereal mixture; toss until evenly coated. Spread in ungreased 15x10x1-inch pan.

3 Bake 15 minutes, stirring twice. Spread on waxed paper. Cool about 30 minutes. Store in tightly covered container at room temperature.

"Keep this easy cereal snack mix that's loaded with nuts and dried fruit on hand. Munch on small amounts often, even if you're not feeling too hungry."—Dr. Ghosh

High in iron and folic acid; good source of fiber

1 Serving: Calories 200 (Calories from Fat 40); Total Fat 4.5g (Saturated Fat 1.5g, Trans Fat 0g); Cholesterol 5mg; Sodium 120mg; Potassium 340mg; Total Carbohydrate 38g (Dietary Fiber 4g); Protein 2g
% Daily Value: Vitamin A 10%; Vitamin C 0%; Calcium 45%; Iron 45%; Folic Acid 40%; Magnesium 8%
Exchanges: ½ Starch, ½ Fruit, 1 ½ Other Carbohydrate, 1 Fat **Carbohydrate Choices:** 2 ½

{Q & A}

Why do I have so much heartburn?

Dr. Ghosh: Heartburn can be a complication of radiation therapy, surgery, chemotherapy and excessive stress. Heartburn causes symptoms of nausea, vomiting, pain, loss of appetite, bloating, acid reflux and belching. Your doctor can prescribe antibiotics, antacids and medications that may lessen your symptoms.

You can try consuming milk, yogurt or rice for some relief, or follow the list of suggestions below:

- Avoid large meals, and refrain from lying down after meals.
- Avoid eating within three hours of retiring.
- No cigarette smoking or alcoholic beverages.
- No caffeine-containing foods or beverages.
- No spices, especially black and red peppers.
- No citrus fruits, juices or soft drinks.
- Avoid peppermint, chocolate and high-fat foods (fried or greasy items).

Lentil-Rice Casserole

Prep Time: 30 Minutes | **Start to Finish:** 35 Minutes | 6 servings

1 tablespoon vegetable oil

1 small onion, chopped
(¼ cup)

1 teaspoon grated gingerroot

1 cup uncooked regular
long-grain rice

1 cup dried red lentils
(8 oz), sorted, rinsed

6 cups boiling water

1 tablespoon ground turmeric

1 teaspoon salt

2 tablespoons safflower or
vegetable oil

2 teaspoons whole allspice

1 dried chile

1 dried bay leaf

1 teaspoon sugar

3 tablespoons butter or
margarine, cut up

1 In 2-quart saucepan, heat vegetable oil over medium-high heat. Add onion and gingerroot; cook 2 to 3 minutes, stirring occasionally, until onion is crisp-tender. Stir in rice and lentils. Cook about 3 minutes, stirring frequently, until rice is browned.

2 Reduce heat to medium. Gradually stir in boiling water. Stir in turmeric and salt. Cover; simmer 15 to 20 minutes, stirring occasionally, until rice and lentils are tender.

3 In 12-inch skillet, heat safflower oil over medium-high heat. Add allspice, chile and bay leaf; heat 1 to 2 minutes, stirring frequently, until allspice pops. Stir in rice and lentil mixture. Stir in sugar. Cook about 5 minutes longer or until heated.

4 Just before serving, stir in butter. Serve casserole with chile and bay leaf left in, but do not eat.

> The Milk and Rice 'Soup' on page 39 can be helpful for heartburn. Or try this ancient Indian recipe to help lessen stomach discomfort. If spicy foods are bothersome, reduce the amount of onion, allspice and dried chili, or omit them altogether."—Dr. Ghosh

High in iron and folic acid; excellent source of fiber

1 Serving: Calories 360 (Calories from Fat 120); Total Fat 14g (Saturated Fat 4.5g, Trans Fat 0g); Cholesterol 15mg; Sodium 450mg; Potassium 480mg; Total Carbohydrate 48g (Dietary Fiber 6g); Protein 11g
% Daily Value: Vitamin A 15%; Vitamin C 2%; Calcium 4%; Iron 25%; Folic Acid 45%; Magnesium 15%
Exchanges: 3 Starch, 1 Vegetable, 2 ½ Fat **Carbohydrate Choices:** 3

{Q & A}

Why does it hurt when I swallow?

Dr. Ghosh: Having difficulty swallowing foods can sometimes feel like foods are sticking in your throat.

If you experience pain or difficulty swallowing, follow these dietary modifications:

- Choose soft or semisolid foods because they are easier to swallow.

- Thicken liquids with cornstarch or powdered milk so they go down easier. Eat mashed potatoes or peas.

- Eat small, frequent meals at room temperature.

- Avoid spicy, acidic or hard, coarse foods.

- Sit up and concentrate on coordinating your breathing and swallowing. Allow one to two minutes between each bite.

- Avoid talking while chewing and swallowing.

Roasted Garlic Mashed Potatoes

Prep Time: 10 Minutes | **Start to Finish:** 40 Minutes | 5 servings

1 bulb garlic

6 medium red or white potatoes (2 lb)

1 medium dark-orange sweet potato or yam

⅓ to ½ cup milk

¼ cup butter or margarine, softened

½ teaspoon salt

¼ teaspoon pepper

1 Heat oven to 350°F. Peel paper-like skin from garlic bulb, leaving just enough to hold cloves of garlic together. Cut ¼-inch slice from top of bulb to expose cloves. Place cut side up on 12-inch square of foil; wrap securely in foil. Place in pie plate or shallow baking pan. Bake about 30 minutes or until garlic is tender when pierced with toothpick or fork. Let stand until cool enough to handle.

2 Meanwhile, in 3-quart saucepan, place red potatoes and sweet potato. Add enough water to cover potatoes. Heat to boiling. Reduce heat; cover and simmer 20 to 25 minutes or until tender. Drain.

3 Peel sweet potato; if desired, leave skins on red potatoes or peel. Gently squeeze soft garlic out of cloves into potatoes. Mash potatoes and garlic in saucepan until no lumps remain.

4 Add milk in small amounts, mashing after each addition. Add butter, salt and pepper. Mash vigorously until light and fluffy. (If running low on energy, blend all ingredients in a food processor.)

> **"**Easy to eat, these tasty potatoes go down easily, even when chewing and swallowing become a chore. If garlic bothers you, omit it from the recipe."—Dr. Ghosh

High in potassium and excellent source of fiber

1 Serving: Calories 320 (Calories from Fat 90); Total Fat 10g (Saturated Fat 6g, Trans Fat 0g); Cholesterol 25mg; Sodium 330mg; Potassium 1490mg; Total Carbohydrate 52g (Dietary Fiber 6g); Protein 5g
% Daily Value: Vitamin A 100%; Vitamin C 30%; Calcium 10%; Iron 25%; Folic Acid 4%; Magnesium 20%
Exchanges: 2 ½ Other Carbohydrate, 3 Vegetable, 2 Fat **Carbohydrate Choices:** 3 ½

Key to Common Side Effects

During treatment, the four most common side effects experienced are nausea, mouth sores, constipation and diarrhea. Listed below are the recipes in this cookbook that are most helpful for soothing each of these side effects. If there is a particular ingredient in any of the recipes that is bothersome to you, just leave it out.

Ⓝ Nausea

- Baking Powder Biscuits (page 68)
- Berry-Banana Smoothie (page 29)
- Blueberry Brunch Cake (page 67)
- Cantaloupe and Chicken Salad (page 121)
- Chicken Soup with Homemade Noodles (page 154)
- Cinnamon-Raisin Morning Mix (page 59)
- Citrus-Peach Smoothie (page 103)
- Cranberry Herbal Tea Granita (page 35)
- Creamy Caramel Dip with Fruit (page 100)
- Easy Brown Bread (page 64)
- Easy Lemon Bars (page 224)
- Extra-Easy Baked Ziti (page 163)
- Fresh Salsa (page 98)
- Fresh Spinach and New Potato Frittata (page 179)
- Fruit Parfaits (page 60)
- Grilled Marinated Vegetables (page 204)
- Layered Chicken Salad (page 145)
- Macaroni Pasta "Soup" (page 135)
- Orange-Pineapple Fruit Salad (page 217)
- Oven-Fried Potato Wedges (page 83)
- Raspberry-Banana Gelatin Dessert (page 230)
- Refreshing Lemon-Lime Drink (page 33)
- Roasted Vegetable Dip (page 80)
- Rosalie's Orange Butter Cookies (page 227)
- Sugar 'n Spice Green Tea (page 107)

Ⓜ Mouth Sores

- Acorn Squash and Apple Soup (page 177)
- Baked Custard (page 234)
- Beef-Barley Stew (page 196)
- Beef-Vegetable Soup (page 158)
- Berry-Banana Smoothie (page 29)
- Blueberry Breakfast Bake (page 55)
- Chai Tea (page 108)
- Cheesy Vegetable Soup (page 178)
- Chicken Soup with Homemade Noodles (page 154)
- Cinnamon Apples (page 73)
- Cranberry Herbal Tea Granita (page 35)
- Cream of Broccoli Soup (page 136)
- Creamy Seafood Risotto (page 41)
- Easy Creamed Vegetables (page 206)
- Easy Lemon Bars (page 224)
- Macaroni Pasta "Soup" (page 135)
- Mashed Potatoes (page 208)
- Milk and Rice "Soup" (page 39)
- Orange-Cream Frosty (page 228)
- Poached Eggs in Milk (page 56)
- Raspberry-Banana Gelatin Dessert (page 230)
- Rice Pudding (page 235)
- Roasted Garlic Mashed Potatoes (page 47)
- Sugar 'n Spice Green Tea (page 107)
- Watermelon-Kiwi-Banana Smoothie (page 104)

Diarrhea

- Baking Powder Biscuits (page 68)
- Banana Bread (page 62)
- Blueberry Brunch Cake (page 67)
- Caramelized Pork Slices (page 139)
- Country Fruit Cobbler (page 222)
- Crab Scramble Casserole (page 169)
- Creamy Caramel Dip with Fruit (page 100)
- Dijon Chicken (page 148)
- Easy Brown Bread (page 64)
- Easy Salmon Spread (page 102)
- Gingerbread with Brown Sugar Meringue (page 231)
- Hot Fruit Compote (page 37)
- Hot Turkey Sandwiches (page 90)
- Lemony Fish over Vegetables and Rice (page 183)
- Macaroni Pasta "Soup" (page 135)
- Make-Ahead Waffles with Peanut Butter Spread (page 76)
- Milk and Rice "Soup" (page 39)
- Orange-Pineapple Smoothie (page 106)
- Potato Pancakes with Cinnamon Apples (page 72)
- Pumpkin Drop Cookies (page 225)
- Raspberry-Banana Gelatin Dessert (page 230)
- Rice Pudding (page 235)
- Rosalie's Orange Butter Cookies (page 230)
- Spaghetti and Meat Squares (page 161)
- Tropical Pancakes (page 70)
- Wild Rice Stuffing (page 215)

Constipation

- Barley and Asparagus (page 216)
- Beef-Barley Stew (page 196)
- Beef Fajita Bowls (page 194)
- Beef and Bean Dinner (page 198)
- Berry-Banana Smoothie (page 29)
- Bulgur Pilaf (page 211)
- Chopped Vegetable and Crabmeat Salad (page 128)
- Corn and Black Bean Salad (page 142)
- Creamy Quinoa Primavera (page 116)
- Crispy Baked Fish with Tropical Fruit Salsa (page 184)
- Crowd-Size Minestrone (page 155)
- Easy Chicken Nuggets (page 91)
- Fiesta Taco Salad (page 131)
- Grilled Marinated Vegetables (page 204)
- Hot Fruit Compote (page 37)
- Layered Beef and Vegetable Dinner (page 160)
- Lentil-Rice Casserole (page 45)
- Mashed Potatoes (page 208)
- Mediterranean Couscous and Beans (page 118)
- Roasted Garlic Mashed Potatoes (page 47)
- Savory Black-Eyed Peas with Bacon (page 214)
- Southwestern Pork Salad (page 146)
- Spaghetti and "Meatballs" (page 173)
- White Turkey Chili (page 156)

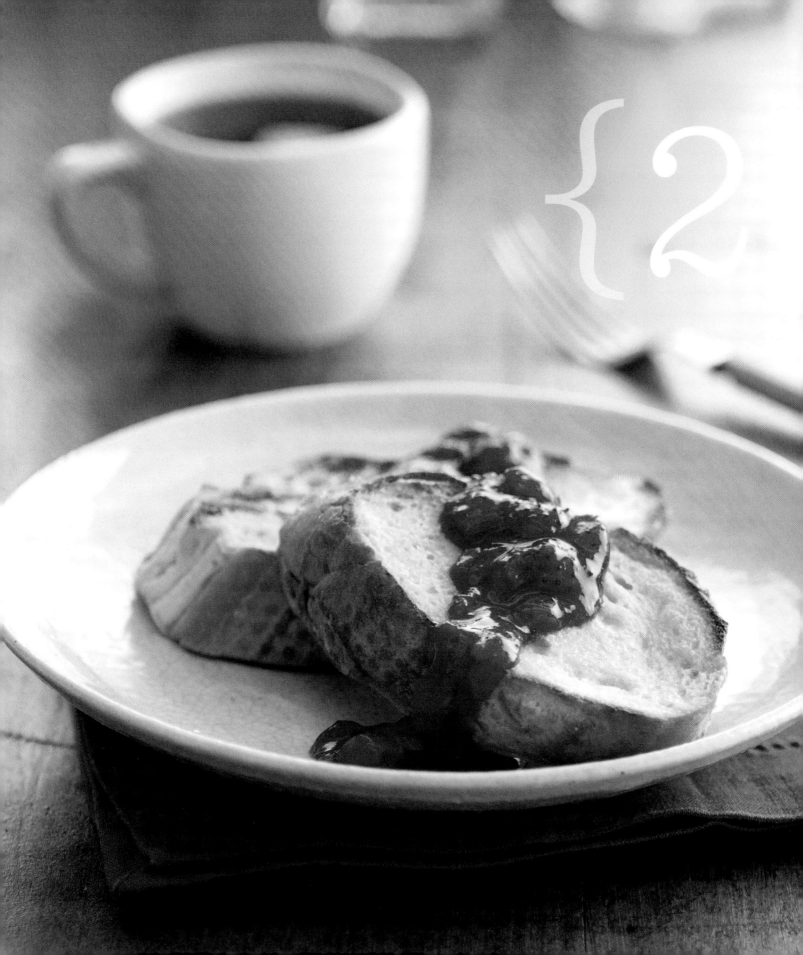

{2

Energy-Boosting Breakfasts

}

52   Country Eggs in Tortilla Cups

54   Cheesy Ham and Asparagus Bake

55   Blueberry Breakfast Bake

56   Poached Eggs in Milk

57   Home-Style Oatmeal with Raisins

58   Cheese Grits

59   Cinnamon-Raisin Snack Mix

60   Fruit Parfaits

62   Banana Bread

64   Easy Brown Bread

65   Rise 'n Shine Muffins with Creamy Orange Glaze

66   Streusel-Topped Fruit Brunch Cake

67   Blueberry Brunch Cake

68   Baking Powder Biscuits

70   Tropical Pancakes

71   Cheesy Pear Oven Pancake

72   Potato Pancakes with Cinnamon Apples

74   Baked French Toast with Strawberry-Rhubarb Sauce

76   Make-Ahead Waffles with Peanut Butter Spread

A Note from Dr. Ghosh The eggs and potatoes are good sources of iron. Try eating an orange, kiwifruit or other food high in vitamin C with this recipe to help you more easily absorb the iron.

Country Eggs in Tortilla Cups

Prep Time: 25 Minutes | **Start to Finish:** 25 Minutes | 4 servings

4 flour tortillas (6 inch)

Cooking spray

4 eggs

¼ cup milk

¼ teaspoon salt

1 tablespoon butter or margarine

3 cups frozen shredded hash brown potatoes (from 32-oz bag)

¼ cup chopped green bell pepper

¼ cup shredded Cheddar cheese (1 oz)

Sour cream, if desired

Salsa, if desired

1 Heat oven to 400°F. Turn 4 (6-oz) custard cups upside down onto cookie sheet. To make tortillas more pliable, warm as directed on package. Spray both sides of each tortilla lightly with cooking spray. Place tortilla over each cup, gently pressing edges toward cup. Bake 8 to 10 minutes or until light golden brown.

2 Meanwhile, in small bowl, beat eggs, milk and salt with fork or whisk until well mixed; set aside. In 10-inch nonstick skillet, melt butter over medium-high heat. Add potatoes and bell pepper; cook 6 to 8 minutes, stirring occasionally, until potatoes are light golden brown. Reduce heat to medium. Push potatoes to one side of skillet; carefully pour eggs into open side of skillet. Cook about 3 minutes, stirring occasionally, until eggs are almost set. Sprinkle with cheese; cover and let stand 1 minute or until cheese melts.

3 Remove tortillas from cups; place upright on serving plates. Spoon ¼ each of the potatoes and eggs into each tortilla cup. Serve with sour cream and salsa.

66 When I have mouth sores, I use chopped low-acid tomatoes and no green peppers. When I don't have mouth sores, I eat salsa because that's what makes these eggs taste 'normal.'"—Anne R.

High in calcium; good source of fiber and iron

1 Serving: Calories 350 (Calories from Fat 140); Total Fat 16g (Saturated Fat 8g, Trans Fat 0.5g); Cholesterol 190mg; Sodium 480mg; Potassium 490mg; Total Carbohydrate 36g (Dietary Fiber 3g); Protein 15g **% Daily Value:** Vitamin A 10%; Vitamin C 15%; Calcium 20%; Iron 10%; Folic Acid 15%; Magnesium 10% **Exchanges:** 2 ½ Starch, 1 Medium-Fat Meat, 2 Fat **Carbohydrate Choices:** 2 ½

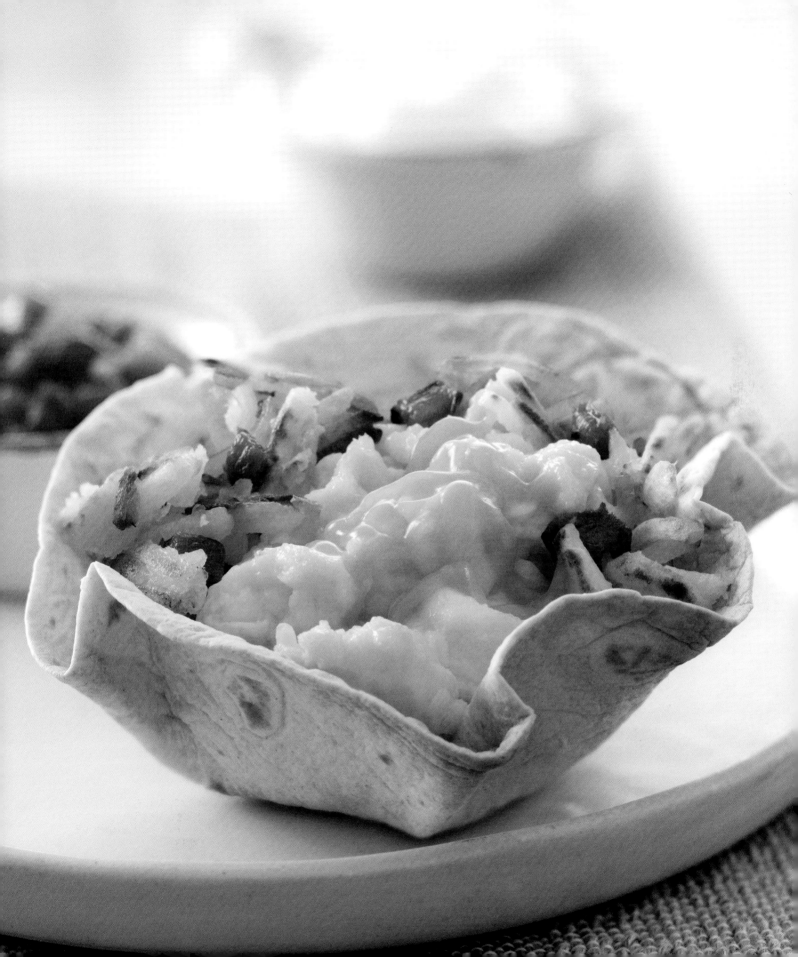

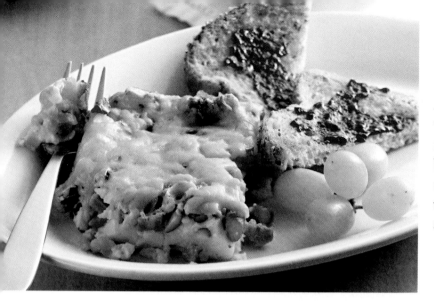

A Note from Dr. Ghosh Loaded with calcium from the cheese and milk, this recipe offers important benefits for cancer healing. Calcium also helps to prevent osteoporosis, the brittle bone disease that often affects us as we age.

Cheesy Ham and Asparagus Bake

Prep Time: 20 Minutes | **Start to Finish:** 50 Minutes | 8 servings

1 ½ cups chopped fully cooked ham

1 medium onion, chopped (½ cup)

¼ cup chopped bell pepper

1 box (9 oz) frozen asparagus cuts or cut broccoli

8 eggs or 2 cups fat-free egg product

2 cups milk

1 cup all-purpose flour

¼ cup grated Parmesan cheese

½ teaspoon salt

½ teaspoon pepper

½ teaspoon dried tarragon leaves

1 cup shredded Cheddar cheese (4 oz)

1 Heat oven to 425°F. Generously spray bottom and sides of 13x9-inch (3-quart) glass baking dish with cooking spray. Sprinkle ham, onion, bell pepper and asparagus into baking dish.

2 In medium bowl, beat eggs, milk, flour, Parmesan cheese, salt, pepper and tarragon with fork or whisk until smooth; pour over ham mixture.

3 Bake about 20 minutes or until knife inserted in center comes out clean. Sprinkle with Cheddar cheese. Bake 3 to 5 minutes longer or until cheese is melted. Let stand 5 minutes before cutting.

❝I sauté green peppers and onions in butter before adding them to recipes. This helps minimize the acid and makes them less bothersome for both mouth sores and gas in the intestine."
—Anne R.

High in calcium and folic acid; low fiber

1 Serving: Calories 290 (Calories from Fat 130); Total Fat 15g (Saturated Fat 7g, Trans Fat 0g); Cholesterol 250mg; Sodium 760mg; Potassium 370mg; Total Carbohydrate 18g (Dietary Fiber 1g); Protein 21g **% Daily Value:** Vitamin A 20%; Vitamin C 10%; Calcium 25%; Iron 10%; Folic Acid 25%; Magnesium 8% **Exchanges:** 1 Starch, ½ Vegetable, 1 Lean Meat, 1 Medium-Fat Meat, ½ High-Fat Meat, ½ Fat **Carbohydrate Choices:** 1

A Note from Dr. Ghosh For a tasty source of vitamin A, you can't beat this breakfast. Vitamin A is vital for proper eyesight and healthy hair and skin.

Blueberry Breakfast Bake

Prep Time: 10 Minutes | **Start to Finish:** 9 Hours 10 Minutes | 8 servings

8 slices white bread, cut into 1-inch pieces (6 cups)

1 package (8 oz) reduced-fat cream cheese (Neufchâtel), chilled, cut into ½-inch pieces

1 cup fresh or frozen (thawed and drained) blueberries

8 eggs or 2 cups fat-free egg product

1 ½ cups milk

1 cup blueberry syrup

1 Spray bottom and sides of 11x7-inch (2-quart) glass baking dish with cooking spray. Spread half of the bread pieces evenly in baking dish. Top with cream cheese. Sprinkle with blueberries. Spread remaining bread over blueberries.

2 In medium bowl, beat eggs and milk with fork or whisk until blended; pour over bread. Cover tightly with foil; refrigerate at least 8 hours but no longer than 24 hours.

3 Heat oven to 350°F. Bake covered 30 minutes. Uncover; bake 25 to 30 minutes longer or until top is puffed and center is set. Serve with blueberry syrup.

❝Berries taste 'normal' even with the common metallic taste during many chemotherapy treatments. I love food that I can cook—or have someone else cook for me—and then reheat in the microwave in single servings for quick, low-odor meals. This dish fills the bill perfectly."—Anne R.

Low fiber

1 Serving: Calories 360 (Calories from Fat 120); Total Fat 14g (Saturated Fat 6g, Trans Fat 0g); Cholesterol 235mg; Sodium 360mg; Potassium 220mg; Total Carbohydrate 46g (Dietary Fiber 1g); Protein 12g **% Daily Value:** Vitamin A 15%; Vitamin C 0%; Calcium 15%; Iron 10%; Folic Acid 15%; Magnesium 6% **Exchanges:** 1 Starch, 2 Other Carbohydrate, ½ Lean Meat, 1 Medium-Fat Meat, 1 ½ Fat **Carbohydrate Choices:** 3

Food for Thought An important source of calories and protein, eggs and egg yolks are great as sandwich spreads and in salads, dressings and casseroles.

Poached Eggs in Milk

Prep Time: 10 Minutes | **Start to Finish:** 15 Minutes | 2 servings

1 ½   cups milk

4   eggs

4   slices bread

1   to 2 tablespoons butter or margarine

1   In 8-inch skillet, heat milk to boiling over medium-high heat. Reduce heat so milk is simmering.

2   Break each egg into custard cup or saucer. Carefully slip egg into milk. Cook about 5 minutes or until whites and yolks are firm and not runny.

3   Meanwhile, lightly toast bread. Spread butter on toast; break into bite-size pieces into individual bowls. Using slotted spoon, remove eggs from milk and place on toast. Pour milk over toast to soften.

66 To keep on keeping on, I had to act like a well person. Even when I didn't feel like it, I got out of bed, showered, got dressed, and smiled. Eating soft foods, like these poached eggs, was a big comfort, and it helped when my mouth was so sore from chemo."— **Carol N. Shares Her Recipe**

High in calcium, vitamin C and folic acid; low fiber

1 Serving: Calories 480 (Calories from Fat 250); Total Fat 27g (Saturated Fat 13g, Trans Fat 1g); Cholesterol 470mg; Sodium 620mg; Potassium 450mg; Total Carbohydrate 35g (Dietary Fiber 1g); Protein 22g **% Daily Value:** Vitamin A 25%; Vitamin C 0%; Calcium 35%; Iron 15%; Folic Acid 25%; Magnesium 10% **Exchanges:** 1 Starch, ½ Other Carbohydrate, 1 Low-Fat Milk, 1 ½ Medium-Fat Meat, 3 Fat **Carbohydrate Choices:** 2

A Note from Dr. Ghosh To make this comfort food low residue, prepare oatmeal with water and leave out the raisins. Sprinkling it with a little brown sugar and a dash of ground cinnamon boosts the flavor level.

Home-Style Oatmeal with Raisins

Prep Time: 5 Minutes | **Start to Finish:** 10 Minutes | 1 serving

¾ cup milk or water

⅓ cup old-fashioned oats

⅓ cup raisins

¼ cup milk, if desired

1 In large microwavable bowl or 4-cup microwavable measuring cup, mix ¾ cup milk and the oats. Microwave uncovered on High about 3 minutes or until boiling.

2 Stir in raisins and up to ¼ cup milk until desired consistency. Let stand about 5 minutes or until cool enough to eat.

66 I found oatmeal, in any form, to be so very comforting during my treatment. Sometimes, I ate just plain oatmeal several times a day. When I couldn't have milk, I cooked the oatmeal with water, and the easiest way to cook it was in the microwave."—Susan S.

High in potassium and calcium; good source of fiber and magnesium

1 Serving: Calories 350 (Calories from Fat 50); Total Fat 6g (Saturated Fat 2.5g, Trans Fat 0g); Cholesterol 15mg; Sodium 80mg; Potassium 730mg; Total Carbohydrate 65g (Dietary Fiber 4g); Protein 11g **% Daily Value:** Vitamin A 6%; Vitamin C 0%; Calcium 25%; Iron 10%; Folic Acid 6%; Magnesium 20% **Exchanges:** 2 Starch, ½ Fruit, 1 ½ Other Carbohydrate, ½ Low-Fat Milk, ½ Fat **Carbohydrate Choices:** 4

A Note from Dr. Ghosh Take time to celebrate treatment milestones. Prepare a nice dinner, if you are up to it, meet friends or family at a favorite restaurant or order a cake to celebrate once in a while! This will help lift your spirits.

Cheese Grits

Prep Time: 20 Minutes | **Start to Finish:** 1 Hour 10 Minutes | 8 servings

2 cups milk

2 cups water

½ teaspoon salt

¼ teaspoon pepper

1 cup uncooked quick-cooking corn grits

1 ½ cups shredded Cheddar cheese (6 oz)

2 medium green onions, sliced (2 tablespoons)

2 eggs, slightly beaten

1 tablespoon butter or margarine

¼ teaspoon paprika

1 Heat oven to 350°F. Spray 1 ½-quart casserole with cooking spray. In 2-quart saucepan, heat milk, water, salt and pepper to boiling. Gradually add grits, stirring constantly. Reduce heat; simmer uncovered about 5 minutes, stirring frequently, until thickened. Stir in cheese and onions.

2 Stir 1 cup of the grits mixture into eggs, then stir back into remaining grits in saucepan. Pour into casserole. Cut butter into small pieces; sprinkle over grits. Sprinkle with paprika.

3 Bake uncovered 35 to 40 minutes or until set. Let stand 10 minutes before serving.

66 Flavorful comfort foods like these cheese grits were a lifesaver for me on days when I was feeling awful. When I wanted more flavor, I added a dash of cayenne pepper or red pepper flakes, and served these grits with salsa for a real flavor kick."—Susan S.

High in calcium; low fiber

1 Serving: Calories 220 (Calories from Fat 100); Total Fat 11g (Saturated Fat 6g, Trans Fat 0g); Cholesterol 85mg; Sodium 340mg; Potassium 160mg; Total Carbohydrate 19g (Dietary Fiber 0g); Protein 11g **% Daily Value:** Vitamin A 10%; Vitamin C 0%; Calcium 20%; Iron 6%; Folic Acid 10%; Magnesium 6% **Exchanges:** 1 Starch, 1 High-Fat Meat, ½ Fat **Carbohydrate Choices:** 1

A Note from Dr. Ghosh Fortified ready-to-eat cereal, such as Chex®, provides a good source of folic acid, a nutrient necessary for all cells to function properly. Folic acid also helps to prevent certain birth defects.

Cinnamon-Raisin Snack Mix

Prep Time: 10 Minutes | **Start to Finish:** 10 Minutes | 10 servings (½ cup each)

¼ cup sugar

1 teaspoon ground cinnamon

¼ cup butter or margarine

1 ½ cups Corn Chex® cereal

1 ½ cups Rice Chex® cereal

1 ½ cups Wheat Chex® cereal

½ cup raisins, sweetened dried cranberries or dried cherries

1 In small bowl, mix sugar and cinnamon; set aside.

2 In large microwavable bowl, microwave butter uncovered on High about 40 seconds or until melted. Stir in cereals until evenly coated. Microwave uncovered 2 minutes, stirring after 1 minute.

3 Sprinkle half of the sugar mixture evenly over cereals; stir. Sprinkle with remaining sugar mixture; stir. Microwave uncovered 1 minute. Stir in raisins. Spread on paper towels to cool.

❝This mix was so easy to make in my microwave, and when I used the dried cranberries, the color was pretty. I kept this snack on hand to munch on whenever I felt like having something crunchy." —Susan S.

High in iron; good source of folic acid

1 Serving: Calories 140 (Calories from Fat 45); Total Fat 5g (Saturated Fat 2.5g, Trans Fat 0g); Cholesterol 10mg; Sodium 180mg; Potassium 95mg; Total Carbohydrate 24g (Dietary Fiber 1g); Protein 2g **% Daily Value:** Vitamin A 8%; Vitamin C 2%; Calcium 6%; Iron 25%; Folic Acid 30%; Magnesium 2% **Exchanges:** ½ Starch, 1 Other Carbohydrate, 1 Fat **Carbohydrate Choices:** 1 ½

Food for Thought Packed with vitamin C, potassium and calcium, this fruit and yogurt combination can't be beat for nutritional benefits geared toward cancer healing!

Fruit Parfaits

Prep Time: 10 Minutes | **Start to Finish:** 10 Minutes | 2 servings

½ cup chopped cantaloupe

½ cup chopped strawberries

½ cup chopped honeydew melon or kiwifruit

½ banana, sliced

1 cup vanilla low-fat yogurt

2 tablespoons sliced almonds, toasted*

1 In 2 goblets or parfait glasses, alternate layers of fruit and yogurt, beginning and ending with fruit.

2 Top with almonds.

*To toast nuts, bake uncovered in ungreased shallow pan in 350°F oven about 10 minutes, stirring occasionally, until golden brown.

❝This 'treat' tastes great and is easy to eat. Even with extremely bad mouth sores, I can eat this by skipping the strawberries and almonds, which don't feel good if your mouth is raw. It is also quick to fix and has very little odor, which is important if you have nausea."—Anne R.

High in calcium, potassium, vitamin C and folic acid; good source of fiber

1 Serving: Calories 220 (Calories from Fat 45); Total Fat 4.5g (Saturated Fat 1.5g, Trans Fat 0g); Cholesterol 5mg; Sodium 95mg; Potassium 680mg; Total Carbohydrate 35g (Dietary Fiber 3g); Protein 8g **% Daily Value:** Vitamin A 30%; Vitamin C 80%; Calcium 25%; Iron 4%; Folic Acid 10%; Magnesium 15% **Exchanges:** 1 Starch, 1 Fruit, ½ Low-Fat Milk, ½ Fat **Carbohydrate Choices:** 2

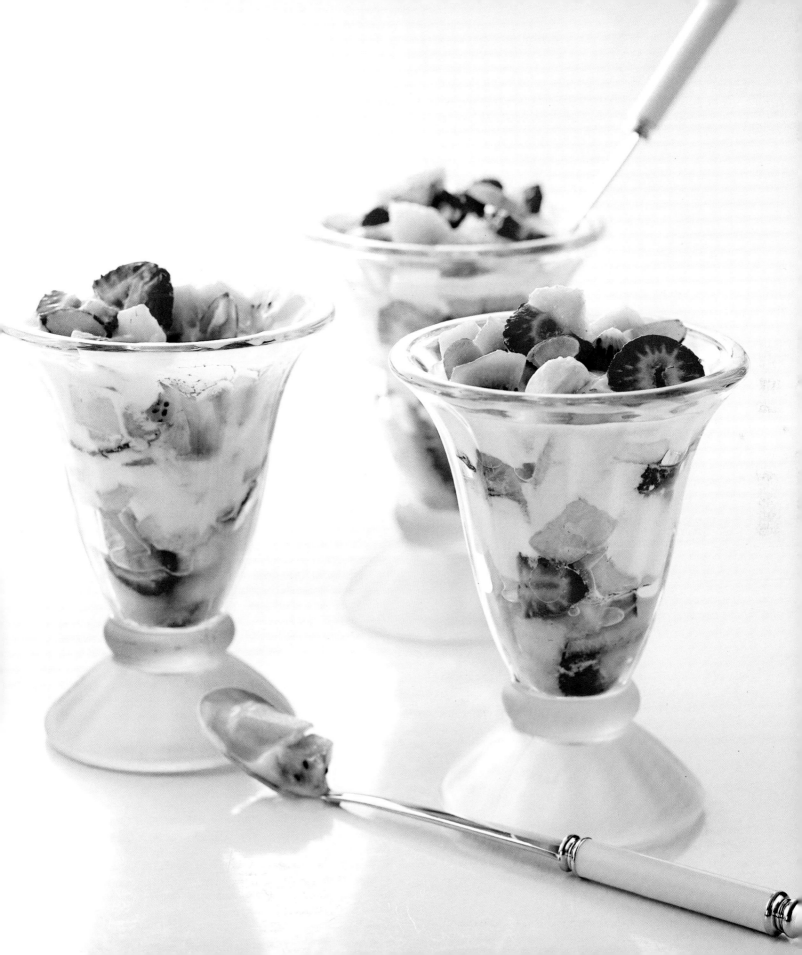

A Note from Dr. Ghosh You may have heard of the BRAT diet. Bananas, the B in BRAT, are a good food source of nutrients when severe diarrhea is a problem. Rice, applesauce and toast make up the rest of the acronym.

Banana Bread

Prep Time: 20 Minutes | **Start to Finish:** 3 Hours 30 Minutes | 1 loaf (24 slices)

3	very ripe medium bananas
1 ¼	cups sugar
½	cup butter or margarine, softened
2	eggs
½	cup buttermilk
1	teaspoon vanilla
2 ½	cups all-purpose flour
1	teaspoon baking soda
1	teaspoon salt
1	cup chopped nuts, if desired

1 Move oven rack to low position so tops of pans will be in center of oven. Heat oven to 350°F. Spray bottom only of 2 (8x4-inch) loaf pans with cooking spray. In medium bowl, mash bananas with potato masher or fork to measure 1 ½ cups.

2 In large bowl, stir together sugar and butter. Stir in eggs until well mixed. Stir in bananas, buttermilk and vanilla until smooth. Stir in flour, baking soda and salt just until moistened. Stir in nuts. Divide batter evenly between pans.

3 Bake 1 hour or until golden brown and toothpick inserted in center comes out clean. Cool in pan 10 minutes.

4 Run knife along sides of pan to loosen bread; remove bread from pan to cooling rack. Cool completely, about 2 hours, before slicing.

❝I learned to be careful when I baked wearing my wig! I didn't know that hot air can burn the hair. I found the best thing to do is open the oven door, stand to the side and let out some of the heat first." **— Patty N. Shares her Recipe**

❝Save your very ripe bananas in the freezer until you're ready to make this recipe. Thaw and mash, using all the liquid."**—Patty N.**

Low fiber; low residue

1 Slice: Calories 150 (Calories from Fat 40); Total Fat 4.5g (Saturated Fat 2.5g, Trans Fat 0g); Cholesterol 30mg; Sodium 190mg; Potassium 85mg; Total Carbohydrate 24g (Dietary Fiber 0g); Protein 2g **% Daily Value:** Vitamin A 4%; Vitamin C 0%; Calcium 0%; Iron 4%; Folic Acid 6%; Magnesium 2% **Exchanges:** ½ Starch, 1 Other Carbohydrate, 1 Fat **Carbohydrate Choices:** 1 ½

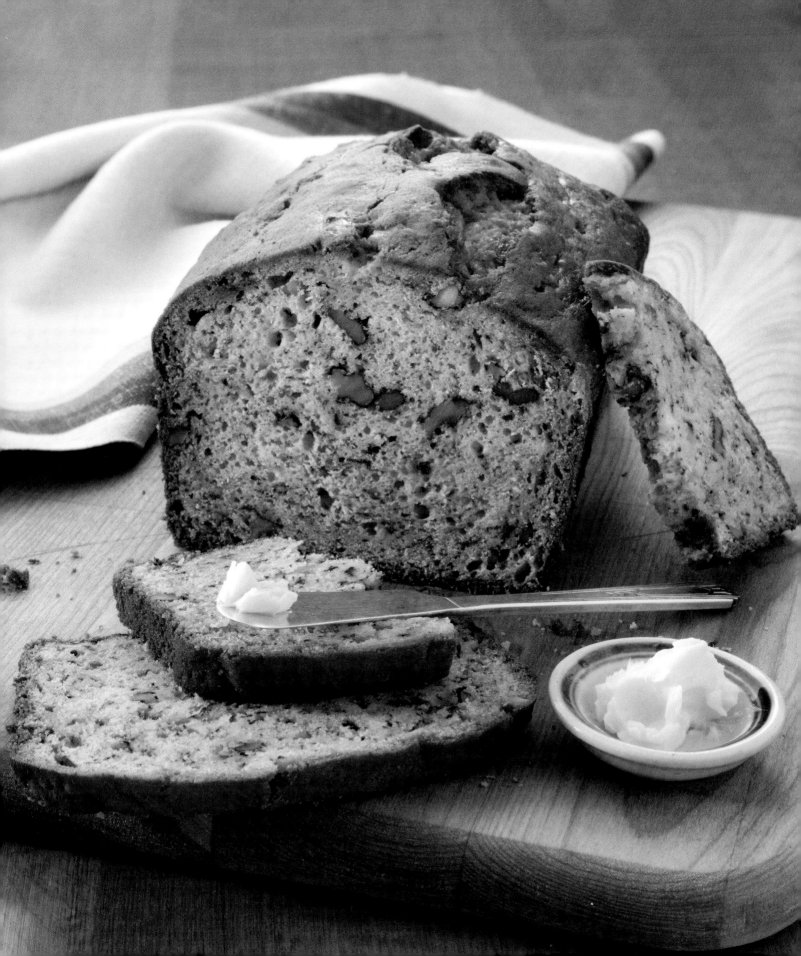

Food for Thought Jump-start your day by eating breakfast. Studies show that people who eat breakfast get a head start on their daily nutrition goals and are better prepared to face the challenges of the day.

Easy Brown Bread

Prep Time: 10 Minutes | **Start to Finish:** 2 Hours 50 Minutes | 2 loaves (24 slices each)

2 cups graham cracker crumbs (about 26 squares)

1 ¾ cups all-purpose flour

2 teaspoons baking soda

½ teaspoon salt

1 cup chopped prunes, dates or raisins

¾ cup full-flavor molasses

⅓ cup vegetable oil

2 eggs

2 cups buttermilk

1 Heat oven to 375°F. Spray bottoms only of 2 (9x5-inch) or 3 (8x4-inch) loaf pans with cooking spray.

2 In large bowl, mix cracker crumbs, flour, baking soda, salt and prunes; set aside. In medium bowl, mix molasses, oil and eggs; stir in buttermilk. Stir molasses mixture into cracker mixture until blended. Divide batter evenly into pans.

3 Bake 30 to 35 minutes or until toothpick inserted in center comes out clean. Cool in pans 5 minutes. Loosen sides of loaves from pans; remove from pans to cooling rack. Cool completely, about 2 hours, before slicing.

66 I like this recipe because it uses so many of the yummy foods I keep in my kitchen. Once I crushed the graham crackers, it went together in no time. I baked this bread and kept it on hand for any time that I was even a little bit hungry. It freezes very well!"—Theresa H.

Low fiber

1 Slice: Calories 80 (Calories from Fat 20); Total Fat 2.5g (Saturated Fat 0g, Trans Fat 0g); Cholesterol 10mg; Sodium 110mg; Potassium 135mg; Total Carbohydrate 13g (Dietary Fiber 0g); Protein 1g **% Daily Value:** Vitamin A 0%; Vitamin C 0%; Calcium 4%; Iron 4%; Folic Acid 2%; Magnesium 4% **Exchanges:** ½ Starch, ½ Other Carbohydrate, ½ Fat **Carbohydrate Choices:** 1

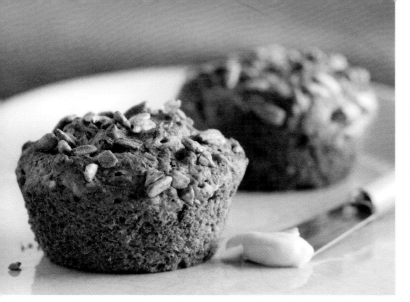

A Note from Dr. Ghosh Grains supply fiber, a nutrient lacking in the diets of most Americans. Daily fiber keeps foods moving through your intestinal tract and can help lessen constipation.

Rise 'n Shine Muffins with Creamy Orange Glaze

Prep Time: 15 Minutes | **Start to Finish:** 35 Minutes | 12 muffins

MUFFINS

⅔   cup orange juice

⅓   cup honey

2   tablespoons vegetable oil

1   egg

1 ½   cups Original Bisquick® mix

1   cup Fiber One® cereal, crushed

½   teaspoon baking soda

½   cup plus 2 tablespoons salted sunflower nuts, toasted

CREAMY ORANGE SPREAD

1   package (3 oz) reduced-fat cream cheese (Neufchâtel), softened

2   tablespoons orange marmalade

1   Heat oven to 400°F. Spray bottoms only of 12 regular-size muffin cups with cooking spray or line with paper baking cups. In medium bowl, mix orange juice, honey, oil and egg.

2   In large bowl, stir together Bisquick mix, cereal, baking soda and ½ cup of the nuts. Stir orange juice mixture into cereal mixture just until moistened. Spoon batter evenly into muffin cups. Sprinkle with remaining nuts.

3   Bake about 20 minutes or until golden brown. Immediately remove from pan.

4   In small bowl, mix cream cheese and marmalade until well blended. Serve muffins with spread.

❝Pain drugs, especially morphine, and some chemos can make a person constipated. These muffins are a really easy way to grab a quick breakfast and help with constipation. The orange glaze makes the muffins taste good even with the metallic taste that's common after some chemotherapy treatments."—**Anne R.**

Good source of fiber and iron

1 Muffin: Calories 220 (Calories from Fat 90); Total Fat 10g (Saturated Fat 2.5g, Trans Fat 0.5g); Cholesterol 25mg; Sodium 330mg; Potassium 125mg; Total Carbohydrate 27g (Dietary Fiber 3g); Protein 4g **% Daily Value:** Vitamin A 2%; Vitamin C 6%; Calcium 4%; Iron 8%; Folic Acid 15%; Magnesium 4% **Exchanges:** 1 Starch, 1 Other Carbohydrate, 2 Fat **Carbohydrate Choices:** 2

A Note from Dr. Ghosh Did you know that breakfast cereals, like Chex®, are a great source of iron? We need iron for proper oxygen transfer in our blood to keep us healthy.

Streusel-Topped Fruit Brunch Cake

Prep Time: 15 Minutes | **Start to Finish:** 1 Hour | 12 servings

CAKE

2	cups Wheat Chex® or Multi-Bran Chex® cereal
1 ½	cups orange juice
¼	cup canola oil
1	egg, slightly beaten
2	small bananas, thinly sliced
1	cup all-purpose flour
½	cup whole wheat flour
¾	cup granulated sugar
½	cup raisins, if desired
1	teaspoon baking soda
1	teaspoon ground cinnamon
½	teaspoon salt

STREUSEL TOPPING

½	cup Wheat Chex® or Multi-Bran Chex® cereal
½	cup chopped nuts, if desired
⅓	cup packed brown sugar
¼	cup all-purpose flour
2	tablespoons butter or margarine, softened
½	teaspoon ground cinnamon

1 Heat oven to 350°F. Grease bottom and sides of 9-inch square pan with shortening or cooking spray. In large bowl, mix 2 cups cereal and the orange juice; let stand about 2 minutes or until cereal is soft.

2 Stir oil, egg and bananas into cereal mixture. Stir in remaining cake ingredients. Spread in pan.

3 Bake 35 to 40 minutes or until top springs back when touched lightly in center. Meanwhile, place ½ cup cereal in resealable food-storage plastic bag or between sheets of waxed paper; coarsely crush with rolling pin. In small bowl, mix crushed cereal and remaining topping ingredients until crumbly.

4 When cake is done, set oven control to broil. Sprinkle topping evenly over warm cake. Broil with top about 5 inches from heat for 1 to 2 minutes or until bubbly (watch carefully to avoid burning).

66 Close friends make coffee cake and bring it over; it makes all of us feel great. I get to enjoy tasty food, and they really are doing me an important favor. My family loves the treats, too."—Anne R.

High in iron; good source of folic acid and fiber

1 Serving: Calories 280 (Calories from Fat 70); Total Fat 7g (Saturated Fat 1.5g, Trans Fat 0g); Cholesterol 25mg; Sodium 340mg; Potassium 230mg; Total Carbohydrate 50g (Dietary Fiber 3g); Protein 4g **% Daily Value:** Vitamin A 6%; Vitamin C 15%; Calcium 4%; Iron 30%; Folic Acid 35%; Magnesium 8% **Exchanges:** 1 ½ Starch, 2 Other Carbohydrate, 1 Fat **Carbohydrate Choices:** 3

Food for Thought Blueberries are a source of antioxidant vitamins. Some research suggests that these components may help reduce risk of certain diseases.

Blueberry Brunch Cake

Prep Time: 15 Minutes | **Start to Finish:** 55 Minutes | 12 servings

CAKE

2	cups all-purpose flour
2	teaspoons baking powder
½	teaspoon salt
½	teaspoon ground ginger
¼	teaspoon baking soda
1	cup sugar
½	cup butter or margarine, softened
2	eggs
¾	cup sour cream or plain fat-free yogurt
1	teaspoon vanilla
2	cups fresh or frozen blueberries

TOPPING

¼	cup sugar
1	teaspoon ground cinnamon

1 Heat oven to 350°F. Grease bottom and sides of 13x9-inch pan with shortening or cooking spray; lightly flour. In medium bowl, stir together flour, baking powder, salt, ginger and baking soda; set aside.

2 In large bowl, mix 1 cup sugar and the butter. Stir in eggs, sour cream and vanilla. Stir in flour mixture. Carefully fold in blueberries. Spoon into pan.

3 In small bowl, mix ¼ cup sugar and the cinnamon; sprinkle over batter.

4 Bake about 40 minutes or until golden brown. Serve warm.

❝I made it a point to cook and eat foods with happy family memories during treatment. I made this cake and shared the recipe with family and friends during the holidays."—**Kathy S. Shares Her Recipe**

Low fiber; low residue

1 Serving: Calories 290 (Calories from Fat 110); Total Fat 12g (Saturated Fat 7g, Trans Fat 0g); Cholesterol 65mg; Sodium 280mg; Potassium 75mg; Total Carbohydrate 41g (Dietary Fiber 1g); Protein 3g
% Daily Value: Vitamin A 8%; Vitamin C 2%; Calcium 8%; Iron 8%; Folic Acid 8%; Magnesium 2%
Exchanges: 1 Starch, 1 ½ Other Carbohydrate, 2 ½ Fat **Carbohydrate Choices:** 3

A Note from Dr. Ghosh If you're on a fiber- and residue-restricted diet, these simple biscuits may be just for you. They're both low fiber and low residue, and can be eaten alone or with a meal.

Baking Powder Biscuits

Prep Time: 10 Minutes | **Start to Finish:** 25 Minutes | 12 biscuits

- 2 cups all-purpose or whole wheat flour
- 1 tablespoon sugar
- 3 teaspoons baking powder
- 1 teaspoon salt
- ½ cup shortening or cold butter, cut into 8 pieces
- ¾ cup milk

1 Heat oven to 450°F. In medium bowl, mix flour, sugar, baking powder and salt. Using pastry blender (or pulling 2 table knives through ingredients in opposite directions), cut in shortening until mixture looks like fine crumbs. Stir in milk until dough leaves side of bowl (dough will be soft and sticky).

2 On lightly floured surface, knead dough lightly 10 times. Roll or pat until ½ inch thick. Cut with floured 2- to 2 ¼-inch round cutter. On ungreased cookie sheet, place biscuits about 1 inch apart for crusty sides, touching for soft sides.

3 Bake 10 to 12 minutes or until golden brown. Immediately remove from cookie sheet to cooling rack. Serve warm.

"To save time, I made drop biscuits with this recipe. I increased the milk to 1 cup and dropped them onto a greased cookie sheet. I liked keeping these on hand and reheating them whenever I needed a little something to eat."—Theresa H.

Low fiber; low residue

1 Biscuit: Calories 160 (Calories from Fat 80); Total Fat 9g (Saturated Fat 2.5g, Trans Fat 1.5g); Cholesterol 0mg; Sodium 330mg; Potassium 45mg; Total Carbohydrate 18g (Dietary Fiber 0g); Protein 3g
% Daily Value: Vitamin A 0%; Vitamin C 0%; Calcium 8%; Iron 6%; Folic Acid 6%; Magnesium 0%
Exchanges: 1 Starch, 2 Fat **Carbohydrate Choices:** 1

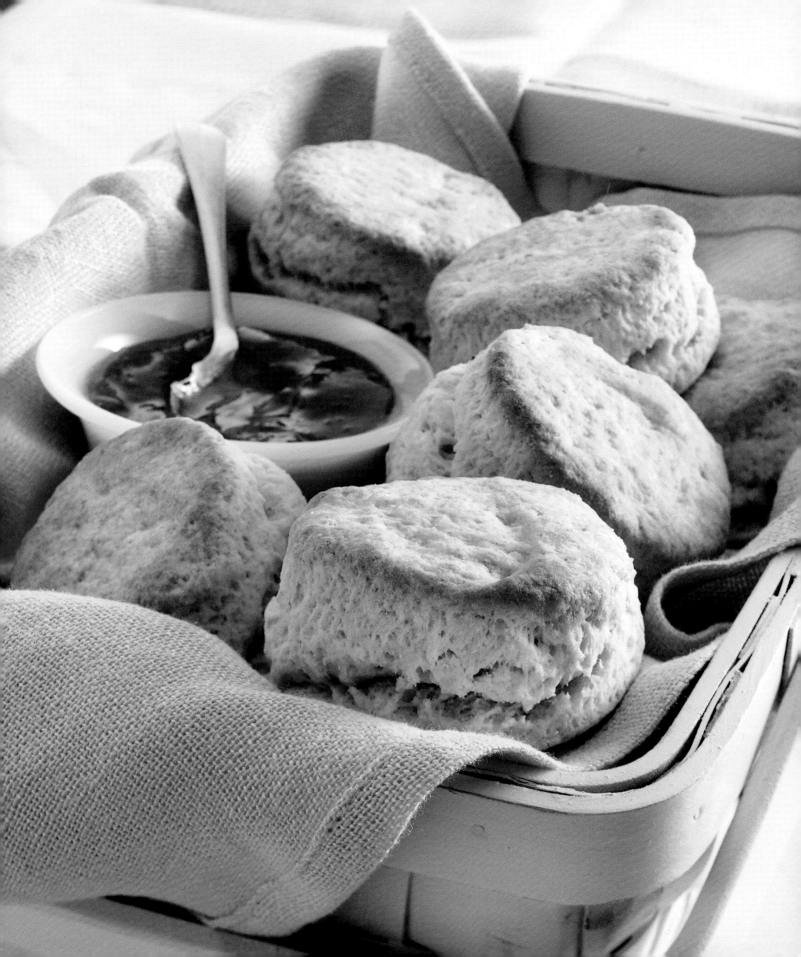

A Note from Dr. Ghosh This whole-grain breakfast is a healthy way to begin your day. Whole grains supply fiber and B vitamins and may help to reduce the risk of heart disease and certain types of cancer.

Tropical Pancakes

Prep Time: 20 Minutes | **Start to Finish:** 20 Minutes | 5 servings (two 4-inch pancakes each)

1 cup Whole Grain Total® or Wheaties® cereal

1 egg

1 medium very ripe banana, mashed (½ cup)

1 cup buttermilk

2 tablespoons vegetable oil

1 cup all-purpose flour

1 tablespoon sugar

1 teaspoon baking powder

½ teaspoon baking soda

½ teaspoon salt

1 Place cereal in plastic bag or between sheets of waxed paper; crush with rolling pin (or crush cereal in blender or food processor); set aside.

2 In medium bowl, beat egg with hand beater or whisk until fluffy. Beat in remaining ingredients until well blended. Gently stir in crushed cereal.

3 Heat griddle or skillet over medium heat or to 375°F. (To test griddle, sprinkle with a few drops of water. If bubbles jump around, heat is just right.) If necessary, grease griddle with butter.

4 For each pancake, pour slightly less than ¼ cup batter from cup or pitcher onto hot griddle. Cook until puffed and full of bubbles; turn before bubbles break. Cook other side until golden brown.

❝Serving these pancakes with honey or real maple syrup, whipped cream (I try to add calories whenever I can) and a few slices of banana makes me feel like I am having a real treat. I freeze the pancakes in individual plastic bags (two per bag) and reheat them in the toaster oven. Then I have an instant, low-odor breakfast.”
—Anne R.

High in iron and folic acid

1 Serving: Calories 240 (Calories from Fat 70); Total Fat 8g (Saturated Fat 2g, Trans Fat 0g); Cholesterol 45mg; Sodium 560mg; Potassium 240mg; Total Carbohydrate 36g (Dietary Fiber 2g); Protein 6g
% Daily Value: Vitamin A 4%; Vitamin C 15%; Calcium 40%; Iron 35%; Folic Acid 40%; Magnesium 6%
Exchanges: 1 ½ Starch, 1 Other Carbohydrate, 1 ½ Fat **Carbohydrate Choices:** 2 ½

Food for Thought Cheese and pears are a wonderful blend of flavors—don't save this oven pancake just for breakfast! The salty richness of the cheese complements the sweetness of the pears.

Cheesy Pear Oven Pancake

Prep Time: 20 Minutes | **Start to Finish:** 30 Minutes | 4 servings

1 cup all-purpose flour

1 cup milk

¼ teaspoon salt

4 eggs

1 tablespoon butter or margarine

2 unpeeled medium pears, thinly sliced (2 cups)

2 tablespoons chopped fresh or 2 teaspoons freeze-dried chives

2 tablespoons sugar

¾ cup shredded Cheddar cheese (3 oz)

1 Heat oven to 450°F. Spray 13x9-inch (3-quart) glass baking dish with cooking spray. In medium bowl, beat flour, milk, salt and eggs with whisk until smooth. Pour into baking dish. Bake 15 to 18 minutes or until puffy and golden brown.

2 Meanwhile, in 10-inch nonstick skillet, melt butter over medium-high heat. Add pears and chives; cook about 5 minutes, stirring frequently, until pears are slightly softened. Stir in sugar.

3 Spoon pear mixture onto pancake. Sprinkle with cheese. Bake about 1 minute or until cheese is melted.

❝After treatment, my energy is really low, so this makes an easy-to-eat breakfast, especially if the pancake- and-pear mixture is already made by my son or husband. If I can't eat it all at once, I can just take it from the refrigerator, reheat and eat."—**Anne R.**

High in calcium; good source of fiber

1 Serving: Calories 410 (Calories from Fat 150); Total Fat 17g (Saturated Fat 9g, Trans Fat 0g); Cholesterol 245mg; Sodium 390mg; Potassium 310mg; Total Carbohydrate 47g (Dietary Fiber 4g); Protein 17g **% Daily Value:** Vitamin A 15%; Vitamin C 4%; Calcium 20%; Iron 15%; Folic Acid 20%; Magnesium 8% **Exchanges:** 2 Starch, ½ Fruit, ½ Other Carbohydrate, 1 ½ Medium-Fat Meat, 1 ½ Fat **Carbohydrate Choices:** 3

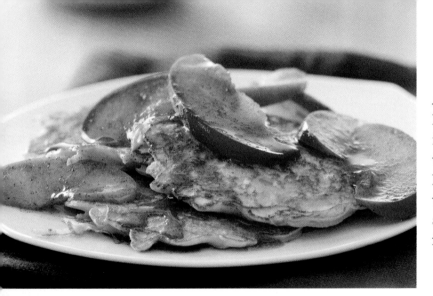

A Note from Dr. Ghosh
Potassium, found in abundance in this recipe, is a nutrient that's helpful in cancer healing. Potassium also helps to maintain the body's natural water balance and aids in nerve and muscle function.

Potato Pancakes with Cinnamon Apples

Prep Time: 20 Minutes | **Start to Finish:** 20 Minutes | 6 servings (three 4-inch pancakes and about ⅓ cup apples each)

Cinnamon Apples (opposite)
½ cup Original Bisquick® mix
½ cup milk
1 teaspoon salt
3 eggs
3 cups finely shredded uncooked potatoes

1 Make Cinnamon Apples. Keep warm.

2 In large bowl, mix Bisquick mix, milk, salt and eggs until blended. Stir in potatoes.

3 Heat griddle or skillet over medium heat or to 375°F. (To test griddle, sprinkle with a few drops of water. If bubbles jump around, heat is just right.) If necessary, grease griddle with butter.

4 For each pancake, pour slightly less than ¼ cup batter from cup or pitcher onto hot griddle, spreading each slightly to make 4-inch pancake. Cook until dry around edges. Turn and cook other side until golden brown. Serve warm Cinnamon Apples with pancakes.

❝I add a very good whey protein powder to increase the protein content of breads, pancakes and cakes. I reduce the flour by the amount of powder that I add. This makes every mouthful count. The carbs give me energy, the protein rebuilds damaged tissue and the fat slows down absorption so it lessens the nausea for me. That way, every meal has some fat, carb and good protein."—**Anne R.**

Excellent source of fiber when eaten with the Cinnamon Apples

1 Serving: Calories 280 (Calories from Fat 40); Total Fat 4.5g (Saturated Fat 1.5g, Trans Fat 0g); Cholesterol 110mg; Sodium 580mg; Potassium 570mg; Total Carbohydrate 53g (Dietary Fiber 4g); Protein 7g
% Daily Value: Vitamin A 4%; Vitamin C 10%; Calcium 8%; Iron 8%; Folic Acid 8%; Magnesium 10%
Exchanges: 2 Starch, ½ Fruit, 1 Other Carbohydrate, ½ Fat **Carbohydrate Choices:** 3 ½

Food for Thought A twist on homemade applesauce, these apples offer a big cinnamon taste. If you prefer, remove the peel. For variety, try adding ¼ teaspoon ground nutmeg and ¼ teaspoon ground cloves in addition to the cinnamon and enjoy this recipe as a snack or dessert.

Cinnamon Apples

Prep Time: 10 Minutes | **Start to Finish:** 10 Minutes | 3 or 4 servings (about ⅔ cup each)

3   medium unpeeled tart cooking apples (Granny Smith, Greening, Rome, Braeburn), sliced (3 cups)

½   cup water

⅓   cup sugar

1   teaspoon ground cinnamon

1   In 2-quart microwavable casserole or large microwavable bowl, place apple slices. Stir in water, sugar and cinnamon.

2   Cover; microwave on High 5 minutes. Uncover; stir. Microwave uncovered about 5 minutes longer or until apples are tender when pierced with fork.

66 These apples are so easy to make and very tasty served with pancakes, waffles or biscuits. I sometimes blend the apples after cooking to make applesauce."—**Lois K. Shares Her Recipe**

Good source of fiber

1 Serving: Calories 200 (Calories from Fat 0); Total Fat 0g (Saturated Fat 0g, Trans Fat 0g); Cholesterol 0mg; Sodium 0mg; Potassium 200mg; Total Carbohydrate 48g (Dietary Fiber 5g); Protein 0g **% Daily Value:** Vitamin A 2%; Vitamin C 8%; Calcium 2%; Iron 0%; Folic Acid 0%; Magnesium 2% **Exchanges:** 1 Fruit, 2 Other Carbohydrate **Carbohydrate Choices:** 3

Food for Thought This combination of healthy ingredients contains nutritional benefits from vitamin C, calcium, iron and folic acid. It also contains magnesium—a nutrient that helps to release energy from foods, particularly from carbohydrate sources.

Baked French Toast with Strawberry-Rhubarb Sauce

Prep Time: 20 Minutes | **Start to Finish:** 8 Hours 25 Minutes | 6 servings (3 slices French toast and ⅓ cup sauce each)

FRENCH TOAST

½	cup all-purpose flour
1 ½	cups milk
1	tablespoon sugar
½	teaspoon vanilla
¼	teaspoon salt
6	eggs
18	slices (1 inch thick) French bread

SAUCE

2	cups medium whole strawberries
2	cups cut-up rhubarb (about 1 ⅓ lb)
⅓	cup water
1	box (4-serving size) strawberry-flavored gelatin

1 Generously grease 15x10x1-inch pan with shortening or cooking spray. In medium bowl, beat flour, milk, sugar, vanilla, salt and eggs with whisk until smooth.

2 Arrange bread slices to fit in single layer in pan. Pour egg mixture over bread slices; turn to coat both sides. Cover; refrigerate at least 8 hours but no longer than 24 hours.

3 Heat oven to 450°F. Uncover; bake 10 to 13 minutes or until golden brown.

4 Meanwhile, in 2-quart saucepan, heat strawberries, rhubarb and water to boiling. Boil 5 minutes, stirring occasionally. Remove from heat; stir in gelatin until dissolved. Boil 2 minutes longer, stirring constantly. Serve warm sauce with French toast.

❝Strawberry-rhubarb sauce really helps me when I'm mildly constipated and don't want to take another medicine. The strawberry-rhubarb combination works for me, and it tastes great, even after chemo!"—Anne R.

Good source of calcium, iron, vitamin C and folic acid

1 Serving: Calories 160 (Calories from Fat 30); Total Fat 3.5g (Saturated Fat 1g, Trans Fat 0g); Cholesterol 70mg; Sodium 270mg; Potassium 150mg; Total Carbohydrate 27g (Dietary Fiber 2g); Protein 7g **% Daily Value:** Vitamin A 4%; Vitamin C 8%; Calcium 8%; Iron 8%; Folic Acid 20%; Magnesium 4% **Exchanges:** 1 ½ Starch, ½ Other Carbohydrate, ½ Fat **Carbohydrate Choices:** 2

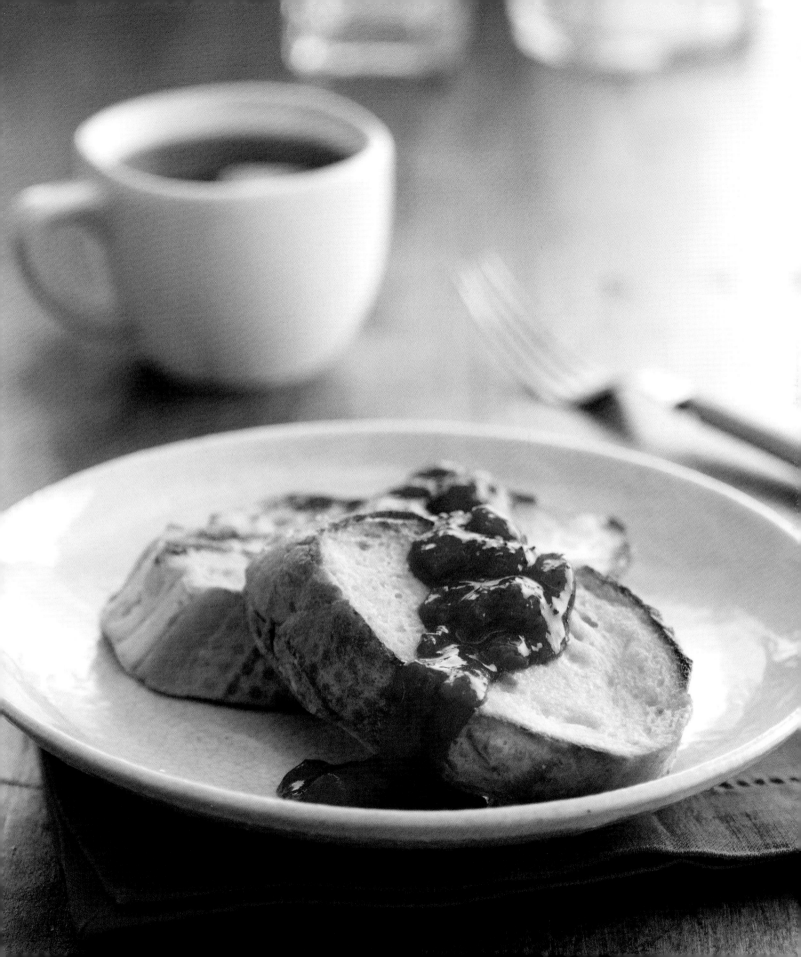

Food for Thought These waffles, made from a blend of peanut butter and flour, provide protein, magnesium and iron. Protein supplies needed nitrogen that's vital for life and the growth of new cells in the body. The waffles supply lots of important calories your body needs for healing. If you can eat only one, save the other for later in the day. For a crisp waffle, pop it into the toaster.

Make-Ahead Waffles with Peanut Butter Spread

Prep Time: 25 Minutes | **Start to Finish:** 9 Hours 55 Minutes | 6 servings (two 4-inch waffle squares and about 3 tablespoons spread each)

WAFFLES

1	package regular active dry yeast
¼	cup warm water (105°F to 115°F)
1 ¾	cups lukewarm milk (scalded then cooled)
2	tablespoons sugar
1	teaspoon salt
3	eggs
¼	cup butter or margarine, softened
2	cups all-purpose flour

PEANUT BUTTER SPREAD

½	cup maple-flavored syrup
½	cup peanut butter

1 In large bowl, dissolve yeast in warm water. Add remaining waffle ingredients; beat with electric mixer on medium speed until smooth. Cover; let rise in warm place 1 hour 30 minutes.

2 Stir down batter. Cover; refrigerate at least 8 hours but no longer than 12 hours.

3 Heat waffle maker. Meanwhile, mix syrup and peanut butter until blended; set aside. If necessary, grease waffle maker with shortening. Stir down batter. Pour about ½ cup batter from cup or pitcher onto center of hot waffle maker. (Waffle makers vary in size; check manufacturer's directions for recommended amount of batter.) Close lid of waffle maker.

4 Bake about 5 minutes or until steaming stops. Carefully remove waffle. Repeat with remaining batter. Serve with peanut butter spread.

66 I make these into pancakes by pouring ¼ cup batter onto a greased hot griddle and cooking until they're puffed and full of bubbles. Then I turn them and cook the other side until golden brown. I freeze them and reheat as needed. Pancakes are so easy to eat; I live on them right after chemo or as soon as I can eat solid food after surgery."—**Anne R.**

High in folic acid; good source of fiber and iron

1 Serving: Calories 520 (Calories from Fat 210); Total Fat 23g (Saturated Fat 9g, Trans Fat 0g); Cholesterol 130mg; Sodium 620mg; Potassium 350mg; Total Carbohydrate 62g (Dietary Fiber 3g); Protein 15g **% Daily Value:** Vitamin A 10%; Vitamin C 0%; Calcium 10%; Iron 15%; Folic Acid 30%; Magnesium 15% **Exchanges:** 2 ½ Starch, 1 ½ Other Carbohydrate, ½ Medium-Fat Meat, ½ High-Fat Meat, 3 Fat **Carbohydrate Choices:** 4

Keep a Lemon in Your Kitchen . . .
and Other Ways to Reduce Nausea

Nausea can be very unpleasant and unsettling. Nausea is a direct side effect for many on chemotherapy or radiation, but there are ways to reduce it. Try these tips:

1. Take nausea medication. Only take what your doctor prescribes, and work with him or her to find the most effective medication for you. The right medication will help you eat better, eat more and stay well hydrated.

2. Keep citrus fruits around. Keep a lemon in your kitchen or at your desk, and pick it up and sniff it every once in a while. For more citrus power, cut the lemon and squeeze a few drops of juice into your water glass. Add ice and water. Every time you take a sip of water, you will feel refreshed! Don't have a lemon? Try a lime or an orange.

3. Eat foods that smell good to you. Aroma is directly linked to taste. If a certain food smells good, it will most likely taste good to you, too.

4. Sip or drink liquids slowly and often throughout the day. Extra liquids are important, and if you drink them slowly, they can help ease the nausea and relax you.

5. Eat dry toast or crackers. Even before getting up, nibble on crackers from your bedside table if you have nausea in the morning.

6. Wear loose-fitting clothes. Anything too tight, particularly around your tummy, may worsen or trigger nausea.

7. Avoid eating for 1 to 2 hours before chemotherapy or radiation.

8. Eat small amounts and more frequently. Eating mini-meals or snacks more often throughout the day instead of three large meals may lessen feelings of nausea.

9. Eat before you get hungry. Hunger can actually make the nausea feel much worse. Try to keep something small in your stomach, even if it's just a cracker.

10. Sit up for about an hour after meals. Lying down too quickly after a meal can increase nausea or discomfort and interfere with digestion

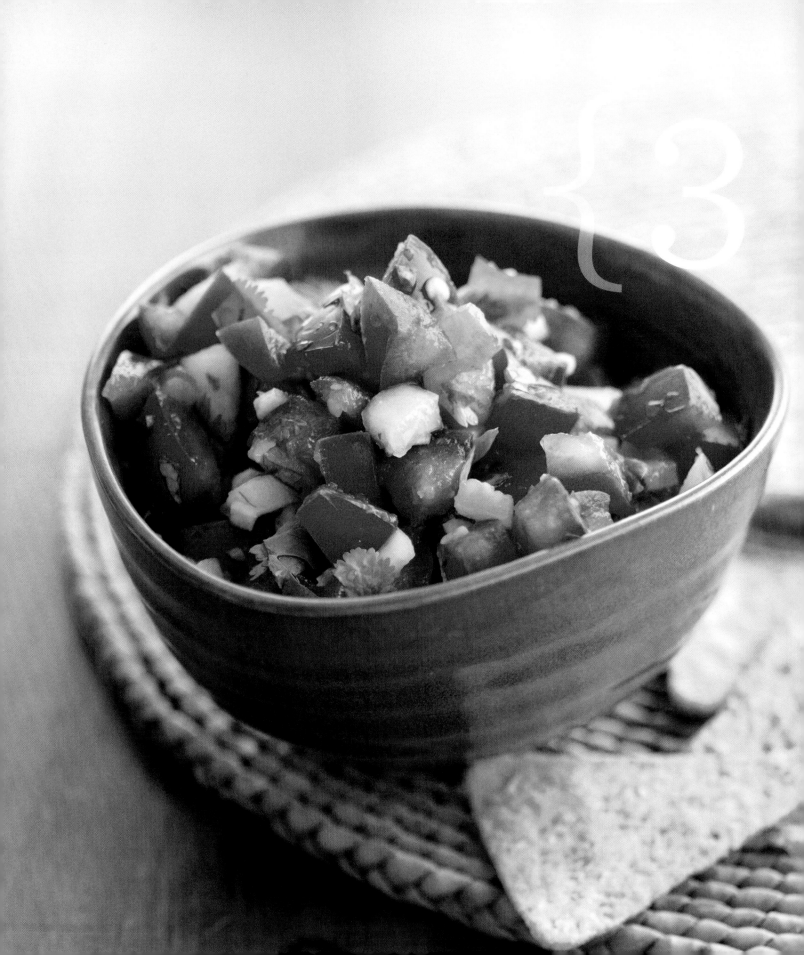

Fatigue-Fighting Snacks }

80   Roasted Vegetable Dip

82   Zucchini Bites

83   Oven-Fried Potato Wedges

84   Onion and Rosemary Focaccia Wedges

85   Tomato Bruschetta

86   String Cheese Sticks with Dipping Sauce

87   Super Grilled Cheese Sandwiches

88   Veggies and Cheese Mini-Pizzas

90   Hot Turkey Sandwiches

91   Easy Chicken Nuggets

92   Philly Beef Sandwiches

93   Quick Quesadillas

94   Chicken Salad in Pitas

96   Snappy Stuffed Tomatoes

97   Mozzarella and Tomatoes

98   Fresh Salsa

100   Creamy Caramel Dip with Fruit

101   Spinach Dip in Bread Bowl

102   Easy Salmon Spread

103   Citrus-Peach Smoothie

104   Watermelon-Kiwi-Banana Smoothie

106   Orange-Pineapple Smoothie

107   Sugar 'n Spice Green Tea

108   Chai Tea

A Note from Dr. Ghosh Dips, especially healthy ones like this, along with plenty of fun dippers make great excuses for sharing. Surround yourself with family and friends to lift your spirits. Your mental health is as important as your physical health.

Roasted Vegetable Dip

Prep Time: 15 Minutes | **Start to Finish:** 45 Minutes | 7 servings (¼ cup each)

1 medium zucchini, sliced (2 cups)

1 medium yellow summer squash, sliced (1 ½ cups)

1 medium red bell pepper, sliced

1 medium red onion, thinly sliced

2 cloves garlic, peeled

Cooking spray

½ teaspoon salt

¼ teaspoon ground red pepper (cayenne)

Dippers (baby-cut carrots, cucumber slices, green bell pepper strips, toasted pita bread wedges, baked tortilla chips), if desired

1 Heat oven to 400°F. In 15x10x1-inch pan, spread zucchini, yellow squash, bell pepper, onion and garlic. Spray vegetables with cooking spray. Sprinkle with salt and red pepper.

2 Bake about 30 minutes, turning vegetables once, until vegetables are tender and lightly browned.

3 Place vegetables in blender or food processor. Cover; blend on high speed about 1 minute, stopping blender occasionally to scrape sides, until smooth.

4 Serve warm, or refrigerate at least 2 hours until chilled. Serve with dippers.

66 Thinking of things that made me smile really helped. My grandson, Nolan, loves to recite from the book, *We're Going on a Bear Hunt,* and emphasize 'It's a beauuutiful day!' I often smile and say to myself, 'It's a beauuutiful day!' Serving this dip was fun for both me and Nolan." —**Judy O. Shares Her Recipe**

High in vitamins A and C; low fiber

1 Serving: Calories 25 (Calories from Fat 0); Total Fat 0g (Saturated Fat 0g, Trans Fat 0g); Cholesterol 0mg; Sodium 170mg; Potassium 210mg; Total Carbohydrate 5g (Dietary Fiber 1g); Protein 1g
% Daily Value: Vitamin A 15%; Vitamin C 25%; Calcium 0%; Iron 0%; Folic Acid 6%; Magnesium 4%
Exchanges: ½ Vegetable **Carbohydrate Choices:** ½

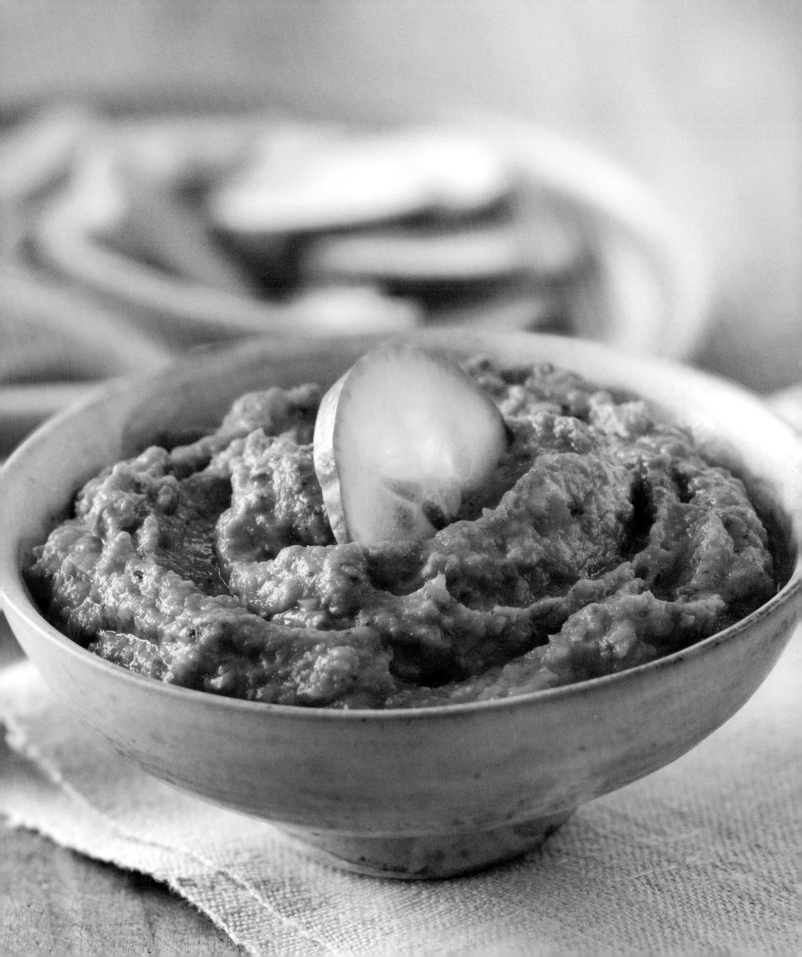

A Note from Dr. Ghosh A good source of vitamin C, this dish will help you maintain healthy gums, muscles, bones and teeth. A powerful antioxidant, vitamin C is also involved in promoting healing.

Zucchini Bites

Prep Time: 10 Minutes | **Start to Finish:** 35 Minutes | 8 servings (6 bites each)

4   eggs, slightly beaten

½   cup vegetable oil

1   cup Original Bisquick® mix

½   cup grated Parmesan cheese

2   tablespoons chopped fresh parsley

½   teaspoon salt

½   teaspoon seasoned salt

½   teaspoon dried marjoram or oregano leaves

4   small unpeeled zucchini, thinly sliced (3 cups)

1   medium onion, finely chopped (½ cup)

1   clove garlic, finely chopped

1   Heat oven to 350°F. Grease bottom and sides of 13x9-inch pan with shortening or cooking spray.

2   In large bowl, stir together all ingredients until blended. Spread in pan.

3   Bake about 25 minutes or until golden brown. Cut into 2-inch squares; cut squares diagonally in half into triangles.

66 Recently I decided to plant a small vegetable and herb garden. It gives me great pleasure to pick something from my garden and then cook with it. I find gardening and enjoying the outdoors very healing."—**Judy O.**

Low fiber; low residue

1 Serving: Calories 270 (Calories from Fat 180); Total Fat 20g (Saturated Fat 4.5g, Trans Fat 0.5g); Cholesterol 110mg; Sodium 570mg; Potassium 240mg; Total Carbohydrate 14g (Dietary Fiber 1g); Protein 7g **% Daily Value:** Vitamin A 8%; Vitamin C 10%; Calcium 15%; Iron 6%; Folic Acid 10%; Magnesium 4% **Exchanges:** ½ Starch, 1 Vegetable, ½ Medium-Fat Meat, 3 ½ Fat **Carbohydrate Choices:** 1

A Note from Dr. Ghosh Some scientific studies suggest that cancer survivors who eat a low-fat diet may live longer. It's important to remember that dieting is not recommended during cancer treatment. Low-fat foods like these potato wedges can be delicious, as well as healthy.

Oven-Fried Potato Wedges

Prep Time: 10 Minutes | **Start to Finish:** 40 Minutes | 4 servings

¾ teaspoon salt

½ teaspoon sugar

½ teaspoon paprika

¼ teaspoon garlic powder

¼ teaspoon ground mustard

3 medium baking potatoes (8 to 10 oz each)

Cooking spray

1 Heat oven to 425°F. In small bowl, mix salt, sugar, paprika, garlic powder and mustard.

2 Gently scrub potatoes, but do not peel. Cut each potato lengthwise in half; cut each half lengthwise into 4 wedges. Place potato wedges, skin sides down, in ungreased 13x9-inch pan.

3 Spray potatoes with cooking spray until lightly coated. Sprinkle with salt mixture.

4 Bake uncovered 25 to 30 minutes or until potatoes are tender when pierced with fork. (Baking time will vary depending on the size and type of the potato used.)

❝On days when I am hungry for potatoes, this recipe is a quick and tasty side dish. To make it low residue, peel the skin from the potatoes before cutting. Peeling is a bit of extra work, but doing it makes the recipe better for me."—**Theresa H.**

Low residue if skins are removed

1 Serving: Calories 130 (Calories from Fat 0); Total Fat 0g (Saturated Fat 0g, Trans Fat 0g); Cholesterol 0mg; Sodium 460mg; Potassium 700mg; Total Carbohydrate 28g (Dietary Fiber 3g); Protein 3g **% Daily Value:** Vitamin A 4%; Vitamin C 10%; Calcium 2%; Iron 8%; Folic Acid 10%; Magnesium 10% **Exchanges:** 1 Starch, ½ Other Carbohydrate, ½ Vegetable **Carbohydrate Choices:** 2

Food for Thought If foods taste bland to you and you need a flavor boost, this snack made with garlic and onions just may do the trick. If you're not fond of the flavor of rosemary, substitute fresh or dried basil in its place.

Onion and Rosemary Focaccia Wedges

Prep Time: 15 Minutes | **Start to Finish:** 30 Minutes | 6 servings (2 wedges each)

Olive oil-flavored cooking spray

1   can (13.8 oz) refrigerated pizza crust

3   cloves garlic, finely chopped

½   teaspoon dried rosemary leaves, crumbled

1   large sweet onion (Bermuda, Maui, Spanish or Walla Walla), thinly sliced, separated into rings

¾   cup grated Parmesan cheese

¼   teaspoon salt, if desired

1 Heat oven 400°F. Spray cookie sheet with cooking spray. Roll or pat pizza dough into 13x9-inch rectangle on cookie sheet. Sprinkle with garlic and rosemary. Arrange onion rings evenly over dough. Sprinkle with cheese.

2 Bake about 12 minutes or until cheese just begins to brown. Lightly spray focaccia with cooking spray; sprinkle with salt. Cut into 12 wedges. Serve immediately.

" Remembering the myth about garlic warding off vampires and evil spirits, I figured I had nothing to lose by adding garlic to my diet to ward off the cancer! It made me chuckle when I decided to call in all the help I could get to fight the cancer—even garlic!"—Catherine H.

Good source of calcium; low fiber

1 Serving: Calories 230 (Calories from Fat 50); Total Fat 6g (Saturated Fat 3g, Trans Fat 0g); Cholesterol 10mg; Sodium 700mg; Potassium 55mg; Total Carbohydrate 34g (Dietary Fiber 1g); Protein 10g **% Daily Value:** Vitamin A 0%; Vitamin C 0%; Calcium 20%; Iron 10%; Folic Acid 0%; Magnesium 2% **Exchanges:** 1 ½ Starch, 1 Other Carbohydrate, ½ Very Lean Meat, 1 Fat **Carbohydrate Choices:** 2

A Note from Dr. Ghosh Skip the feta cheese during neutropenic times when your resistance is down. Try substituting a cooked cheese, such as shredded mozzarella.

Tomato Bruschetta

Prep Time: 10 Minutes | **Start to Finish:** 25 Minutes | 10 servings (2 slices each)

1   loaf (1 lb) French or Italian bread

2   tablespoons butter or margarine, softened

4   medium plum (Roma) tomatoes, thinly sliced

¼   cup sliced ripe olives

½   teaspoon dried basil leaves

¾   cup crumbled feta cheese (3 oz)

2   cloves garlic, finely chopped

¼   cup olive or vegetable oil

1   Heat oven to 375°F. Cut bread loaf horizontally in half. Place halves, cut sides up, on ungreased cookie sheet. Brush with butter. Top with tomatoes, olives, basil and cheese.

2   In small bowl, mix garlic and oil. Drizzle oil mixture over cheese.

3   Bake 12 to 15 minutes or until cheese just begins to brown. Cut into 2-inch slices.

66 When I was really fatigued, I turned to the easiest recipes possible, like these tasty bruschetta. Eating small amounts of foods more often throughout the day helped me be able to eat more overall."
—**Joan K. Shares Her Recipe**

Low fiber

1 Serving: Calories 230 (Calories from Fat 100); Total Fat 11g (Saturated Fat 4g, Trans Fat 0g); Cholesterol 15mg; Sodium 440mg; Potassium 120mg; Total Carbohydrate 27g (Dietary Fiber 1g); Protein 6g
% Daily Value: Vitamin A 6%; Vitamin C 2%; Calcium 6%; Iron 10%; Folic Acid 20%; Magnesium 4%
Exchanges: 1 ½ Starch, ½ Other Carbohydrate, 2 Fat **Carbohydrate Choices:** 2

Food for Thought There's something about eating with your fingers that brings on a smile. These tasty cheese sticks make a happy snack that's loaded with calcium.

String Cheese Sticks with Dipping Sauce

Prep Time: 10 Minutes | **Start to Finish:** 20 Minutes | 4 servings (2 cheese sticks each)

2 ¼ cups Original Bisquick® mix

⅔ cup milk

1 package (8 oz) plain or smoked string cheese

1 can (8 oz) pizza sauce

1 tablespoon butter or margarine, melted

¼ teaspoon garlic powder

1 Heat oven to 450°F. In medium bowl, stir Bisquick mix and milk until soft dough forms; beat 30 seconds with spoon. On surface sprinkled with Bisquick mix, gently roll dough in Bisquick mix to coat. Shape into a ball; knead 10 times.

2 Roll dough into 12x8-inch rectangle, ¼ inch thick. Cut into 8 (6x2-inch) rectangles. Roll each rectangle around 1 piece of cheese. Pinch edge into roll to seal; seal ends. Roll on surface to completely enclose cheese sticks. On ungreased cookie sheet, place sticks seam sides down.

3 Bake 8 to 10 minutes or until golden brown. Meanwhile, in 1-quart saucepan, heat pizza sauce over low heat until warm. In small bowl, mix butter and garlic powder.

4 Before removing warm cheese sticks from cookie sheet, brush with butter mixture. Serve warm with pizza sauce for dipping.

❝The smell of bread baking, as in these cheese sticks, reminds me of my mother's kitchen and stimulates my appetite—very therapeutic!"—Judy O.

High in calcium; low fiber

1 Serving: Calories 500 (Calories from Fat 220); Total Fat 24g (Saturated Fat 12g, Trans Fat 2g); Cholesterol 40mg; Sodium 1540mg; Potassium 420mg; Total Carbohydrate 50g (Dietary Fiber 2g); Protein 22g **% Daily Value:** Vitamin A 10%; Vitamin C 2%; Calcium 60%; Iron 20%; Folic Acid 20%; Magnesium 8% **Exchanges:** 2 ½ Starch, 1 Other Carbohydrate, 2 High-Fat Meat, 1 Fat **Carbohydrate Choices:** 3

Food for Thought Read the Nutrition Facts labels on the foods you buy, and check the recipes you make to be sure you're getting enough calcium daily. If you add up all the percentages for the day, you should reach at least 100 percent Daily Value for calcium. This recipe, with 20 percent, is a great start.

Super Grilled Cheese Sandwiches

Prep Time: 5 Minutes | **Start to Finish:** 15 Minutes | 4 sandwiches

4 slices (1 oz each) Cheddar, mozzarella, Colby or Monterey Jack cheese

8 slices Italian sourdough, white or whole wheat bread

2 medium green onions, sliced (2 tablespoons)

1 medium tomato, seeded, chopped (¾ cup)

8 teaspoons butter or margarine, softened

1 Place cheese slices on 4 slices of bread. Top with onions and tomato, then remaining bread. Spread 1 teaspoon butter over each top slice of bread.

2 In 12-inch skillet, place sandwiches, butter sides down. Spread remaining butter over top slices of bread.

3 Cook uncovered over medium heat about 5 minutes or until bottoms are golden brown. Turn and cook 2 to 3 minutes longer or until bottoms are golden brown and cheese is melted. Using pizza cutter, cut sandwiches into wedges or sticks.

66 If I cut sandwiches into smaller pieces, like quarters or eighths, I can eat one or two pieces now and one or two later. These are super dunked in tomato soup!"—Theresa H.

High in calcium

1 Sandwich: Calories 300 (Calories from Fat 170); Total Fat 19g (Saturated Fat 11g, Trans Fat 1g); Cholesterol 50mg; Sodium 470mg; Potassium 160mg; Total Carbohydrate 22g (Dietary Fiber 1g); Protein 11g **% Daily Value:** Vitamin A 15%; Vitamin C 4%; Calcium 20%; Iron 8%; Folic Acid 20%; Magnesium 6% **Exchanges:** 1 ½ Starch, 1 High-Fat Meat, 2 Fat **Carbohydrate Choices:** 1 ½

Food for Thought Vegetables are loaded with nutrients you need each day to be healthy. MyPlate recommends eating 2 ½ to 4 cups of veggies every day.

Veggies and Cheese Mini-Pizzas

Prep Time: 15 Minutes | **Start to Finish:** 25 Minutes | 4 mini-pizzas

2 pita (pocket) breads (6 inch)

3 medium plum (Roma) tomatoes, chopped (1 cup)

2 small zucchini, chopped (2 cups)

1 small onion, chopped (¼ cup)

2 tablespoons sliced ripe olives

1 teaspoon chopped fresh or ¼ teaspoon dried basil leaves

¼ cup spaghetti sauce or pizza sauce

¾ cup shredded mozzarella cheese (3 oz)

1 Heat oven to 425°F. Split each pita bread around edge with knife to make 2 rounds. Place rounds on ungreased cookie sheet. Bake about 5 minutes or just until crisp.

2 In medium bowl, mix tomatoes, zucchini, onion, olives and basil. Spread spaghetti sauce evenly over pita rounds. Top with vegetable mixture. Sprinkle with cheese.

3 Bake 5 to 7 minutes or until cheese is melted. Cut into wedges.

❝Pizza is a family favorite, and with this recipe, we are also sure to get our vegetables."—Judy O.

High in vitamin A

1 Mini-Pizza: Calories 130 (Calories from Fat 45); Total Fat 5g (Saturated Fat 2g, Trans Fat 0.5g); Cholesterol 10mg; Sodium 260mg; Potassium 50mg; Total Carbohydrate 19g (Dietary Fiber 2g); Protein 2g **% Daily Value:** Vitamin A 2%; Vitamin C 0%; Calcium 0%; Iron 4%; Folic Acid 6%; Magnesium 4% **Exchanges:** 1 ½ Starch, ½ High-Fat Meat **Carbohydrate Choices:** 1

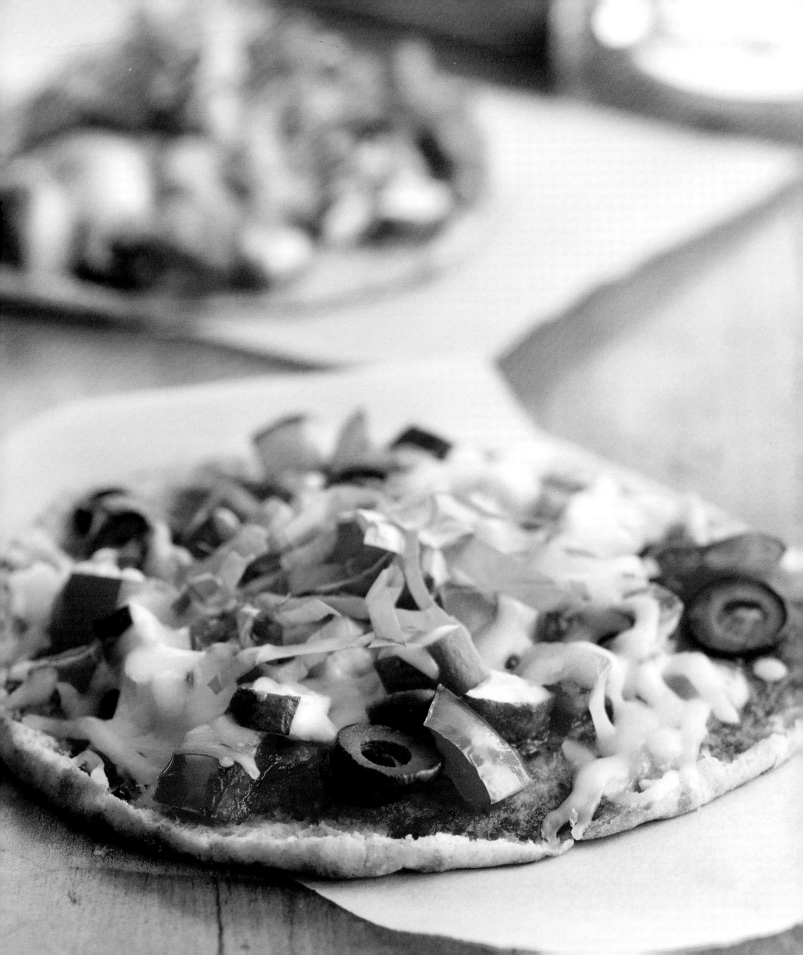

Food for Thought Slow cookers make meal preparation easy and can be a lifesaver at times when you're really fatigued. If you start cooking the turkey midmorning when you are likely to have more energy, you can enjoy a no-fuss, high-carbohydrate dinner later. Freeze leftovers for an easy dinner another day.

Hot Turkey Sandwiches

Prep Time: 10 Minutes | **Start to Finish:** 4 Hours 10 Minutes | 12 sandwiches

1 boneless whole turkey breast (4 to 5 lb)

½ teaspoon salt

½ teaspoon pepper

1 can (10 ¾ oz) condensed cream of chicken soup

12 medium wheat or white burger buns, split

Cranberry sauce, if desired

1 Spray inside of 4- to 5-quart slow cooker with cooking spray. Place turkey in slow cooker; sprinkle with salt and pepper. Cover; cook on Low heat setting 4 to 5 hours or until juice is no longer pink when center is cut.

2 Remove turkey from slow cooker; reserve ⅔ cup broth in 1-quart saucepan. Cool turkey slightly; cut into slices.

3 Add soup to reserved turkey broth in saucepan. Cook over medium heat about 5 minutes, stirring occasionally, until thoroughly heated.

4 Place turkey on bottom halves of buns. Pour gravy over turkey; add top halves of buns. Serve with cranberry sauce. Refrigerate remaining turkey.

"I looked for foods that would boost my energy, and high-protein foods like these turkey sandwiches seemed to work best for me."
—**Marilyn T. Shares Her Recipe**

Low fiber; low residue

1 Sandwich: Calories 330 (Calories from Fat 45); Total Fat 5g (Saturated Fat 1.5g, Trans Fat 0g); Cholesterol 125mg; Sodium 510mg; Potassium 500mg; Total Carbohydrate 23g (Dietary Fiber 1g); Protein 48g **% Daily Value:** Vitamin A 2%; Vitamin C 0%; Calcium 8%; Iron 20%; Folic Acid 10%; Magnesium 15% **Exchanges:** 1 ½ Starch, 5 ½ Very Lean Meat, ½ Lean Meat **Carbohydrate Choices:** 1 ½

A Note from Dr. Ghosh When this easy chicken coating is made with Total® cereal, it provides 100 percent of the folic acid and iron you need daily. Folic acid is a B vitamin that helps protect against nerve damage and birth defects. Iron is a mineral that's crucial for oxygen uptake by cells in the bloodstream.

Easy Chicken Nuggets

Prep Time: 15 Minutes | **Start to Finish:** 25 Minutes | 4 servings

4 cups Whole Grain Total® cereal

1 lb boneless skinless chicken breasts, cut into 1-inch pieces

½ cup Italian dressing, honey mustard or red pepper sauce

1 Heat oven to 425°F. Spray 15x10x1-inch pan with cooking spray. Place cereal in plastic bag or between sheets of waxed paper; crush with rolling pin (or crush cereal in blender or food processor). Place cereal in bowl or plastic food-storage bag.

2 Dip chicken pieces into dressing; roll in cereal until well coated. Place in pan.

3 Bake about 10 minutes or until no longer pink in center.

❝When you're tired, having simple recipes that are easy to prepare like these chicken nuggets is so important."—**Susan S.**

High in iron, calcium, folic acid and vitamin C; good source of fiber

1 Serving: Calories 310 (Calories from Fat 70); Total Fat 8g (Saturated Fat 1.5g, Trans Fat 0g); Cholesterol 70mg; Sodium 380mg; Potassium 330mg; Total Carbohydrate 31g (Dietary Fiber 3g); Protein 28g **% Daily Value:** Vitamin A 15%; Vitamin C 70%; Calcium 140%; Iron 140%; Folic Acid 130%; Magnesium 15% **Exchanges:** 2 Starch, 3 Lean Meat **Carbohydrate Choices:** 2

Food for Thought Beef is an important source of iron, and cheese is an important source of calcium. Combined in this recipe, they give you an excellent source of both nutrients. Following a low-residue diet? Just omit the mushrooms, bell pepper and cheese.

Philly Beef Sandwiches

Prep Time: 10 Minutes | **Start to Finish:** 20 Minutes | 4 sandwiches

2	tablespoons butter or margarine
1	medium onion, coarsely chopped (½ cup)
1 ½	cups sliced fresh mushrooms (4 oz) or 1 jar (4.5 oz) sliced mushrooms, drained
⅓	cup chopped green bell pepper
4	kaiser rolls, split
¾	lb thinly sliced cooked roast beef
4	slices (1 oz each) provolone cheese

1 In 10-inch skillet, melt butter over medium-high heat. Add onion, mushrooms and bell pepper; cook about 5 minutes, stirring occasionally, until vegetables are tender.

2 Set oven control to broil. Place bottom halves of rolls on ungreased cookie sheet. Top with vegetable mixture, beef and cheese. Broil with tops 4 to 6 inches from heat 2 to 3 minutes or just until cheese is melted. Top with tops of rolls.

❝This recipe is rather high in fat, but I needed to make an exception sometimes and add extra calories and fat. Knowing that fat was helping my body heal made giving myself permission to eat it easier. 'Just enjoy it' was what I kept telling myself."—**Judy O.**

High in calcium, iron and folic acid

1 Sandwich: Calories 520 (Calories from Fat 260); Total Fat 28g (Saturated Fat 14g, Trans Fat 1.5g); Cholesterol 100mg; Sodium 610mg; Potassium 530mg; Total Carbohydrate 31g (Dietary Fiber 2g); Protein 36g **% Daily Value:** Vitamin A 10%; Vitamin C 10%; Calcium 30%; Iron 20%; Folic Acid 15%; Magnesium 10% **Exchanges:** 2 Starch, ½ Vegetable, 3 Lean Meat, 1 High-Fat Meat, 2 Fat **Carbohydrate Choices:** 2

A Note from Dr. Ghosh For some patients, early in the day is often the best time to eat. Eating can become more of a challenge as the day progresses due to increased fatigue. If that's the case with you, try a few quesadilla wedges with salsa for lunch or as a midmorning snack.

Quick Quesadillas

Prep Time: 15 Minutes | **Start to Finish:** 15 Minutes | 4 servings

4   flour tortillas (8 to 10 inch)

1   cup shredded Mexican 4-cheese blend (4 oz)

¼   cup medium chunky-style salsa

¼   cup sour cream

1   Heat 10-inch skillet over medium heat 1 to 2 minutes. Place tortilla in skillet; sprinkle ½ cup of the cheese over tortilla. Top with second tortilla. Heat about 2 minutes or until bottom is lightly browned. Turn and cook other side until lightly browned. Repeat with remaining tortillas and cheese.

2   Cut quesadillas into wedges. Serve with salsa and sour cream.

66 The lighter the meal, the easier I found it to eat. Making this quesadilla recipe was perfect—it's light, tasty and nutritious."
—Theresa H. Shares Her Recipe

High in calcium

1 Serving: Calories 280 (Calories from Fat 130); Total Fat 15g (Saturated Fat 8g, Trans Fat 1g); Cholesterol 35mg; Sodium 580mg; Potassium 180mg; Total Carbohydrate 25g (Dietary Fiber 1g); Protein 11g
% Daily Value: Vitamin A 8%; Vitamin C 0%; Calcium 30%; Iron 10%; Folic Acid 15%; Magnesium 6%
Exchanges: 1 ½ Starch, 1 High-Fat Meat, 1 Fat **Carbohydrate Choices:** 1 ½

Food for Thought Chicken with fruits and vegetables gives you a hefty dose of vitamins, minerals and protein in one tasty combination. The mango adds color, a bit of sweetness and vitamin C to this dish.

Chicken Salad in Pitas

Prep Time: 15 Minutes | **Start to Finish:** 15 Minutes | 4 sandwiches

2 pita (pocket) breads (6 inch)

2 cups chopped cooked chicken breast

1 cup frozen sweet peas, thawed, drained

½ cup mayonnaise or salad dressing

¼ teaspoon salt

¼ teaspoon pepper

1 medium stalk celery, chopped (½ cup)

4 medium green onions, sliced (¼ cup)

1 small mango, peeled, pitted and diced (¾ cup)

1 Cut pita breads in half; open to form pockets. In medium bowl, mix remaining ingredients.

2 Divide chicken mixture among pita bread halves.

❝I tried to stimulate my appetite by trying a new twist on an old favorite, which this recipe does in an easy way.”—**Judy O.**

High in vitamin C; good source of fiber

1 Sandwich: Calories 460 (Calories from Fat 230); Total Fat 25g (Saturated Fat 4g, Trans Fat 0g); Cholesterol 70mg; Sodium 550mg; Potassium 370mg; Total Carbohydrate 32g (Dietary Fiber 3g); Protein 26g **% Daily Value:** Vitamin A 25%; Vitamin C 30%; Calcium 6%; Iron 15%; Folic Acid 15%; Magnesium 10% **Exchanges:** 1 ½ Starch, ½ Fruit, ½ Vegetable, 3 Very Lean Meat, 4 ½ Fat **Carbohydrate Choices:** 2

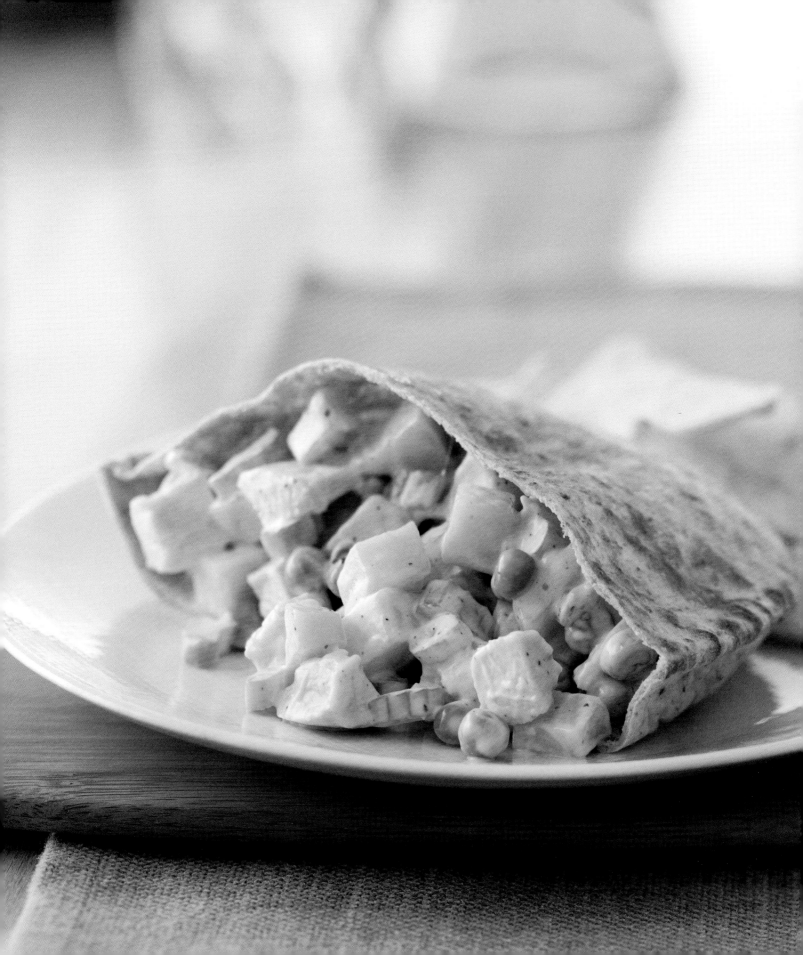

Food for Thought When you're tired, any new thing can seem like a daunting task. To make filling the tomatoes easier, fill 5 or 6 plum (Roma) tomatoes instead of the cherry tomatoes. No need to scoop out the seeds; just make a hole in the tomato by making a cone-shaped cut near the stem end and removing the stem. Fill the tomatoes with the cheese mixture, and you're all set.

Snappy Stuffed Tomatoes

Prep Time: 25 Minutes | **Start to Finish:** 2 Hours 25 Minutes | 5 servings (4 tomatoes each)

20   cherry tomatoes (1 ¼ to 1 ½ inch)

⅔   cup shredded reduced-fat Cheddar cheese

½   cup whole kernel corn

2   packages (3 oz each) reduced-fat cream cheese (Neufchâtel), softened

2   medium green onions, sliced (2 tablespoons)

1   teaspoon ground red chiles or chili powder, if desired

1   Cut thin slice from stem ends of tomatoes. Using melon baller or spoon, remove pulp and seeds.

2   In medium bowl, mix remaining ingredients. Fill tomatoes with cheese mixture. If desired, sprinkle with additional ground red chiles and sliced green onions. Cover; refrigerate to blend flavors before serving, at least 2 hours but no longer than 48 hours.

66 "Tomatoes make a wonderful snack because they taste the same no matter where I am on my treatment plan."—Anne R.

High in vitamins A and C; low fiber

1 Serving: Calories 140 (Calories from Fat 80); Total Fat 9g (Saturated Fat 5g, Trans Fat 0g); Cholesterol 30mg; Sodium 260mg; Potassium 270mg; Total Carbohydrate 7g (Dietary Fiber 1g); Protein 7g **% Daily Value:** Vitamin A 20%; Vitamin C 15%; Calcium 15%; Iron 2%; Folic Acid 6%; Magnesium 4% **Exchanges:** ½ Other Carbohydrate, ½ Vegetable, ½ Medium-Fat Meat, 1 ½ Fat **Carbohydrate Choices:** ½

A Note from Dr. Ghosh Tomatoes are a good source of lycopene, a phytochemical or naturally-occuring plant chemical in foods that may be helpful in reducing the risk of certain types of cancer in some people.

Mozzarella and Tomatoes

Prep Time: 10 Minutes | **Start to Finish:** 3 Hours 10 Minutes | 4 servings

4 medium tomatoes, cut into ¼-inch slices

¼ cup olive or vegetable oil

1 tablespoon chopped fresh or 1 teaspoon dried basil leaves

3 tablespoons red wine vinegar

1 tablespoon water

⅛ teaspoon salt

3 drops red pepper sauce

2 large cloves garlic, finely chopped

4 oz fresh mozzarella cheese, sliced

Salad greens, if desired

1 Place tomatoes in glass or plastic dish. In tightly covered container, shake remaining ingredients except cheese and salad greens. Pour over tomatoes.

2 Cover; refrigerate at least 3 hours, turning occasionally, to blend flavors.

3 To serve, layer tomatoes alternately with cheese on salad greens.

66 I love appetizers. And when I didn't feel up to going out, my daughter-in-law would stop over with this tasty dish, made with fresh tomatoes from her garden. So flavorful!"—Catherine H.

High in calcium and vitamins A and C; low fiber

1 Serving: Calories 240 (Calories from Fat 190); Total Fat 21g (Saturated Fat 6g, Trans Fat 0g); Cholesterol 25mg; Sodium 200mg; Potassium 330mg; Total Carbohydrate 6g (Dietary Fiber 1g); Protein 7g **% Daily Value:** Vitamin A 25%; Vitamin C 25%; Calcium 20%; Iron 4%; Folic Acid 6%; Magnesium 6% **Exchanges:** 1 Vegetable, 1 High-Fat Meat, 2 ½ Fat **Carbohydrate Choices:** ½

Food for Thought For a snack, dip tortilla chips or cut-up veggies into this special salsa. For breakfast, use it to sauce up any kind of eggs. You can even try salsa and eggs in a flour tortilla for a zesty pick-me-up!

Fresh Salsa

Prep Time: 15 Minutes | **Start to Finish:** 1 Hour 15 Minutes | 20 servings (¼ cup each)

4   large tomatoes, seeded, chopped and drained (4 cups)

1   medium onion, chopped (½ cup)

2   cloves garlic, finely chopped

1   can (4.5 oz) chopped green chiles, drained, or ½ cup chopped seeded fresh jalapeño chiles

½   cup chopped fresh cilantro

2   tablespoons fresh lime juice

½   teaspoon salt

¼   teaspoon pepper

1   In glass or plastic bowl, mix all ingredients.

2   Cover; refrigerate to blend flavors before serving, at least 1 hour but no longer than 1 week.

66 Though I was told bland foods were better, I preferred stronger seasonings like garlic and herbs. As it turned out, foods with more flavor—like this salsa—worked better for me."—**Theresa H. Shares Her Recipe**

Low fiber

1 Serving: Calories 10 (Calories from Fat 0); Total Fat 0g (Saturated Fat 0g, Trans Fat 0g); Cholesterol 0mg; Sodium 80mg; Potassium 100mg; Total Carbohydrate 2g (Dietary Fiber 0g); Protein 0g **% Daily Value:** Vitamin A 6%; Vitamin C 10%; Calcium 0%; Iron 0%; Folic Acid 0%; Magnesium 0% **Exchanges:** Free **Carbohydrate Choices:** 0

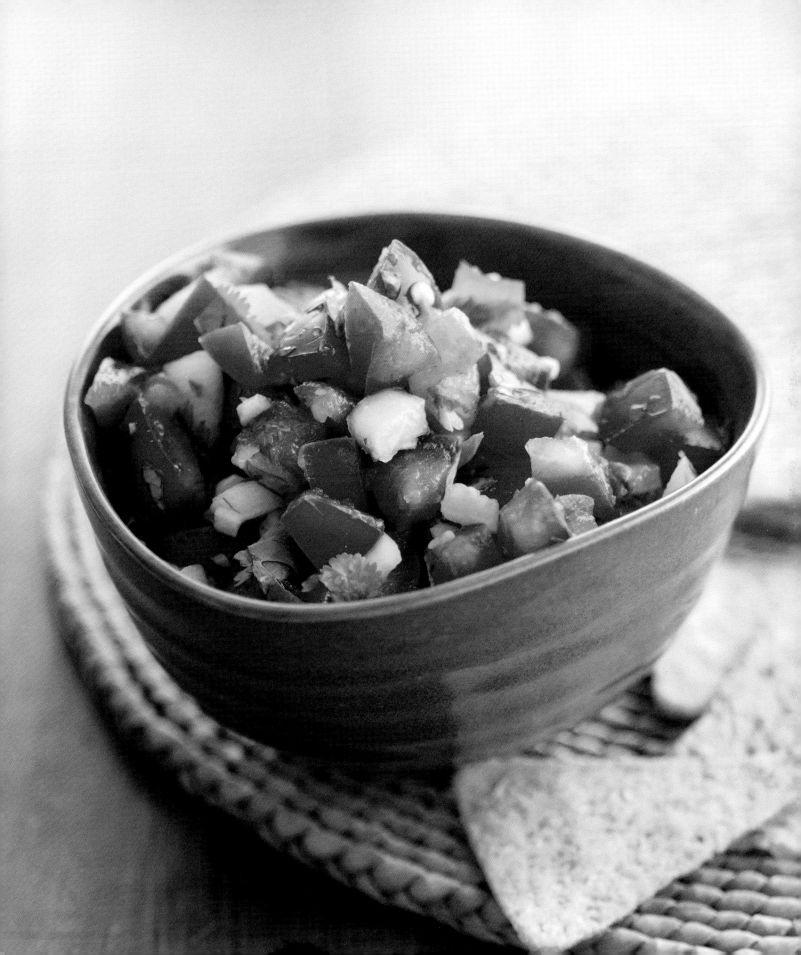

Food for Thought Experts recommend you eat at least 1 ½ to 2 cups of fruits daily to be sure you're getting all the nutrients you need to be healthy. Add this flavorful dip to make eating fruit even more enjoyable.

Creamy Caramel Dip with Fruit

Prep Time: 10 Minutes | **Start to Finish:** 40 Minutes | 4 servings (¼ cup each)

4 oz (half 8-oz package) cream cheese, softened

½ cup vanilla low-fat yogurt

¼ cup plus 1 to 2 teaspoons caramel topping

1 tablespoon chopped crystallized ginger, if desired

1 medium apple, sliced

1 medium pear, sliced

1 medium banana, sliced

1 In medium bowl, beat cream cheese with electric mixer on medium speed until creamy. Beat in yogurt and ¼ cup of the caramel topping until smooth. Cover; refrigerate at least 30 minutes until chilled.

2 Spoon dip into small serving bowl. Drizzle with 1 to 2 teaspoons caramel topping; swirl with tip of knife. Sprinkle with ginger. Serve with apple, pear and banana slices for dipping.

66 This recipe has a great 'treat yourself' feel to it. Sometimes it's nice to treat yourself. My kids also love dipping. Having a variety of tasty, healthy dips that are easy for me to make and easy for all of us to eat makes mealtime easier."—**Judy O.**

Good source of fiber

1 Serving: Calories 270 (Calories from Fat 90); Total Fat 10g (Saturated Fat 6g, Trans Fat 0g); Cholesterol 35mg; Sodium 190mg; Potassium 330mg; Total Carbohydrate 40g (Dietary Fiber 3g); Protein 4g **% Daily Value:** Vitamin A 8%; Vitamin C 10%; Calcium 10%; Iron 2%; Folic Acid 4%; Magnesium 6% **Exchanges:** 1 Starch, ½ Fruit, 1 Other Carbohydrate, 2 Fat **Carbohydrate Choices:** 2 ½

Food for Thought Spinach is a super source of folic acid. Necessary for all cells to function normally, folic acid is lacking in the diets of many people. Recent studies show that as much as 40 percent of the American population don't meet their folic acid requirement.

Spinach Dip in Bread Bowl

Prep Time: 15 Minutes | **Start to Finish:** 1 Hour 15 Minutes | 8 servings (½ cup dip and 1 oz bread each)

1 box (9 oz) frozen chopped spinach, thawed, squeezed to drain

1 can (4 oz) sliced water chestnuts, drained, chopped

5 medium green onions, chopped (5 tablespoons)

1 clove garlic, finely chopped

½ cup reduced-fat or regular sour cream

½ cup plain yogurt

¼ teaspoon salt

¼ teaspoon ground mustard

⅛ teaspoon pepper

1 loaf (1 lb) unsliced round whole wheat, white or rye bread

1 In large bowl, mix spinach, water chestnuts, onions and garlic. Stir in sour cream, yogurt, salt, mustard and pepper. Cover; refrigerate at least 1 hour to blend flavors.

2 Just before serving, cut 1- to 2-inch slice from top of bread loaf. Hollow out bread loaf by cutting along edge with serrated knife, leaving about 1-inch shell, and pulling out large chunks of bread. Cut or tear top slice and hollowed-out bread into bite-size pieces.

3 Fill bread loaf with spinach dip; place on serving plate. Arrange bread pieces around loaf to use for dipping.

"A very easy recipe using two of my favorites: bread and spinach. Besides using the bread as a dipper, I used baby carrots, colorful peppers and any other veggies I had on hand. Eating colorful foods like fresh veggies just made me feel like I was doing something really good for myself."—**Judy O.**

High in folic acid and vitamin A; excellent source of fiber

1 Serving: Calories 200 (Calories from Fat 45); Total Fat 5g (Saturated Fat 2g, Trans Fat 0.5g); Cholesterol 10mg; Sodium 380mg; Potassium 300mg; Total Carbohydrate 28g (Dietary Fiber 5g); Protein 10g **% Daily Value:** Vitamin A 50%; Vitamin C 4%; Calcium 15%; Iron 10%; Folic Acid 15%; Magnesium 20% **Exchanges:** 1 Starch, ½ Other Carbohydrate, ½ Vegetable, ½ Very Lean Meat, 1 Fat **Carbohydrate Choices:** 2

Food for Thought Salmon is a fabulous source of the mineral phosphorus. You need phosphorus to build strong bones and help your muscles function properly when they relax and contract. If you crush up and eat the bones in canned salmon, you'll get some extra calcium, too.

Easy Salmon Spread

Prep Time: 15 Minutes | **Start to Finish:** 2 Hours 15 Minutes | 16 servings (2 tablespoons dip and 4 crackers each)

1 package (8 oz) reduced-fat (Neufchâtel) or fat-free cream cheese, softened

1 can (14 ¾ oz) red or pink salmon, drained, flaked

3 tablespoons finely chopped red onion

2 tablespoons chopped fresh or ¼ teaspoon dried dill weed

1 tablespoon Dijon mustard

2 tablespoons capers

64 whole-grain crackers

1 Line 2-cup bowl or mold with plastic wrap. In medium bowl, beat cream cheese with electric mixer on medium speed until smooth. Stir in salmon, 2 tablespoons of the red onion, 1 tablespoon of the dill weed and the mustard. Spoon into plastic-lined bowl, pressing firmly.

2 Cover; refrigerate to chill and blend flavors before serving, at least 2 hours but no longer than 24 hours.

3 Turn bowl upside down onto serving plate; remove bowl and plastic wrap. Garnish with remaining 1 tablespoon red onion, 1 tablespoon dill weed and the capers. Serve with crackers.

❝I don't eat many meals while I'm on chemo. I usually graze all day long, so a few crackers with salmon spread and two of the Snappy Stuffed Tomatoes (page 96) would make a great snack or mini-meal for me.❞—**Anne R.**

Low fiber

1 Serving: Calories 120 (Calories from Fat 35); Total Fat 4g (Saturated Fat 1g, Trans Fat 0.5g); Cholesterol 15mg; Sodium 380mg; Potassium 135mg; Total Carbohydrate 13g (Dietary Fiber 0g); Protein 9g **% Daily Value:** Vitamin A 4%; Vitamin C 0%; Calcium 8%; Iron 6%; Folic Acid 6%; Magnesium 4% **Exchanges:** 1 Starch, 1 Very Lean Meat **Carbohydrate Choices:** 1

A Note from Dr. Ghosh Orange juice is a well-known source of vitamin C. When eaten with a food containing iron, the vitamin C in foods can improve iron absorption to help prevent anemia. Having a diet high in vitamin C also decreases the risk of infections and helps heal wounds.

Citrus-Peach Smoothie

Prep Time: 5 Minutes | **Start to Finish:** 5 Minutes | 3 servings (1 cup each)

1   container (8 oz) lemon fat-free yogurt

1   cup unsweetened frozen, fresh or canned (drained) sliced peaches

¾   cup calcium-fortified orange juice

3   tablespoons blueberries, if desired

1   In blender, place yogurt, peaches and orange juice. Cover; blend on high speed about 30 seconds or until smooth.

2   Pour mixture into glasses. Garnish with blueberries.

66 When I was very fatigued, I used any fruit I had on hand to make this quick smoothie. Dropping fresh blueberries into the glass on top of the smoothie adds extra color and flavor that is so good with the lemon and peach."—Susan S. Shares Her Recipe

High in calcium and vitamin C

1 Serving: Calories 120 (Calories from Fat 0); Total Fat 0g (Saturated Fat 0g, Trans Fat 0g); Cholesterol 0mg; Sodium 50mg; Potassium 340mg; Total Carbohydrate 26g (Dietary Fiber 1g); Protein 4g **% Daily Value:** Vitamin A 10%; Vitamin C 160%; Calcium 20%; Iron 2%; Folic Acid 6%; Magnesium 6% **Exchanges:** ½ Fruit, 1 Other Carbohydrate, ½ Skim Milk **Carbohydrate Choices:** 2

A Note from Dr. Ghosh Smoothies make a great solution for mouth sores, as they are soothing. Because citrus foods can make the discomfort worse, kiwifruit, watermelon and bananas are good choices.

Watermelon-Kiwi-Banana Smoothie

Prep Time: 10 Minutes | **Start to Finish:** 10 Minutes | 2 servings (1 cup each)

1   cup coarsely chopped seeded watermelon

1   kiwifruit, peeled, cut into pieces

2   ice cubes

1   ripe banana, frozen, peeled and cut into chunks

¼   cup chilled apple juice

1   In blender, place all ingredients. Cover; blend on high speed about 30 seconds or until smooth.

2   Pour mixture into glasses.

66 When I didn't feel like eating a meal, smoothies were quick, easy to swallow and nutritious. I keep ripe bananas in the freezer—then they're always ready for this refreshing shake."—**Judy O. Shares Her Recipe**

High in vitamin C; good source of fiber

1 Serving: Calories 130 (Calories from Fat 0); Total Fat 0.5g (Saturated Fat 0g, Trans Fat 0g); Cholesterol 0mg; Sodium 0mg; Potassium 450mg; Total Carbohydrate 29g (Dietary Fiber 3g); Protein 1g
% Daily Value: Vitamin A 10%; Vitamin C 80%; Calcium 2%; Iron 4%; Folic Acid 6%; Magnesium 8%
Exchanges: 1 Fruit, 1 Other Carbohydrate **Carbohydrate Choices:** 2

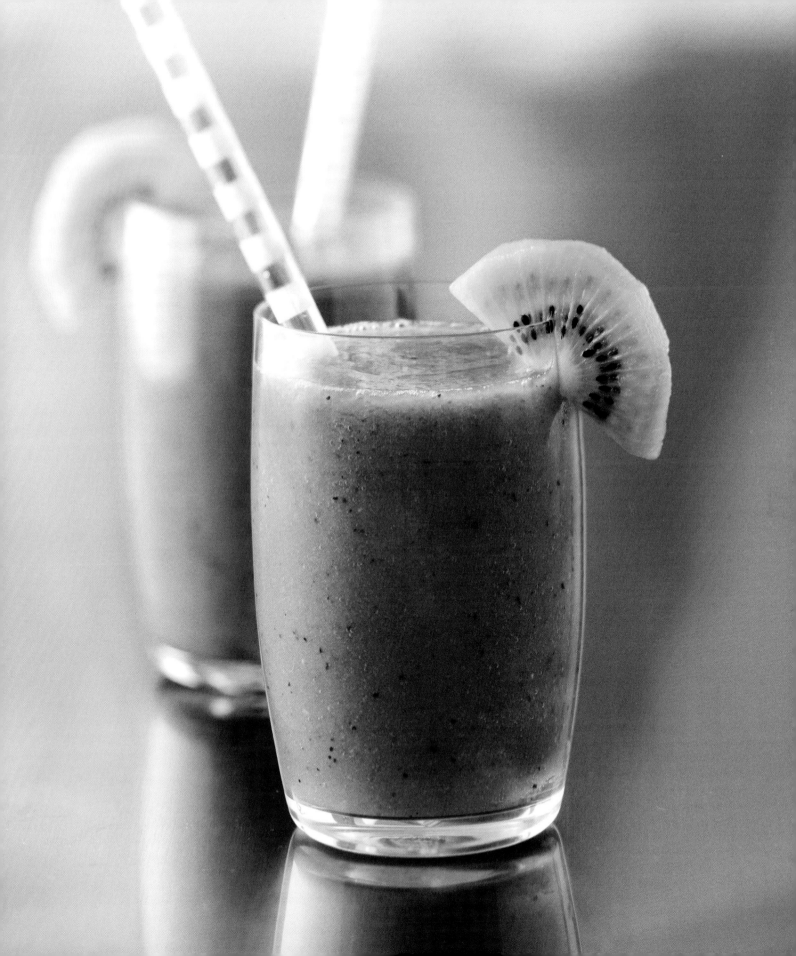

A Note from Dr. Ghosh This smoothie is a great choice during chemotherapy when you may be experiencing nausea, vomiting or diarrhea or having difficulty chewing. Staying well-hydrated can be half the battle.

Orange-Pineapple Smoothie

Prep Time: 10 Minutes | **Start to Finish:** 10 Minutes | 3 servings (1 cup each)

1 ½ cups calcium-fortified orange juice

½ cup fresh or canned pineapple chunks

1 ripe banana, frozen, cut into chunks

2 tablespoons vanilla-protein powder or ¼ cup orange yogurt

3 ice cubes

1 In blender, place all ingredients. Cover; blend on high speed about 30 seconds or until smooth.

2 Pour mixture into glasses.

❝The two changes I've made to my diet are drinking more water and eating more fruits and vegetables. Now I never get in my car without my water bottle, and this smoothie is an easy way to load up on fruit."—**Judy O. Shares Her Recipe**

High in calcium and vitamin C

1 Serving: Calories 140 (Calories from Fat 5); Total Fat 0.5g (Saturated Fat 0g, Trans Fat 0g); Cholesterol 0mg; Sodium 20mg; Potassium 440mg; Total Carbohydrate 30g (Dietary Fiber 2g); Protein 2g **% Daily Value:** Vitamin A 6%; Vitamin C 90%; Calcium 20%; Iron 0%; Folic Acid 10%; Magnesium 8% **Exchanges:** 1 Fruit, 1 Other Carbohydrate, ½ Very Lean Meat **Carbohydrate Choices:** 2

A Note from Dr. Ghosh This fruity tea is helpful if you have a metallic taste in your mouth. The combination of citrus and spices can help to disguise an off taste. Don't forget that green tea is not an herbal tea; like black tea, it contains caffeine.

Sugar 'n Spice Green Tea

Prep Time: 10 Minutes | **Start to Finish:** 10 Minutes | 4 servings (about 1 cup each)

4	cups boiling water
4	tea bags green tea
¼	teaspoon ground cinnamon
6	whole cloves, broken into pieces
¼	cup sugar
¼	cup orange juice
2	tablespoons lemon juice
2	orange slices, cut in half

1 In heatproof container, pour boiling water over tea bags. Add cinnamon and cloves. Cover; let steep 3 to 5 minutes.

2 Remove tea bags; strain tea to remove cloves. Stir sugar, orange juice and lemon juice into tea. Serve hot with orange slice half in each cup.

❝I have always enjoyed coffee, but now I'm trying to drink more tea— green tea especially. This spicy, sweet tea is a great alternative to plain green tea, and it's good when served chilled. Sometimes, I'd make it up hot and refrigerate the rest to drink later as iced tea, especially in the summer."—**Judy O.**

Low fiber

1 Serving: Calories 60 (Calories from Fat 0); Total Fat 0g (Saturated Fat 0g, Trans Fat 0g); Cholesterol 0mg; Sodium 10mg; Potassium 125mg; Total Carbohydrate 15g (Dietary Fiber 0g); Protein 0g **% Daily Value:** Vitamin A 0%; Vitamin C 6%; Calcium 0%; Iron 0%; Folic Acid 4%; Magnesium 2% **Exchanges:** 1 Fruit **Carbohydrate Choices:** 1

A Note from Dr. Ghosh Tea has long been linked to relaxation. Chai, popular in India, is black tea mixed with fragrant spices such as nutmeg and cinnamon, milk and a sweetener. This warming tea is especially comforting on cool mornings. It's also good served iced on warm days.

Chai Tea

Prep Time: 10 Minutes | **Start to Finish:** 10 Minutes | 4 servings (1 cup each)

2	cups water
4	tea bags black tea
2	½ cups milk
2	tablespoons honey
½	teaspoon ground ginger
½	teaspoon ground nutmeg
¼	teaspoon ground cinnamon

1 In 2-quart saucepan, heat water to boiling. Add tea bags; reduce heat and simmer 2 minutes.

2 Remove tea bags. Stir remaining ingredients into tea. Heat to boiling. Stir with whisk to foam milk. Pour into cups.

66 I found hot tea to be a lifesaver during treatment; it went down very easily. The honey and spices in this tea are very soothing. If black tea doesn't sound good to you right now, use any herbal tea."
—Lois K.

Good source of calcium

1 Serving: Calories 110 (Calories from Fat 30); Total Fat 3g (Saturated Fat 2g, Trans Fat 0g); Cholesterol 10mg; Sodium 70mg; Potassium 240mg; Total Carbohydrate 16g (Dietary Fiber 0g); Protein 5g **% Daily Value:** Vitamin A 6%; Vitamin C 0%; Calcium 20%; Iron 0%; Folic Acid 2%; Magnesium 4% **Exchanges:** ½ Starch, ½ Low-Fat Milk **Carbohydrate Choices:** 1

Snack Busters

At times, you may not feel up to eating a full meal and instead may find that eating more often throughout the day is better. If a regular-sized meal is too much for you, try eating mini-meals or snacks instead of large meals. For good snack choices, check out the list below:

- Fresh fruits and vegetables provide many needed nutrients. Keep baby carrots, celery sticks, fresh or frozen grapes, bananas and apples on hand.

- String cheese, cheese chunks and cottage cheese, eaten with or without fresh fruit, provide much-needed calcium.

- Graham and saltine crackers are easy to digest and are low in residue. Eat them plain, or spread them with peanut butter, cheese or jam.

- Cereal with or without milk contains many nutrients from fortification. Cereal is very convenient to snack on right from the box or to add to salted peanuts or pretzels, as well as to eat with milk.

- Nuts, snack mixes, popcorn and granola bars work well for those not needing to follow a low-residue diet. Quick energy and convenience are key to these tasty snacks.

- Canned and dried fruits. Mandarin oranges, applesauce, dried plums or apricots and dates are great snacks on their own, or team them up with nuts, popcorn or cheese crackers.

- Small sandwiches, such as grilled cheese or turkey, cut into fourths, work well as mini-meals. Eat one piece now, then if you're up to it, eat another; otherwise save the rest for later.

- Soup and crackers. For convenience, use canned soup and serve yourself a small bowl. Miniature crackers, such as oyster crackers or fish-shaped cheese crackers, may not seem as overwhelming as larger crackers, so start with them first.

- Shakes and smoothies containing milk or yogurt can be a source of extra calcium and other important nutrients. Because no chewing is required, beverages are particularly soothing if you have mouth sores.

- Make the most of leftovers. Reheat mashed potatoes, pizza or pasta. Turn yesterday's salad into a filling for sandwiches. For flavor boosters, see page 127.

- Something sweet. Small cookies or cakes may provide necessary carbohydrates to boost your energy in a pinch, but save room for more sustaining foods, too.

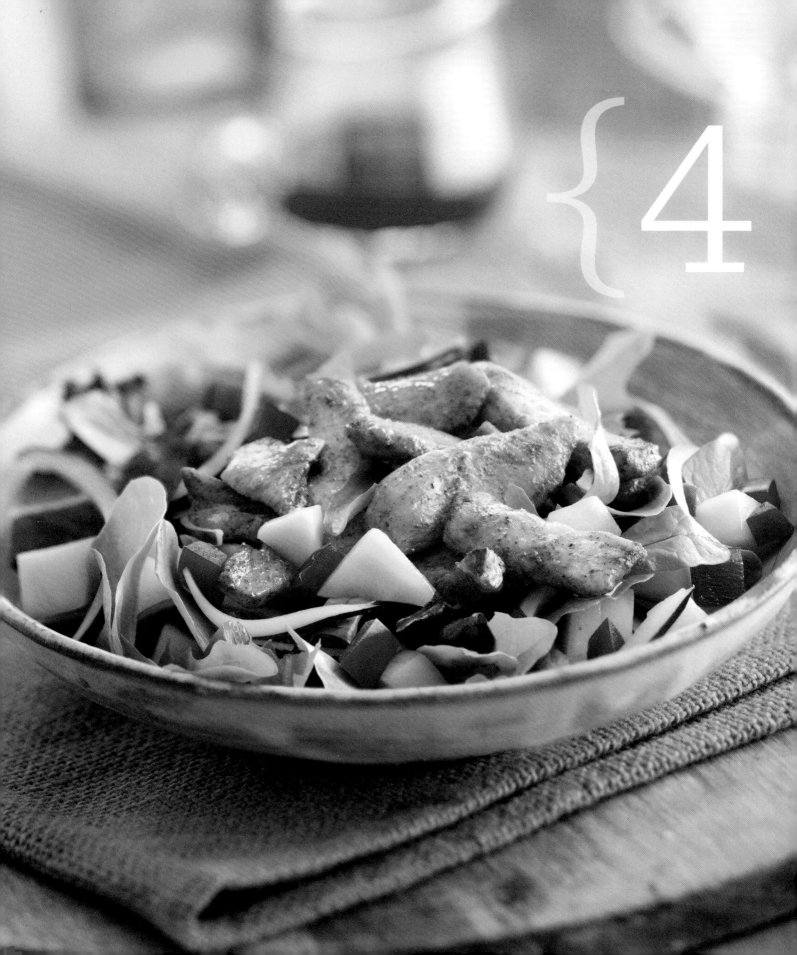

20-Minute Main Dishes }

112 Fettuccine with Asparagus and Mushrooms

114 Angel Hair Pasta with Avocado and Tomatoes

116 Creamy Quinoa Primavera

118 Mediterranean Couscous and Beans

119 Pasta with Chicken in Chili Sauce

120 Honey-Mustard Turkey with Snap Peas

121 Cantaloupe and Chicken Salad

122 Caribbean Chicken Salad

124 Spinach-Shrimp Salad with Hot Bacon Dressing

125 Chutney-Salmon Salad

126 Savory Scallops and Shrimp

128 Chopped Vegetable and Crabmeat Salad

130 Carrot-Tuna Salad

131 Fiesta Taco Salad

132 Potato-Tomato-Tofu Dinner

134 Loaded Potatoes

135 Macaroni Pasta "Soup"

136 Cream of Broccoli Soup

138 Easy Beef Stroganoff

139 Caramelized Pork Slices

A Note from Dr. Ghosh The pasta (grain), pine nuts and cheese make this recipe a good choice for vegetarians with cancer.

Fettuccine with Asparagus and Mushrooms

Prep Time: 10 Minutes | **Start to Finish:** 20 Minutes | 6 servings (1 ⅓ cups each)

¼ cup sun-dried tomatoes (not oil-packed)

8 oz uncooked fettuccine

1 teaspoon olive or vegetable oil

1 lb thin fresh asparagus spears, broken into 2-inch pieces

1 lb fresh mushrooms, sliced (6 cups)

2 cloves garlic, finely chopped

3 tablespoons chopped fresh parsley

2 tablespoons chopped fresh basil leaves

1 cup dry white wine or chicken broth

1 cup chicken broth

2 tablespoons cornstarch

½ teaspoon salt

¼ teaspoon pepper

2 tablespoons pine nuts

¼ cup freshly grated Parmesan cheese

1 Cover dried tomatoes with boiling water. Let stand 10 minutes; drain. Chop tomatoes.

2 Cook and drain fettuccine as directed on package.

3 Meanwhile, in 12-inch skillet, heat oil over medium heat. Add asparagus, mushrooms, garlic, parsley and basil; cook 5 minutes, stirring occasionally. Stir in tomatoes. Simmer 2 to 3 minutes, until tomatoes are heated.

4 In small bowl, place wine and broth; beat in cornstarch, salt and pepper with whisk until blended. Stir into vegetable mixture. Heat to boiling over medium heat, stirring constantly, until mixture is smooth and bubbly. Boil and stir 1 minute. Serve over fettuccine. Sprinkle with nuts and cheese.

> ❝A good friend, well known for her healthy eating habits, shared this recipe with me. I found it to be very soothing, tasty and colorful.”
> —Joan K. Shares Her Recipe

High in folic acid; good source of fiber

1 Serving: Calories 250 (Calories from Fat 60); Total Fat 6g (Saturated Fat 1.5g, Trans Fat 0g); Cholesterol 30mg; Sodium 660mg; Potassium 590mg; Total Carbohydrate 36g (Dietary Fiber 4g); Protein 11g **% Daily Value:** Vitamin A 15%; Vitamin C 8%; Calcium 10%; Iron 25%; Folic Acid 35%; Magnesium 15% **Exchanges:** ½ Starch, ½ Other Carbohydrate, 4 Vegetable, ½ Lean Meat, 1 Fat **Carbohydrate Choices:** 2 ½

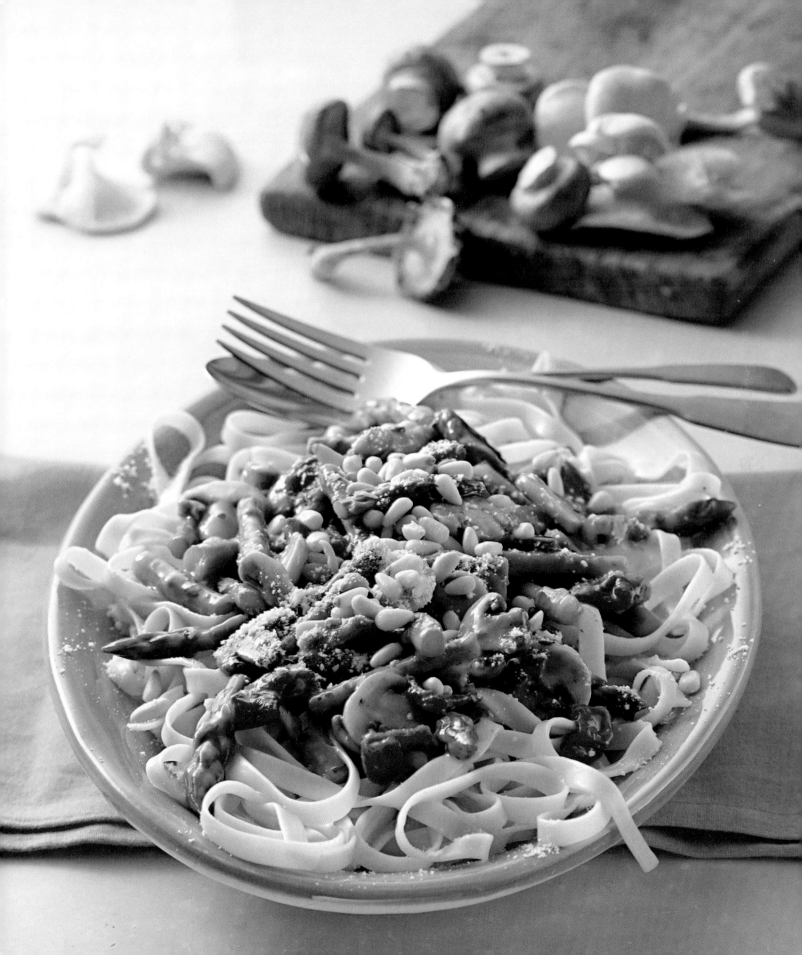

A Note from Dr. Ghosh Coconut oil can be substituted for soy, corn, olive or safflower oil. Coconut oil is a source of medium-chain fatty acids, which for some, may be more easily digested.

Angel Hair Pasta with Avocado and Tomatoes

Prep Time: 20 Minutes | **Start to Finish:** 20 Minutes | 6 servings (1 ⅓ cups each)

8 oz uncooked angel hair pasta

2 tablespoons olive or vegetable oil

2 cloves garlic, finely chopped

¾ cup chopped fresh basil leaves

½ to ¾ large avocado, peeled, pitted and cut into small cubes

4 medium tomatoes, cut into small cubes

½ teaspoon salt

¼ teaspoon pepper

1 Cook and drain pasta as directed on package.

2 Meanwhile, in 3-quart saucepan, heat oil over medium heat. Add garlic; cook 1 to 2 minutes, stirring occasionally, until garlic is tender but not brown. Remove from heat.

3 Stir basil, avocado and tomatoes into garlic in saucepan. Toss vegetable mixture and pasta. Sprinkle with salt and pepper.

66 There is something so appealing about the flavor combination of tomato, avocado and basil with pasta that was very comforting to me and satisfied my cravings."—Susan S. Shares Her Recipe

High in vitamin A and folic acid; good source of fiber

1 Serving: Calories 260 (Calories from Fat 70); Total Fat 8g (Saturated Fat 1g, Trans Fat 0g); Cholesterol 0mg; Sodium 350mg; Potassium 350mg; Total Carbohydrate 38g (Dietary Fiber 4g); Protein 7g **% Daily Value:** Vitamin A 20%; Vitamin C 10%; Calcium 2%; Iron 10%; Folic Acid 25%; Magnesium 10% **Exchanges:** 2 Starch, 1 Vegetable, 1 ½ Fat **Carbohydrate Choices:** 2 ½

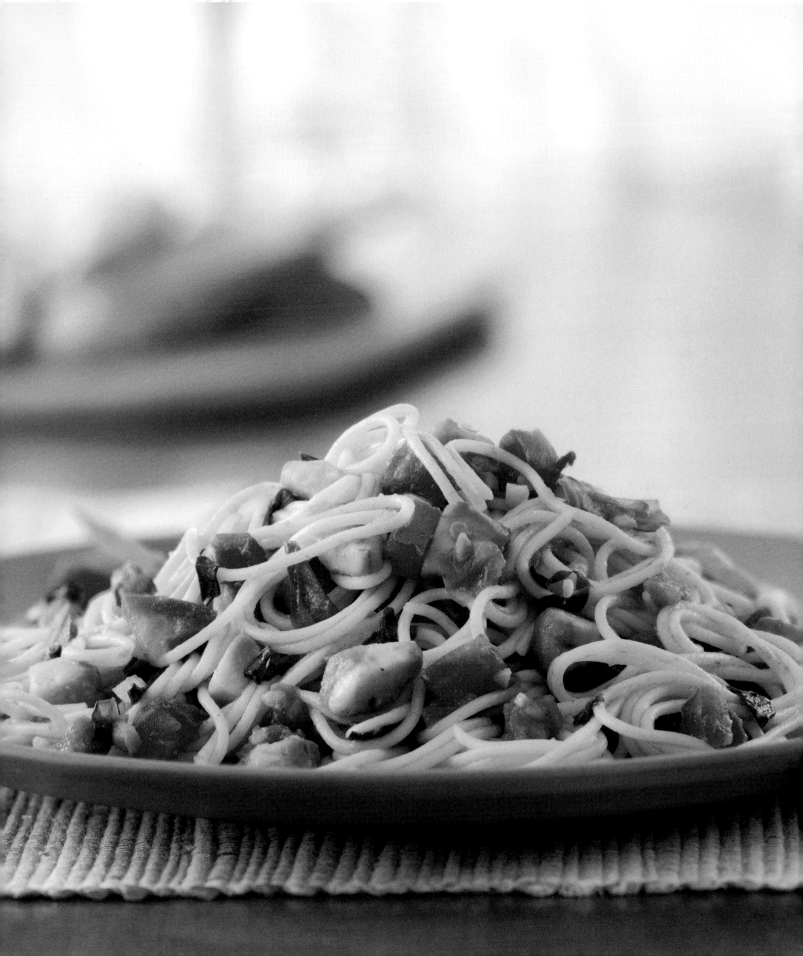

Food for Thought Quinoa, pronounced "keen-wa," was a staple grain of the Incas of Peru. Loaded with nutrients, quinoa has a sweet, slightly nutty flavor. Be sure to rinse quinoa to remove the natural bitter coating of the grain.

Creamy Quinoa Primavera

Prep Time: 20 Minutes | **Start to Finish:** 20 Minutes | 6 servings

1 ½ cups uncooked quinoa

3 cups chicken broth

1 package (3 oz) cream cheese

1 tablespoon chopped fresh or 1 teaspoon dried basil leaves

2 teaspoons butter or margarine

2 cloves garlic, finely chopped

5 cups thinly sliced or bite-size pieces assorted uncooked vegetables (asparagus, broccoli, carrot or zucchini)

2 tablespoons grated Romano cheese

1 Rinse quinoa thoroughly; drain. In 2-quart saucepan, heat quinoa and broth to boiling. Reduce heat; cover and simmer 10 to 15 minutes or until all broth is absorbed. Stir in cream cheese and basil.

2 Meanwhile, in 10-inch nonstick skillet, melt butter over medium-high heat. Add garlic; cook about 30 seconds, stirring frequently, until golden. Stir in vegetables. Cook about 2 minutes, stirring frequently, until vegetables are crisp-tender.

3 Toss vegetables and quinoa mixture. Sprinkle with Romano cheese.

66 Quinoa is such a great source of protein and tastes great! I cooked quinoa for my kids when they were 8 and 11 and for my nieces and nephews (now ages 4 through 9), and they loved it! They didn't even know they were eating something healthy!"—**Anne R.**

High in potassium, vitamins A and C, iron, folic acid and magnesium; excellent source of fiber

1 Serving: Calories 280 (Calories from Fat 90); Total Fat 10g (Saturated Fat 4.5g, Trans Fat 0g); Cholesterol 20mg; Sodium 620mg; Potassium 630mg; Total Carbohydrate 35g (Dietary Fiber 5g); Protein 11g **% Daily Value:** Vitamin A 110%; Vitamin C 15%; Calcium 10%; Iron 20%; Folic Acid 30%; Magnesium 25% **Exchanges:** 1 Starch, ½ Other Carbohydrate, 2 Vegetable, ½ Medium-Fat Meat, 1 ½ Fat **Carbohydrate Choices**: 2

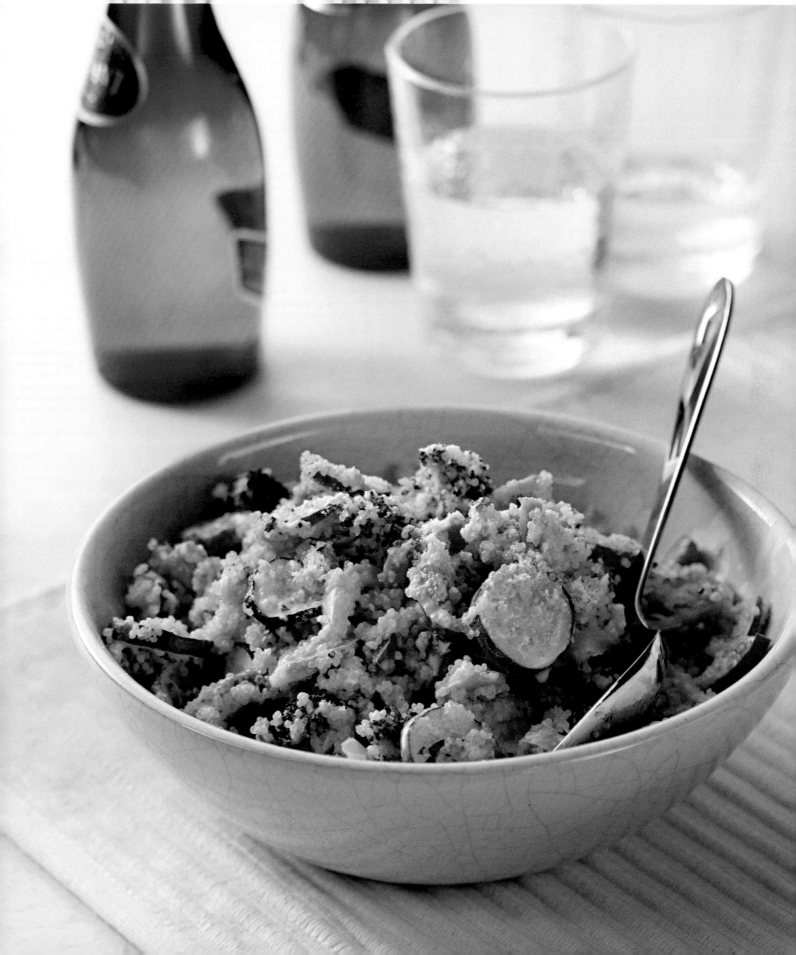

A Note from Dr. Ghosh Legumes, such as dried beans, peas and garbanzo beans, are a great source of fiber. Eating plenty of fiber helps keep the digestive tract moving. This, in turn, lessens the amount of time the intestinal tract is exposed to foods and breakdown products of foods, some of which may contain toxins.

Mediterranean Couscous and Beans

Prep Time: 15 Minutes | **Start to Finish:** 20 Minutes | 4 servings

3 cups chicken broth

2 cups uncooked couscous

½ cup raisins or currants

¼ teaspoon pepper

⅛ teaspoon ground red pepper (cayenne)

1 small tomato, chopped (½ cup)

1 can (15 to 16 oz) garbanzo beans, drained, rinsed

⅓ cup crumbled feta cheese

1 In 3-quart saucepan, heat broth to boiling. Stir in remaining ingredients except cheese; remove from heat.

2 Cover; let stand about 5 minutes or until liquid is absorbed. Stir gently. Sprinkle each serving with cheese.

66 This great main dish has the added benefit of containing fruit and vegetables and is quick to cook. Best of all, my family loves couscous!"—Judy O.

High in potassium, iron, magnesium and folic acid; excellent source of fiber

1 Serving: Calories 590 (Calories from Fat 60); Total Fat 7g (Saturated Fat 2.5g, Trans Fat 0g); Cholesterol 10mg; Sodium 1040mg; Potassium 750mg; Total Carbohydrate 107g (Dietary Fiber 10g); Protein 24g **% Daily Value:** Vitamin A 6%; Vitamin C 4%; Calcium 15%; Iron 25%; Folic Acid 45%; Magnesium 25% **Exchanges:** 3 ½ Starch, ½ Fruit, 3 Other Carbohydrate, 1 Vegetable, 1 Very Lean Meat, ½ Lean Meat, ½ Fat **Carbohydrate Choices:** 7

Food for Thought This recipe supplies a good source of potassium, a nutrient needed to help the body maintain its fluid balance. Potassium also helps with nerve and muscle function.

Pasta with Chicken in Chili Sauce

Prep Time: 15 Minutes | **Start to Finish:** 20 Minutes | 4 servings

4 oz uncooked spinach fettuccine, vermicelli or other pasta

2 tablespoons vegetable oil

4 boneless skinless chicken breasts (about 1 ¼ lb)

1 medium onion, sliced

1 cup chicken broth

½ cup chili sauce

Grated Parmesan cheese, if desired

1 Cook and drain fettuccine as directed on package.

2 Meanwhile, in a 10-inch skillet, heat oil over medium-high heat. Add chicken and onion; cook 10 to 12 minutes, turning chicken once and stirring onions occasionally, until brown.

3 Stir broth and chili sauce into chicken and onion. Cook about 5 minutes or until sauce is thickened and juice of chicken is no longer pink when centers of thickest pieces are cut.

4 Place fettuccine on serving platter. Top with chicken and sauce. Sprinkle with cheese.

66I needed to eat low-residue foods, so having this simple recipe really helped me!"—Theresa H. Shares Her Recipe

Low residue

1 Serving: Calories 380 (Calories from Fat 120); Total Fat 13g (Saturated Fat 3g, Trans Fat 0g); Cholesterol 110mg; Sodium 920mg; Potassium 500mg; Total Carbohydrate 27g (Dietary Fiber 4g); Protein 38g **% Daily Value:** Vitamin A 6%; Vitamin C 6%; Calcium 4%; Iron 15%; Folic Acid 15%; Magnesium 15% **Exchanges:** 1 ½ Starch, ½ Vegetable, 4 ½ Very Lean Meat, 2 Fat **Carbohydrate Choices:** 2

Food for Thought This zesty turkey recipe cooks in a flash. Just marinate the turkey as described below, throw in some carrots and pea pods for vitamins A and C and you're ready to go.

Honey-Mustard Turkey with Snap Peas

Prep Time: 20 Minutes | **Start to Finish:** 40 Minutes | 4 servings

1   **lb uncooked turkey breast cutlets, about ¼ inch thick**

½   **cup honey-Dijon dressing**

1   **cup ready-to-eat baby-cut carrots, cut in half lengthwise**

¼   **cup water**

2   **cups fresh sugar snap peas, strings removed**

1   Place turkey in shallow glass or plastic dish. Pour dressing over turkey; turn turkey to coat evenly. Cover dish; let stand 20 minutes at room temperature.

2   Spray 12-inch skillet with cooking spray; heat over medium heat. Drain dressing from turkey; pat turkey dry. Cook turkey in skillet 3 to 5 minutes, turning once, until brown.

3   Add carrots and water. Top turkey and carrots with sugar snap peas. Cover; cook 7 to 9 minutes or until carrots are tender and turkey is no longer pink in center.

❝ The thin slices of turkey make it easy to eat a small portion and still get a well-balanced and pretty-looking plate. It is very important for food to be appetizing and yet served in small enough quantities so I am not overwhelmed."—Anne R.

High in iron and vitamins A and C; good source of fiber

1 Serving: Calories 240 (Calories from Fat 100); Total Fat 11g (Saturated Fat 2g, Trans Fat 0g); Cholesterol 75mg; Sodium 260mg; Potassium 410mg; Total Carbohydrate 8g (Dietary Fiber 2g); Protein 27g **% Daily Value:** Vitamin A 80%; Vitamin C 15%; Calcium 4%; Iron 10%; Folic Acid 4%; Magnesium 10% **Exchanges:** 1 Vegetable, 3 ½ Very Lean Meat, 2 Fat **Carbohydrate Choices:** ½

A **Note from Dr. Ghosh** Cantaloupe and grapes are moist, tasty fruits that blend well with this tangy dressing. Sometimes eating fruits that contain a lot of water can help soothe dry mouth. The vitamin C helps boost the immune system and fight infection.

Cantaloupe and Chicken Salad

Prep Time: 20 Minutes | **Start to Finish:** 2 Hours 20 Minutes | 6 servings

¼ cup plain yogurt

¼ cup mayonnaise or salad dressing

1 tablespoon lemon juice

1 tablespoon chopped fresh chives

¼ teaspoon salt

5 cups cut-up (1 ½ inch) cantaloupe

2 ½ cups cut-up cooked chicken

1 cup red or green grapes, cut in half

1 medium cucumber, cut into 1 ¼-inch strips

1 In large bowl, mix yogurt and mayonnaise. Stir in lemon juice, chives and salt.

2 Stir in remaining ingredients. Cover; refrigerate until chilled before serving, at least 2 hours but no longer than 24 hours.

66 A very easy chicken and fruit salad, this recipe has always been a hit for me and with family and friends."—**Marie E. Shares Her Recipe**

High in vitamins A and C; good source of potassium

1 Serving: Calories 200 (Calories from Fat 50); Total Fat 5g (Saturated Fat 1.5g, Trans Fat 0g); Cholesterol 50mg; Sodium 250mg; Potassium 620mg; Total Carbohydrate 18g (Dietary Fiber 1g); Protein 19g **% Daily Value:** Vitamin A 90%; Vitamin C 90%; Calcium 4%; Iron 6%; Folic Acid 10%; Magnesium 10% **Exchanges:** 1 Fruit, ½ Vegetable, 2 ½ Very Lean Meat, 1 Fat **Carbohydrate Choices:** 1

Food for Thought Loaded with mango and bell pepper, this salad is a tasty source of vitamins A and C. Vitamin C helps promote healthy gums, blood vessels, bones and teeth, and can also help us to absorb iron better.

Caribbean Chicken Salad

Prep Time: 20 Minutes　|　**Start to Finish:** 20 Minutes　|　4 servings

1　lb boneless skinless chicken breasts, cut into ½-inch strips

2　tablespoons blackened seasoning blend

1　tablespoon canola or vegetable oil

1　bag (5 oz) mixed baby salad greens (4 cups)

1　medium mango, peeled, pitted and diced (1 cup)

½　medium red onion, sliced (¾ cup)

1　small red bell pepper, chopped (½ cup)

⅔　cup raspberry vinaigrette

1　Place chicken in heavy-duty resealable food-storage plastic bag. Sprinkle seasoning blend over chicken; seal bag and shake until chicken is evenly coated.

2　In 10-inch nonstick skillet, heat oil over medium-high heat. Add chicken; cook 7 to 10 minutes, stirring frequently, until no longer pink in center. Remove chicken from skillet; drain on paper towels.

3　In large bowl, toss salad greens, mango, onion and bell pepper; divide among 4 plates. Top with chicken. Drizzle with vinaigrette.

❝I always have boneless, skinless chicken breasts on hand, ready for an easy, quick meal.❞—Judy O.

High in vitamins A and C; good source of fiber

1 Serving: Calories 270 (Calories from Fat 70); Total Fat 7g (Saturated Fat 1.5g, Trans Fat 0g); Cholesterol 70mg; Sodium 440mg; Potassium 530mg; Total Carbohydrate 25g (Dietary Fiber 3g); Protein 26g **% Daily Value:** Vitamin A 70%; Vitamin C 80%; Calcium 6%; Iron 10%; Folic Acid 20%; Magnesium 10% **Exchanges:** 1 ½ Other Carbohydrate, 3 ½ Very Lean Meat, 1 Fat **Carbohydrate Choices:** 1 ½

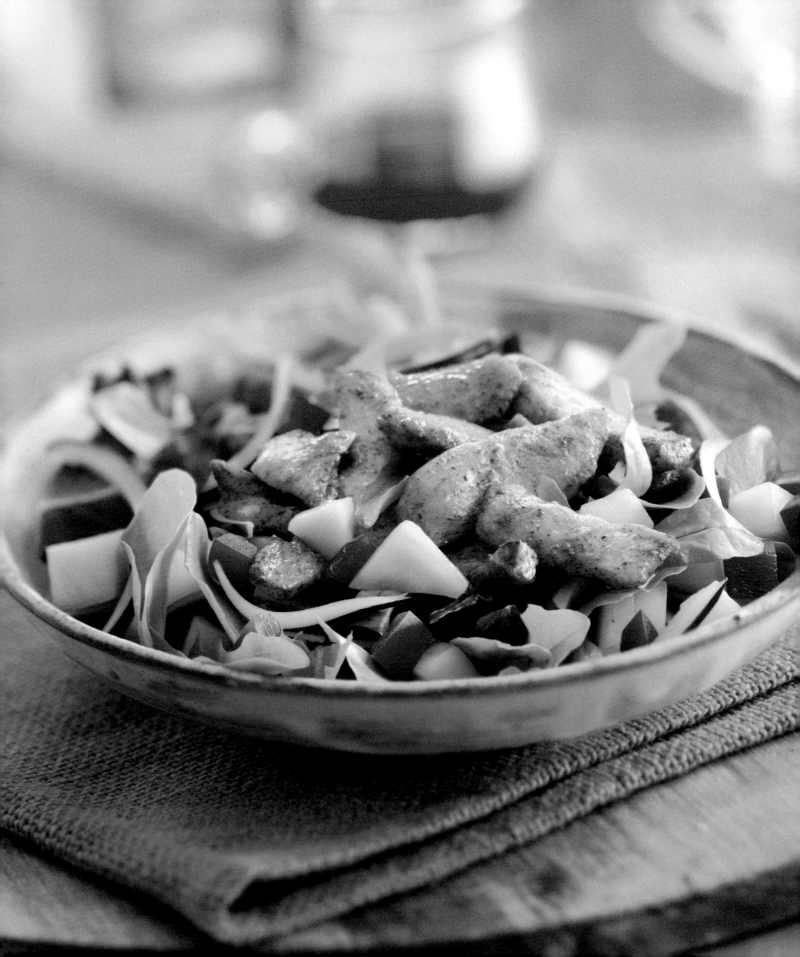

Food for Thought Spinach is an excellent source of magnesium and iron. Magnesium helps with energy release from foods; iron is key for bringing oxygen to cells.

Spinach-Shrimp Salad with Hot Bacon Dressing

Prep Time: 20 Minutes | **Start to Finish:** 20 Minutes | 4 servings

4 slices bacon, cut into 1-inch pieces

¼ cup white vinegar

1 tablespoon sugar

¼ teaspoon ground mustard

4 cups lightly packed bite-size pieces spinach leaves

1 cup sliced fresh mushrooms (3 oz)

1 cup crumbled feta cheese (4 oz)

½ lb cooked peeled deveined medium shrimp

1 In 10-inch skillet, cook bacon over medium-high heat, stirring occasionally, until crisp. Stir in vinegar, sugar and mustard; continue stirring until sugar is dissolved.

2 In large bowl, toss spinach, mushrooms, cheese and shrimp. Drizzle hot bacon dressing over spinach mixture; toss to coat. Serve immediately.

66 I'm trying to eat more spinach, and this recipe makes it easy as it uses three of my favorite foods: mushrooms, cheese and shrimp." —Judy O.

High in calcium and vitamin A; good source of folic acid and iron; low fiber

1 Serving: Calories 200 (Calories from Fat 90); Total Fat 10g (Saturated Fat 6g, Trans Fat 0g); Cholesterol 145mg; Sodium 650mg; Potassium 390mg; Total Carbohydrate 6g (Dietary Fiber 0g); Protein 20g **% Daily Value:** Vitamin A 60%; Vitamin C 8%; Calcium 20%; Iron 15%; Folic Acid 20%; Magnesium 15% **Exchanges:** 1 Vegetable, 1 Very Lean Meat, ½ Medium-Fat Meat, 1 High-Fat Meat **Carbohydrate Choices:** ½

Food for Thought Salmon is a super source of vitamin B_{12}. We need vitamin B_{12} for all body cells to function properly. Other sources of vitamin B_{12} include lean cuts of beef and pork loin.

Chutney-Salmon Salad

Prep Time: 10 Minutes | **Start to Finish:** 10 Minutes | 4 servings

2   cans (6 oz each) boneless skinless salmon, drained, flaked

3   cups broccoli slaw

⅔   cup mayonnaise or salad dressing

⅓   cup chutney

¼   cup dry-roasted peanuts, chopped

1   In glass or plastic bowl, mix salmon, broccoli slaw, mayonnaise and chutney.

2   Just before serving, stir in peanuts.

❝When I'm tired, I like to use shortcuts. Broccoli slaw is one of my favorites."—Judy O.

High in calcium, vitamin C and folic acid; good source of potassium

1 Serving: Calories 460 (Calories from Fat 330); Total Fat 36g (Saturated Fat 5g, Trans Fat 0g); Cholesterol 65mg; Sodium 610mg; Potassium 330mg; Total Carbohydrate 15g (Dietary Fiber 2g); Protein 19g **% Daily Value:** Vitamin A 40%; Vitamin C 50%; Calcium 20%; Iron 8%; Folic Acid 15%; Magnesium 10% **Exchanges:** ½ Starch, ½ Other Carbohydrate, ½ Vegetable, 2 ½ Lean Meat, 5 ½ Fat **Carbohydrate Choices:** 1

A Note from Dr. Ghosh Broth or apple juice can often be substituted for the wine used to flavor a recipe. Use your judgment to determine which flavor would work best with the recipe. Some studies have shown that small amounts of alcohol, such as wine, may lessen the risk of developing coronary heart disease in middle-aged men and women.

Savory Scallops and Shrimp

Prep Time: 20 Minutes | **Start to Finish:** 20 Minutes | 4 servings

2 tablespoons olive or vegetable oil

1 clove garlic, finely chopped

2 medium green onions, sliced (2 tablespoons)

2 medium carrots, thinly sliced (1 cup)

1 tablespoon chopped fresh or 1 teaspoon parsley flakes

1 lb uncooked deveined peeled medium shrimp, thawed if frozen, tail shells removed

1 lb sea scallops, cut in half

½ cup dry white wine or chicken broth

1 tablespoon lemon juice

¼ to ½ teaspoon crushed red pepper flakes

1 In 12-inch nonstick skillet, heat oil over medium heat. Add garlic, onions, carrots and parsley; cook about 5 minutes, stirring occasionally, until carrots are crisp-tender.

2 Stir in remaining ingredients. Cook 4 to 5 minutes, stirring frequently, until shrimp are pink and scallops are white and opaque.

66 I'm using more fresh herbs in my cooking, which enhances the aroma and flavor of foods. This makes me feel more like eating."
—Judy O.

High in vitamin C; low fiber

1 Serving: Calories 220 (Calories from Fat 80); Total Fat 9g (Saturated Fat 1.5g, Trans Fat 0g); Cholesterol 190mg; Sodium 490mg; Potassium 570mg; Total Carbohydrate 4g (Dietary Fiber 1g); Protein 31g **% Daily Value:** Vitamin A 110%; Vitamin C 6%; Calcium 10%; Iron 25%; Folic Acid 6%; Magnesium 15% **Exchanges:** 4 Lean Meat **Carbohydrate Choices:** 0

Flavor Boosters

"Food just tastes different during chemotherapy, not like it used to." Sound familiar? Due to chemotherapy or radiation and the effect these treatments have on the way food tastes, finding ways to enjoy your food can be a real challenge.

What works for one person may not work for another; some patients find that eating bland or plain foods is best, and some find they tolerate highly seasoned or spicy foods and even crave them. Try a few of these ideas to boost the flavor of your foods.

1. Add grated lemon, lime or orange, or the juice from these fruits, to cookies, cakes, chicken and fish.

2. Marinate chicken breasts or turkey breast slices in soy sauce, teriyaki sauce or sauté sauce (such as Dijon chicken sauté sauce) for 30 minutes before cooking.

3. Add pesto or salsa to pasta, fish and main dishes.

4. Use fresh herbs when cooking chicken and fish.

5. Use small amounts of foods that pack a lot of flavor: Kalamata olives, anchovies, capers, roasted garlic, blue cheese, feta cheese, Dijon mustard, toasted walnuts, crushed red pepper.

6. Use garlic to boost the flavor of meats, side dishes, pilafs, salads and soups.

7. Cook rice in broth or apple juice instead of water.

8. Sprinkle toasted nuts over fish, salads and main and side dishes.

9. Caramelize meat by sprinkling brown sugar, drizzling with orange juice or molasses and cooking until the mixture thickens and coats the meat.

10. Experiment with balsamic, raspberry, tarragon, white wine and seasoned rice vinegars to add zing to cooked vegetables, pasta, soups, salads and cooked meats.

11. Use curry powder and coriander in chicken salads and casseroles and to add a jolt of exotic flavor to soups and stews.

Food for Thought This salad is a great source of the mineral magnesium. Considered one of the healing nutrients, magnesium is important in helping to release carbohydrate energy from foods. Magnesium also works to transmit nerve impulses through muscles.

Chopped Vegetable and Crabmeat Salad

Prep Time: 20 Minutes | **Start to Finish:** 20 Minutes | 4 servings

DRESSING

⅓ cup frozen (thawed) limeade concentrate

¼ cup vegetable oil

1 tablespoon rice or white vinegar

1 teaspoon grated gingerroot

¼ teaspoon salt

SALAD

2 cups torn escarole

2 cans (6 oz each) crabmeat, drained and flaked, or 2 cups chopped cooked turkey or chicken

1 small jicama, peeled, chopped (1 cup)

1 large papaya, peeled, seeded and chopped (1 cup)

1 large yellow or red bell pepper, chopped (1 cup)

½ cup dry-roasted peanuts

¼ cup chopped fresh cilantro

1 In tightly covered container, shake dressing ingredients.

2 In large bowl, place remaining ingredients except peanuts and cilantro. Pour dressing over salad; toss to coat. Top with peanuts and cilantro.

❝Me first—that's my new motto. Most of my life I have been caring for other people. During chemo, I allowed myself and my family to put me first on the care list."—**Judy O.**

High in potassium, magnesium, folic acid and vitamin C; good source of fiber

1 Serving: Calories 400 (Calories from Fat 210); Total Fat 24g (Saturated Fat 3.5g, Trans Fat 0g); Cholesterol 55mg; Sodium 520mg; Potassium 660mg; Total Carbohydrate 29g (Dietary Fiber 4g); Protein 18g **% Daily Value:** Vitamin A 20%; Vitamin C 200%; Calcium 10%; Iron 8%; Folic Acid 25%; Magnesium 20% **Exchanges:** ½ Starch, ½ Fruit, ½ Other Carbohydrate, 1 Vegetable, 2 Very Lean Meat, 4 ½ Fat **Carbohydrate Choices:** 2

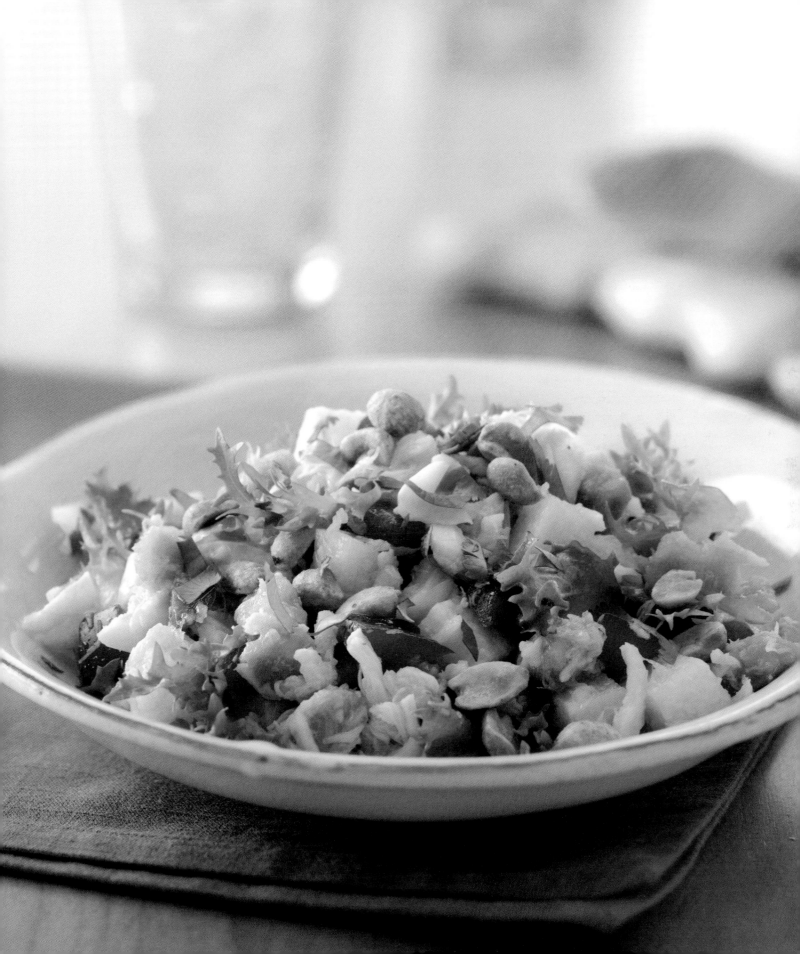

Food for Thought Carrots are a great source of beta-carotene, a form of vitamin A. You need vitamin A daily for proper vision in dim light and for healthy hair and skin.

Carrot-Tuna Salad

Prep Time: 20 Minutes | **Start to Finish:** 1 Hour 20 Minutes | 6 servings (1 cup each)

½ cup mayonnaise or salad dressing

¼ teaspoon salt

¼ teaspoon pepper

2 medium carrots, shredded (1 cup)

2 medium stalks celery, diced (1 cup)

1 small onion, chopped (¼ cup)

2 hard-cooked eggs, sliced

2 cans (5 oz each) tuna in water, drained

1 can (4 oz) shoestring potatoes

1 In large bowl, mix all ingredients except tuna and potatoes. Stir in tuna. Cover; refrigerate about 1 hour or until chilled.

2 Just before serving, stir in potatoes.

"It was important to me to keep things on a routine and prepare foods that my family would eat, like this easy salad."—Joyce K. Shares Her Recipe

High in vitamins A and C

1 Serving: Calories 230 (Calories from Fat 150); Total Fat 17g (Saturated Fat 3g, Trans Fat 0g); Cholesterol 90mg; Sodium 420mg; Potassium 270mg; Total Carbohydrate 7g (Dietary Fiber 1g); Protein 12g **% Daily Value:** Vitamin A 70%; Vitamin C 6%; Calcium 2%; Iron 6%; Folic Acid 6%; Magnesium 4% **Exchanges:** ½ Starch, ½ Vegetable, ½ Very Lean Meat, 1 Lean Meat, 2 ½ Fat **Carbohydrate Choices:** ½

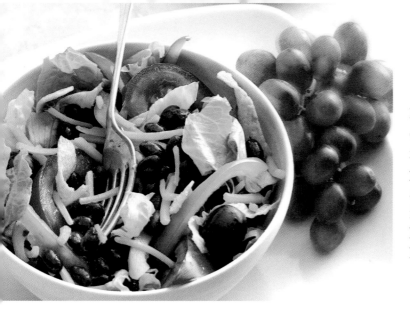

Food for Thought This nutrient-dense recipe is a powerhouse! That means for the amount of calories it provides, it's loaded with vitamins and minerals such as fiber, calcium, iron, magnesium and vitamin C—key nutrients important to the healing process.

Fiesta Taco Salad

Prep Time: 20 Minutes │ **Start to Finish:** 20 Minutes │ 5 servings

1	can (15 oz) black beans, drained, rinsed
½	cup taco sauce
6	cups bite-size pieces lettuce
1	medium green bell pepper, cut into strips
2	medium tomatoes, cut into wedges
½	cup pitted ripe olives, drained
1	cup corn chips
1	cup shredded Cheddar cheese (4 oz)
½	cup Thousand Island dressing

1 In 2-quart saucepan, heat beans and taco sauce over medium heat 2 to 3 minutes, stirring occasionally, until heated.

2 In large bowl, toss lettuce, bell pepper, tomatoes, olives and corn chips. Spoon bean mixture over lettuce mixture; toss. Sprinkle with cheese. Serve immediately with dressing.

66 The beans replace the hamburger in this taco salad. It's a great 'new' way to serve a family favorite."—Judy O.

High in calcium, iron and vitamin C; excellent source of fiber

1 Serving: Calories 370 (Calories from Fat 190); Total Fat 21g (Saturated Fat 7g, Trans Fat 0g); Cholesterol 30mg; Sodium 990mg; Potassium 610mg; Total Carbohydrate 31g (Dietary Fiber 9g); Protein 13g **% Daily Value:** Vitamin A 25%; Vitamin C 25%; Calcium 20%; Iron 15%; Folic Acid 30%; Magnesium 15% **Exchanges:** ½ Starch, 1 Other Carbohydrate, 2 Vegetable, ½ Very Lean Meat, ½ High-Fat Meat, 3 ½ Fat **Carbohydrate Choices:** 2

A Note from Dr. Ghosh Tofu is a great alternative to meat. Made from soybeans, it provides protein, iron and calcium. Tofu can be comforting when mouth sores or dry mouth are a bother, because it's so very easy to chew!

Potato-Tomato-Tofu Dinner

Prep Time: 20 Minutes | **Start to Finish:** 20 Minutes | 5 servings

2   tablespoons olive or vegetable oil

½   cup coarsely chopped red onion

5   small red potatoes, sliced (2 ½ cups)

2   cups frozen cut green beans

½   teaspoon Italian seasoning

½   teaspoon garlic salt

1   package (14 oz) firm tofu, cut into ½-inch cubes

2   plum (Roma) tomatoes, thinly sliced

1   hard-cooked egg, chopped

1   In 12-inch skillet, heat oil over medium-high heat. Add onion; cook 2 minutes, stirring frequently. Stir in potatoes. Reduce heat to medium-low; cover and cook about 8 minutes, stirring occasionally, until potatoes are tender.

2   Stir in green beans, Italian seasoning and garlic salt. Cover; cook about 5 minutes, stirring occasionally, until beans are tender and potatoes are light golden brown.

3   Stir in tofu and tomatoes. Cook 2 to 3 minutes, stirring occasionally and gently, just until hot. Sprinkle each serving with egg.

❝I love tofu when I'm on chemo because it doesn't have the metallic taste that meat has. I used it in mock chicken enchiladas and three-color lasagna, and even my dad didn't notice that he wasn't eating meat!"—Anne R.

Good source of fiber

1 Serving: Calories 210 (Calories from Fat 90); Total Fat 10g (Saturated Fat 2g, Trans Fat 0g); Cholesterol 40mg; Sodium 125mg; Potassium 600mg; Total Carbohydrate 20g (Dietary Fiber 4g); Protein 10g **% Daily Value:** Vitamin A 10%; Vitamin C 10%; Calcium 20%; Iron 15%; Folic Acid 15%; Magnesium 15% **Exchanges:** ½ Starch, ½ Other Carbohydrate, 1 ½ Vegetable, ½ Lean Meat, 1 ½ Fat **Carbohydrate Choices:** 1

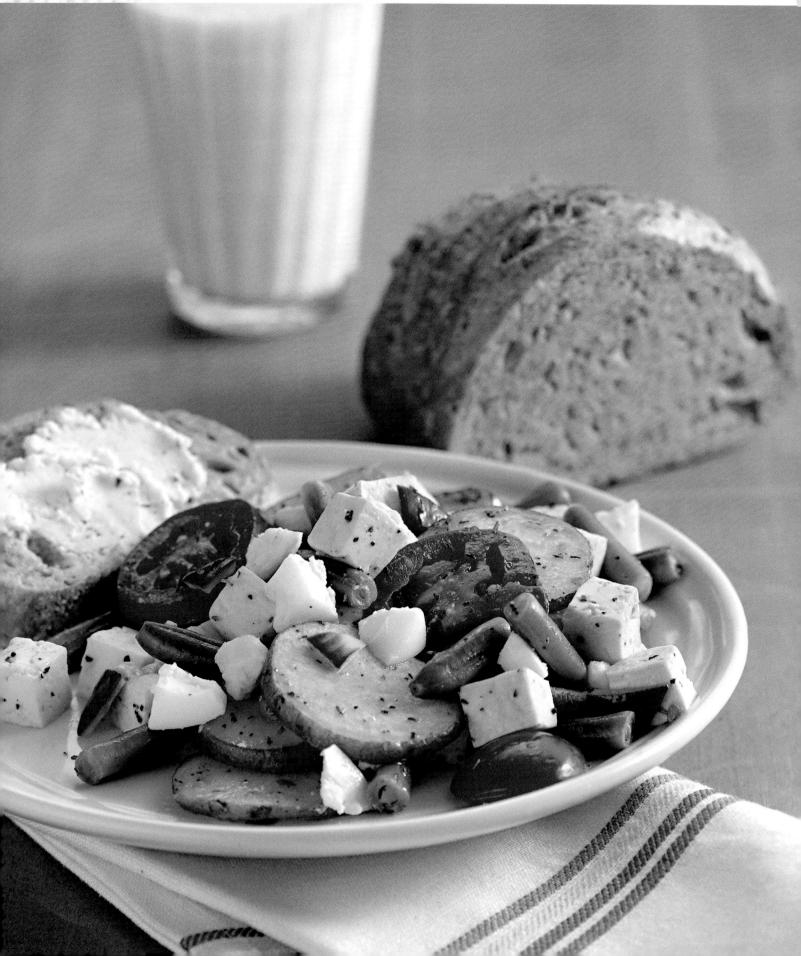

Food for Thought These loaded potatoes are a tasty comfort food. If you don't like the taste of green onions or ham, leave them out for a creamy-textured topping that may help soothe mouth sores. If you find sharp Cheddar is too strong right now, try ricotta or mozzarella.

Loaded Potatoes

Prep Time: 15 Minutes | **Start to Finish:** 20 Minutes | 4 servings

4 medium unpeeled red potatoes

1 package (8 oz) sliced fresh mushrooms (3 cups)

¾ cup chopped fully cooked ham

8 medium green onions, sliced (½ cup)

⅛ teaspoon ground red pepper (cayenne)

½ cup reduced-fat sour cream

½ cup shredded reduced-fat sharp Cheddar cheese (2 oz)

1 Pierce potatoes with fork. On microwavable paper towel in microwave oven, arrange potatoes about 1 inch apart in circle. Microwave uncovered on High 8 to 10 minutes or until tender. (Or bake potatoes in 375°F oven 1 hour to 1 hour 30 minutes.) Let potatoes stand until cool enough to handle.

2 Meanwhile, spray 4-quart Dutch oven with cooking spray; heat over medium-high heat. Add mushrooms; cook 1 minute, stirring frequently. Reduce heat to medium; cover and cook 3 minutes. Remove from heat. Stir in ham, green onions and red pepper. Cover; let stand 4 minutes.

3 Split baked potatoes in half lengthwise; fluff with fork. Spread 1 tablespoon sour cream over each potato half. Top each with ham mixture and cheese.

❝Baked potatoes are a major comfort food, so doctoring them up to make a meal really helps keep my appetite up. Plus, I can add as much butter and cheese and sour cream as I want without any guilt because I need the calories."—Anne R.

High in potassium; excellent source of fiber

1 Serving: Calories 300 (Calories from Fat 70); Total Fat 7g (Saturated Fat 4g, Trans Fat 0g); Cholesterol 30mg; Sodium 550mg; Potassium 1300mg; Total Carbohydrate 41g (Dietary Fiber 5g); Protein 16g **% Daily Value:** Vitamin A 6%; Vitamin C 15%; Calcium 15%; Iron 15%; Folic Acid 20%; Magnesium 15% **Exchanges:** 2 Starch, 2 Vegetable, ½ Lean Meat, ½ High-Fat Meat **Carbohydrate Choices:** 3

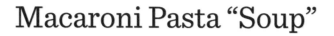

A Note from Dr. Ghosh Macaroni soup helps to relieve digestive discomfort and dry mouth. Mashed potatoes, noodles and cooked cereals are other choices that may help, as well. When suffering from dry mouth, try making your food moist by adding sauces or soaking dry, crisp foods like cereal until they get soggy.

Macaroni Pasta "Soup"

Prep Time: 5 Minutes | **Start to Finish:** 15 Minutes | 4 servings (1 cup each)

1   package (7 oz) elbow macaroni (2 cups)

1 ½   cups whole milk

½   teaspoon salt

¼   teaspoon pepper

¼   cup butter or margarine, softened

½   cup shredded Cheddar cheese (2 oz)

1   In 2-quart saucepan, cook macaroni as directed on package—except cook 2 minutes less than recommended time; drain.

2   Return macaroni to saucepan. Stir in milk, salt and pepper. Heat just until mixture begins to simmer; do not boil. Remove from pan. Pour into heatproof bowl. Stir in butter until melted.

3   Just before serving, sprinkle cheese over top.

❝I had this soup often when I was a kid, and it is still a comfort food for my four grown children and grandchildren. I made it when other food didn't appeal and many times during and after radiation treatments when my digestive tract was in turmoil."—Lois K. Shares Her Recipe

High in calcium and folic acid; low fiber

1 Serving: Calories 430 (Calories from Fat 180); Total Fat 20g (Saturated Fat 12g, Trans Fat 0.5g); Cholesterol 55mg; Sodium 690mg; Potassium 210mg; Total Carbohydrate 47g (Dietary Fiber 2g); Protein 14g **% Daily Value:** Vitamin A 10%; Vitamin C 0%; Calcium 20%; Iron 10%; Folic Acid 25%; Magnesium 10% **Exchanges:** 2 ½ Starch, ½ Milk, ½ High-Fat Meat, 2 Fat **Carbohydrate Choices:** 3

Food for Thought Broccoli, in the cruciferous family of vegetables along with Brussels sprouts, cabbage and kale, is a nutrition powerhouse. Broccoli provides a source of vitamin K, a nutrient that assists the body with blood clotting, particularly important after surgery.

Cream of Broccoli Soup

Prep Time: 10 Minutes | **Start to Finish:** 20 Minutes | 4 servings (1 cup each)

2 tablespoons butter or margarine

1 medium onion, chopped (½ cup)

2 medium carrots, thinly sliced (1 cup)

2 teaspoons mustard seed

½ teaspoon salt

¼ teaspoon pepper

¾ lb fresh broccoli, coarsely chopped (3 ½ cups) or 2 boxes (9 oz) frozen broccoli cuts

1 can (14 oz) chicken broth

1 cup water

2 teaspoons lemon juice

¼ cup sour cream

1 In 3-quart saucepan, melt butter over medium heat. Add onion and carrots; cook about 5 minutes, stirring occasionally, until onion is tender. Stir in mustard seed, salt and pepper. Stir in broccoli, broth and water. Heat to boiling. Reduce heat; cover and simmer about 10 minutes or until broccoli is tender.

2 Place one-third of the broccoli mixture in blender. Cover; blend on high speed until smooth. Pour into bowl. Continue to blend in small batches until all soup is pureed.

3 Return blended mixture to saucepan. Stir in lemon juice. Heat over low heat just until hot. Stir in sour cream.

❝I like this recipe because it's another way to use broccoli and it satisfies my desire for cream soups without all the fat. I use fat-free sour cream for a low-fat soup."—Judy O. Shares Her Recipe

High in vitamins A and C; good source of fiber and folic acid

1 Serving: Calories 170 (Calories from Fat 90); Total Fat 10g (Saturated Fat 6g, Trans Fat 0g); Cholesterol 25mg; Sodium 820mg; Potassium 530mg; Total Carbohydrate 12g (Dietary Fiber 3g); Protein 6g **% Daily Value:** Vitamin A 120%; Vitamin C 70%; Calcium 8%; Iron 6%; Folic Acid 15%; Magnesium 8% **Exchanges:** 3 Vegetable, 2 Fat **Carbohydrate Choices:** 1

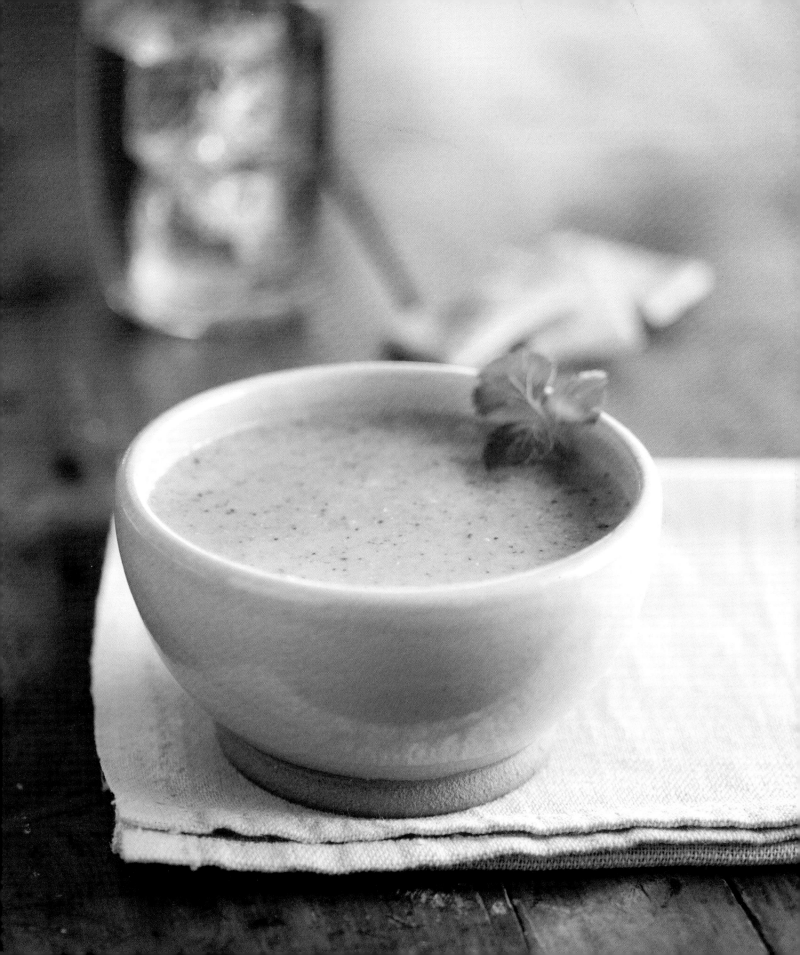

Food for Thought This easy recipe is a good choice because of the high iron and folic acid nutrients it provides. Both folic acid and iron are nutrients that are necessary for good health.

Easy Beef Stroganoff

Prep Time: 20 Minutes | **Start to Finish:** 20 Minutes | 4 servings

1 lb beef sirloin or round steak

2 tablespoons butter or margarine

⅔ cup water

1 jar (4.5 oz) sliced mushrooms, drained

½ package (2-oz size) onion soup mix (1 envelope)

1 cup sour cream

4 cups hot cooked rice or noodles

Chopped fresh parsley, if desired

1 Remove fat from beef. Cut beef across grain into about 1 ½x½-inch strips. (Beef is easier to cut if partially frozen, 30 to 60 minutes.)

2 In 10-inch skillet, melt butter over medium-high heat. Add beef; cook about 10 minutes, stirring occasionally, until brown. Stir in water, mushrooms and soup mix. Cook about 10 minutes, stirring occasionally, until beef is tender.

3 Stir in sour cream; heat until hot. Serve over rice. Sprinkle with parsley.

❝Eating my main meal at noon was a good solution for me because my food settled better when I had more energy; in the evening I was too tired for a big meal. This recipe was one of my favorites.”
—Pat Y. Shares Her Recipe

High in iron and folic acid

1 Serving: Calories 550 (Calories from Fat 200); Total Fat 22g (Saturated Fat 12g, Trans Fat 0.5g); Cholesterol 120mg; Sodium 1440mg; Potassium 510mg; Total Carbohydrate 52g (Dietary Fiber 1g); Protein 36g **% Daily Value:** Vitamin A 10%; Vitamin C 2%; Calcium 10%; Iron 30%; Folic Acid 15%; Magnesium 15% **Exchanges:** 3 ½ Starch, 3 ½ Lean Meat, 2 Fat **Carbohydrate Choices:** 3 ½

A Note from Dr. Ghosh Pork is a good source of iron. Helping with proper oxygen transfer in the bloodstream, iron is crucial for life. Iron also helps prevent anemia and is helpful with immune functions.

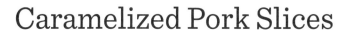

Caramelized Pork Slices

Prep Time: 20 Minutes | **Start to Finish:** 20 Minutes | 4 servings

1	pork tenderloin (1 lb)
2	cloves garlic, finely chopped
2	tablespoons packed brown sugar
1	tablespoon orange juice
1	tablespoon molasses or maple-flavored syrup
½	teaspoon salt
¼	teaspoon pepper
4	cups hot cooked rice

1 Trim fat from pork. Cut pork into ½-inch slices. (Pork is easier to cut if partially frozen, 30 to 60 minutes.)

2 Heat 10-inch nonstick skillet over medium-high heat. Add pork and garlic; cook 6 to 8 minutes, turning pork occasionally, until pork is light brown on outside and no longer pink in center. Drain if necessary.

3 Stir in remaining ingredients except rice. Cook, stirring occasionally, until mixture thickens and coats pork. Serve with rice.

"Pork tenderloin is lean, cooks quickly and is becoming a family favorite. The fact that it is low residue, which works for me, makes it even more appealing."—Theresa H.

High in iron and folic acid; low fiber; low residue

1 Serving: Calories 370 (Calories from Fat 45); Total Fat 5g (Saturated Fat 1.5g, Trans Fat 0g); Cholesterol 50mg; Sodium 950mg; Potassium 630mg; Total Carbohydrate 56g (Dietary Fiber 0g); Protein 26g
% Daily Value: Vitamin A 0%; Vitamin C 0%; Calcium 4%; Iron 15%; Folic Acid 10%; Magnesium 15%
Exchanges: 2 ½ Starch, 1 Other Carbohydrate, 1 ½ Very Lean Meat, 1 Lean Meat **Carbohydrate Choices:** 4

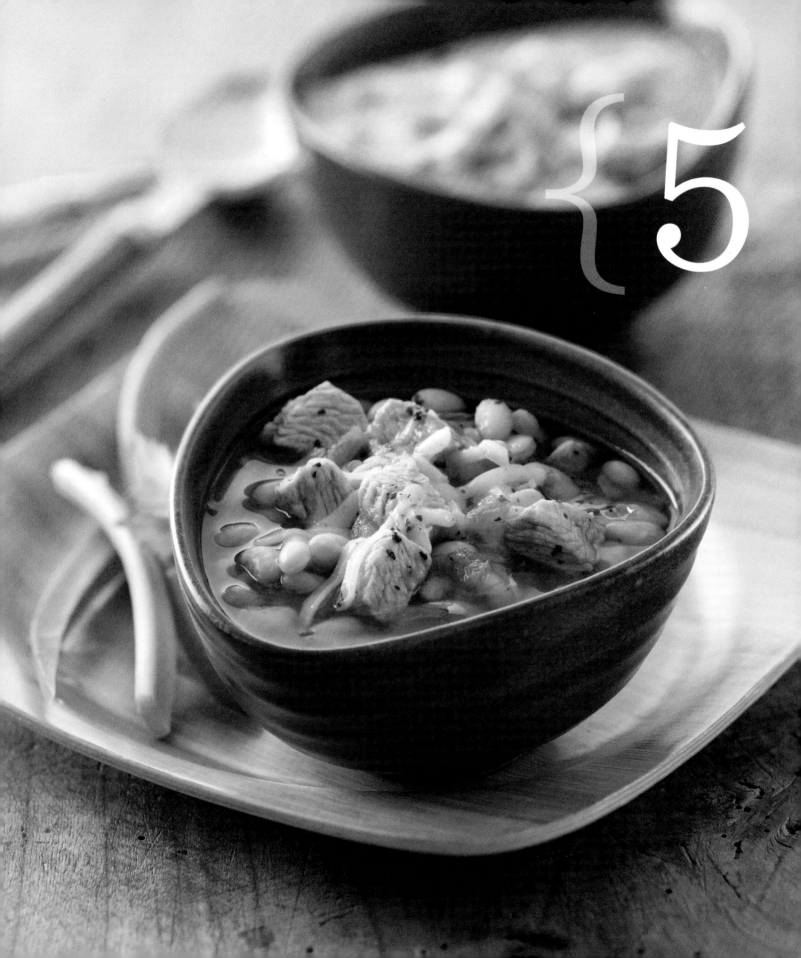

{5

Make-Ahead Meals

}

142   Corn and Black Bean Salad

144   Seven-Layer Pasta Salad

145   Layered Chicken Salad

146   Southwestern Pork Salad

148   Dijon Chicken with Orzo Rice

149   Italian Chicken Rolls

150   Chicken Noodle Casserole

152   The Ultimate Chicken Casserole

154   Chicken Soup with Homemade Noodles

155   Crowd-Size Minestrone

156   White Turkey Chili

158   Beef-Vegetable Soup

160   Layered Beef and Vegetable Dinner

161   Spaghetti and Meat Squares

162   Almond-Stuffed Pork Chops

163   Extra-Easy Baked Ziti

164   Easy Lasagna

165   Italian Spaghetti Sauce

166   Sausage, Vegetable and Cheese Strata

168   Wild Rice, Sausage and Mushroom Casserole

169   Crab Scramble Casserole

A Note from Dr. Ghosh A good source of protein, this recipe delivers some of the necessities for rebuilding strength. However, legumes, beans and other gas-producing foods such as broccoli and cabbage should be avoided after surgery, especially surgery involving the intestines.

Corn and Black Bean Salad

Prep Time: 5 Minutes | **Start to Finish:** 2 Hours 5 Minutes | 6 servings

1   can (15 oz) black beans, drained, rinsed

1   can (7 oz) whole kernel corn, drained

1   can (4.5 oz) chopped green chiles, drained

½   cup medium chunky-style salsa

¼   cup chopped onion

2   tablespoons chopped fresh cilantro

1   In medium bowl, mix all ingredients. Cover; refrigerate until chilled, at least 2 hours but no longer than 24 hours.

66 Because of my fatigue, I sometimes made dinner in steps. I could make this salad ahead of time and chill it while I was making the rest of the meal."—**Theresa H. Shares Her Recipe**

High in folic acid; excellent source of fiber

1 Serving: Calories 110 (Calories from Fat 5); Total Fat 0.5g (Saturated Fat 0g, Trans Fat 0g); Cholesterol 0mg; Sodium 520mg; Potassium 250mg; Total Carbohydrate 22g (Dietary Fiber 6g); Protein 5g **% Daily Value:** Vitamin A 4%; Vitamin C 15%; Calcium 4%; Iron 8%; Folic Acid 20%; Magnesium 8% **Exchanges:** ½ Starch, ½ Other Carbohydrate, 1 Vegetable **Carbohydrate Choices:** 1 ½

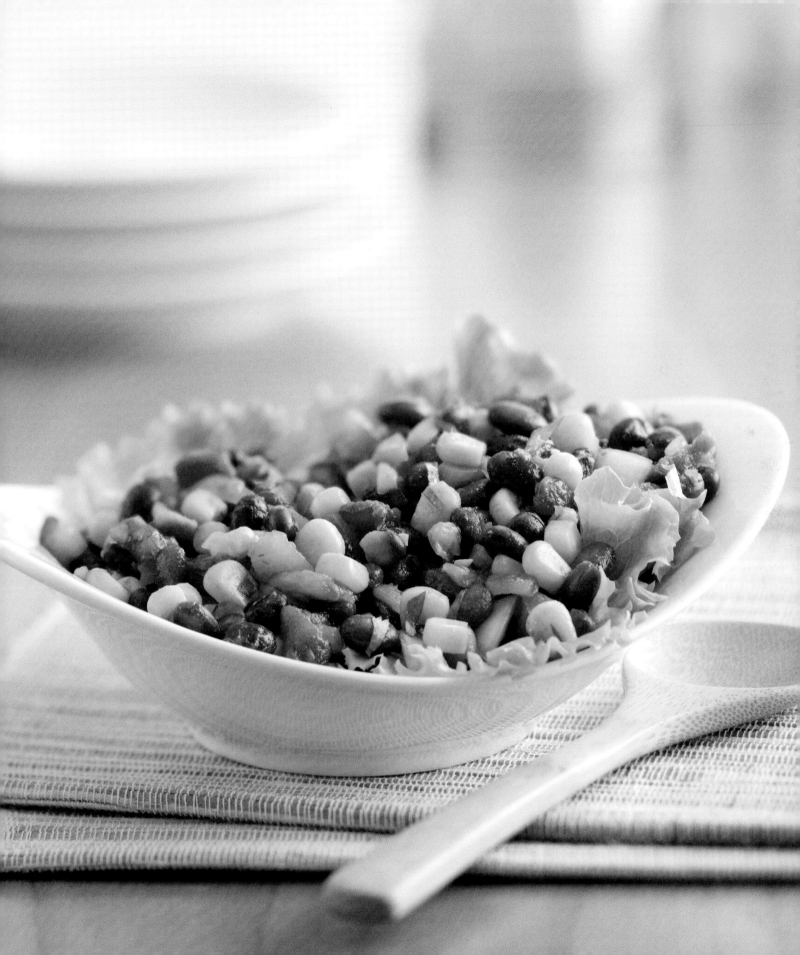

Food for Thought You can get quite an assortment of phytochemicals, which are naturally-occurring plant chemicals, by eating the whole food. It's also important to eat a variety of different foods, especially fruits and vegetables.

Seven-Layer Pasta Salad

Prep Time: 30 Minutes | **Start to Finish:** 8 Hours 30 Minutes | 8 servings (1 cup each)

2	cups uncooked bow-tie (farfalle) pasta (4 oz)
2	cups fresh broccoli florets
2	medium tomatoes, chopped (1 ½ cups)
1	medium yellow bell pepper, chopped (1 cup)
⅓	cup diced red onion
¾	cup mayonnaise or salad dressing
¾	cup plain yogurt
2	tablespoons sugar
½	teaspoon curry powder
1 ½	cups shredded Cheddar cheese (6 oz)
1	tablespoon bacon flavor bits or chips
2	tablespoons finely chopped fresh parsley

1 Cook and drain pasta as directed on package. Meanwhile, in 2-quart saucepan, place broccoli in boiling water. Cover; cook 1 minute. Drain; immediately rinse with cold water and drain again.

2 In 2-quart glass serving bowl, layer tomatoes, broccoli, bell pepper and onion.

3 In medium bowl, mix mayonnaise, yogurt, sugar and curry powder. Stir in pasta. Layer pasta mixture evenly over onion in serving bowl. Sprinkle with cheese. Top with bacon bits and parsley.

4 Cover; refrigerate at least 8 hours but no longer than 24 hours before serving.

❝This is a really tasty and colorful salad. I made it in the morning when I had more energy. Then I could take a nap during the day and serve it for an easy dinner when I felt a little more rested.❞
—Susan S.

High in vitamin C; good source of calcium and vitamin A

1 Serving: Calories 350 (Calories from Fat 220); Total Fat 25g (Saturated Fat 8g, Trans Fat 0g); Cholesterol 35mg; Sodium 330mg; Potassium 260mg; Total Carbohydrate 21g (Dietary Fiber 2g); Protein 9g **% Daily Value:** Vitamin A 15%; Vitamin C 40%; Calcium 15%; Iron 6%; Folic Acid 15%; Magnesium 6% **Exchanges:** ½ Other Carbohydrate, ½ Milk, 1 Vegetable, ½ High-Fat Meat, 3 ½ Fat **Carbohydrate Choices:** 1 ½

A Note from Dr. Ghosh This recipe is higher in fat than many in this cookbook. But not all fat is bad! We need fat to provide energy, insulation and protection for the body. For some cancer patients, though, high-fat foods may cause intestinal distress or nausea and should be avoided.

Layered Chicken Salad

Prep Time: 15 Minutes | **Start to Finish:** 2 Hours 15 Minutes | 5 servings

1 bag (10 oz) mixed salad greens (about 8 cups)

1 small zucchini, thinly sliced

1 can (10 oz) chunk chicken, drained

¼ cup chopped red onion

½ cup pimiento-stuffed salad olives

½ cup mayonnaise or salad dressing

¾ cup shredded reduced-fat Cheddar cheese (3 oz)

1 cup frozen sweet peas, drained, rinsed

1 medium tomato, cut into wedges

1 In large bowl, layer salad greens, zucchini, chicken, onion and olives.

2 Spread mayonnaise over olives, sealing to edge of bowl. Sprinkle with cheese and peas. Cover; refrigerate at least 2 hours but no longer than 24 hours.

3 Just before serving, add tomato and toss salad.

❝When I needed to reduce the fat in this or any recipe, I used less mayonnaise and cheese than was called for. Though I know some fat in our diets is important, I felt better during treatments when I knew my diet was not high in fat."—**Mary W.**

High in vitamins A and C and folic acid; good source of fiber

1 Serving: Calories 290 (Calories from Fat 200); Total Fat 22g (Saturated Fat 4g, Trans Fat 0g); Cholesterol 30mg; Sodium 710mg; Potassium 410mg; Total Carbohydrate 10g (Dietary Fiber 3g); Protein 14g **% Daily Value:** Vitamin A 80%; Vitamin C 30%; Calcium 20%; Iron 10%; Folic Acid 25%; Magnesium 10% **Exchanges:** 1 ½ Vegetable, 1 Very Lean Meat, ½ High-Fat Meat, 3 ½ Fat **Carbohydrate Choices:** ½

A Note from Dr. Ghosh This recipe is loaded with plenty of vitamins and minerals. One of them, magnesium, is a healing nutrient that is important for releasing energy from food so the body can use it properly.

Southwestern Pork Salad

Prep Time: 15 Minutes | **Start to Finish:** 55 Minutes | 4 servings

PORK

- 1 pork tenderloin (¾ lb)
- ¼ teaspoon salt
- ¼ teaspoon pepper

DRESSING

- ½ cup fat-free sour cream or plain yogurt
- ¼ cup chopped fresh cilantro
- 2 tablespoons lime juice
- 2 tablespoons vegetable oil
- ¼ teaspoon salt

SALAD

- 8 cups bite-size pieces mixed salad greens or 1 package (4 oz) mixed salad greens
- 1 medium yellow bell pepper, sliced
- 1 package (8 oz) sliced fresh mushrooms (about 3 cups)
- 1 can (15 to 16 oz) black-eyed peas, drained, rinsed

1 Heat oven to 350°F. Place pork on rack in shallow roasting pan. Sprinkle with salt and pepper. Insert meat thermometer so tip is in thickest part of pork.

2 Bake uncovered 30 to 40 minutes or until pork has slight blush of pink in center and meat thermometer reads 160°F.

3 Meanwhile, in small bowl, mix dressing ingredients; set aside.

4 Cool pork; cut into slices. On large serving plate, arrange greens, bell pepper, mushrooms and peas. Top with pork. Serve with dressing.

To Make Ahead: Cook pork and cool. Make the dressing and prepare vegetables. Refrigerate all ingredients no longer than 48 hours. Just before serving, continue as directed in Step 4.

"Lime juice really helps meat taste great. It covers up the metallic taste that I get from chemotherapy. I've found that ethnic foods, especially Southwestern, Mexican and Italian are often so flavorful that I don't notice the metallic taste."—Anne R.

High in potassium, iron, calcium, magnesium, vitamins A and C and folic acid; excellent source of fiber

1 Serving: Calories 330 (Calories from Fat 100); Total Fat 11g (Saturated Fat 2.5g, Trans Fat 0g); Cholesterol 40mg; Sodium 620mg; Potassium 1210mg; Total Carbohydrate 30g (Dietary Fiber 7g); Protein 28g **% Daily Value:** Vitamin A 130%; Vitamin C 60%; Calcium 10%; Iron 25%; Folic Acid 80%; Magnesium 25% **Exchanges:** 1 Starch, 3 ½ Vegetable, 2 ½ Lean Meat, ½ Fat **Carbohydrate Choices:** 2

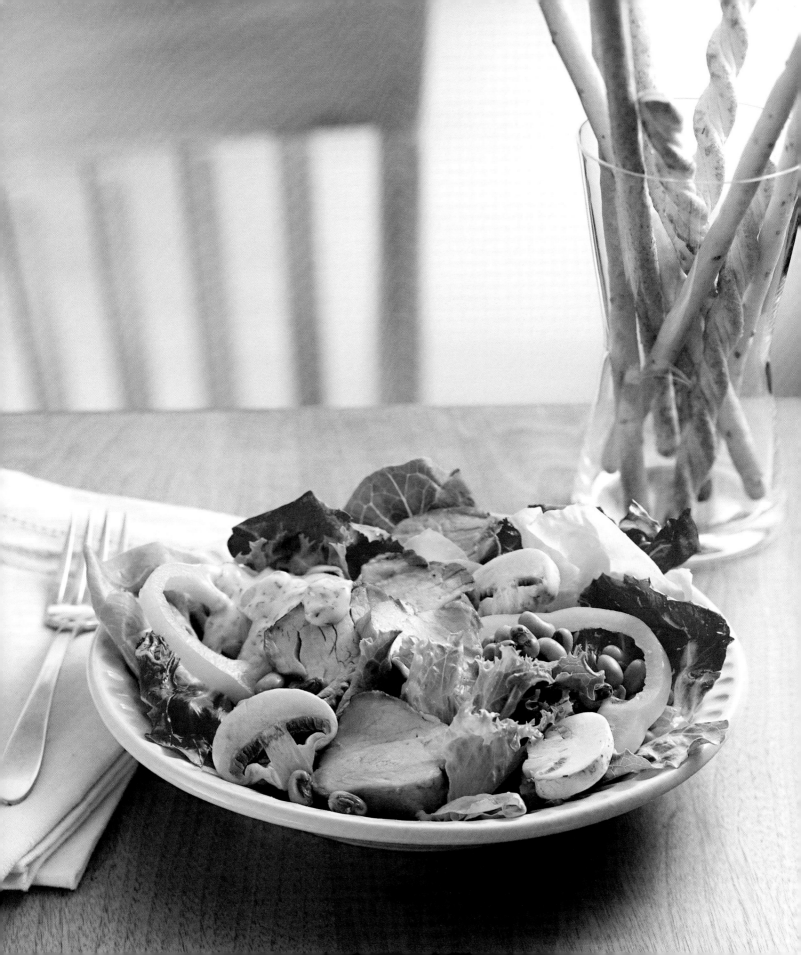

D

A Note from Dr. Ghosh Low in fiber and residue, this recipe is a great choice among survivors who have had intestinal trouble. All ingredients are easy to digest. For a different spin, substitute mashed potatoes or yams for the pasta or rice.

Dijon Chicken with Orzo Rice

Prep Time: 40 Minutes | **Start to Finish:** 40 Minutes | 4 servings

4 boneless skinless chicken breasts (about 1 ¼ lb)

¼ cup Dijon mustard

1 tablespoon olive or vegetable oil

1 tablespoon lemon juice

½ teaspoon dried rosemary leaves, crumbled

¼ teaspoon pepper

1 ⅓ cups uncooked orzo pasta (8 oz)

Chopped fresh parsley, if desired

1 Heat oven to 375°F. Spray 11x7-inch (2-quart) glass baking dish with cooking spray. Place chicken in baking dish.

2 In small bowl, mix remaining ingredients except pasta and parsley. Spread mustard mixture over chicken to coat thoroughly.

3 Bake uncovered 25 to 30 minutes or until juice of chicken is clear when center of thickest part is cut (at least 165°F).

4 Meanwhile, cook and drain pasta as directed on package. Garnish chicken with parsley. Serve with pasta.

To Make Ahead: Mix all ingredients except chicken, parsley and pasta in heavy-duty plastic food-storage bag. Add chicken, turning to coat. Freeze no longer than 2 months. At least 12 hours before serving, place frozen chicken in refrigerator to thaw. Heat oven to 375°. Place chicken in rectangular baking dish and continue as directed in Step 3.

❝Using crushed dried tarragon instead of rosemary is also good in this mustardy chicken. Whenever I made this dish, I made two batches, and kept one on hand in the freezer for another meal.”
—**Catherine H. Shares Her Recipe**

Low fiber; low residue

1 Serving: Calories 400 (Calories from Fat 80); Total Fat 9g (Saturated Fat 2g, Trans Fat 0g); Cholesterol 75mg; Sodium 440mg; Potassium 280mg; Total Carbohydrate 46g (Dietary Fiber 2g); Protein 35g **% Daily Value:** Vitamin A 0%; Vitamin C 0%; Calcium 4%; Iron 20%; Folic Acid 30%; Magnesium 15% **Exchanges:** 3 Starch, 4 Very Lean Meat, 1 Fat **Carbohydrate Choices:** 3

Food for Thought Chicken is a good source of vitamin B$_6$, pyridoxine. Vitamin B$_6$ is important for helping the body break down proteins to free the smaller protein components, called amino acids, that the body needs.

Italian Chicken Rolls

Prep Time: 20 Minutes | **Start to Finish:** 50 Minutes | 4 servings

4   boneless skinless chicken breasts (about 1 ¼ lb)

2   slices (½ oz each) provolone cheese, cut in half

4   thin slices pastrami

⅓   cup seasoned dry bread crumbs

¼   cup grated Romano or Parmesan cheese

2   tablespoons finely chopped fresh parsley

¼   cup milk

1   Heat oven to 425°F. Spray 8-inch square pan with cooking spray. Between sheets of plastic wrap or waxed paper, place each chicken breast smooth side down; gently pound with flat side of meat mallet or rolling pin until about ¼ inch thick.

2   Place piece of provolone cheese and slice of pastrami on each chicken piece. Fold long sides of each chicken piece over pastrami. Roll up chicken from short side; secure with toothpick.

3   Mix bread crumbs, Romano cheese and parsley. Dip chicken rolls into milk, then coat evenly with bread crumb mixture. Place seam sides down in pan.

4   Bake uncovered about 30 minutes or until chicken is no longer pink in center.

To Make Ahead: Freeze unbaked chicken rolls uncovered about 1 hour or until firm. Wrap tightly and label. Freeze no longer than 2 months. About 1 ¼ hours before serving, heat oven to 375°F. Bake uncovered about 50 minutes or until chicken is no longer pink in center.

❝A meal that I can serve to my family or company and eat with them helps me feel like I am still able to be a normal mom. This meal doesn't take a lot of energy to prepare, which is important when you get fatigued from cancer treatments."—**Anne R.**

High in calcium; low fiber

1 Serving: Calories 280 (Calories from Fat 90); Total Fat 10g (Saturated Fat 4.5g, Trans Fat 0g); Cholesterol 105mg; Sodium 420mg; Potassium 340mg; Total Carbohydrate 8g (Dietary Fiber 0g); Protein 39g **% Daily Value:** Vitamin A 6%; Vitamin C 2%; Calcium 20%; Iron 10%; Folic Acid 4%; Magnesium 10% **Exchanges:** ½ Starch, 4 Very Lean Meat, 1 ½ Medium-Fat Meat **Carbohydrate Choices:** ½

A Note from Dr. Ghosh Recipes that are higher in fiber, such as this one, can help with constipation. Increase fluid intake and activity level, if you can tolerate it, to help relieve severe constipation. At times, you may need a stool softener or laxative—consult your doctor.

Chicken Noodle Casserole

Prep Time: 15 Minutes | **Start to Finish:** 1 Hour | 6 servings (1 ½ cups each)

4 cups uncooked egg noodles (8 oz)

1 tablespoon vegetable oil

1 medium onion, chopped (½ cup)

2 medium stalks celery, sliced (1 cup)

3 cups cut-up cooked chicken

½ teaspoon salt

¼ teaspoon pepper

1 can (14 oz) chicken broth

1 can (10 ¾ oz) condensed cream of chicken soup

1 box (10 oz) frozen sweet peas

1 jar (4.5 oz) sliced mushrooms, drained

1 Heat oven to 350°F. Grease 3-quart casserole with butter. Cook noodles as directed on package—except cook 2 minutes less than package directions.

2 Meanwhile, in 10-inch skillet, heat oil over medium-high heat. Add onion and celery; cook about 5 minutes, stirring occasionally, until tender. Stir in remaining ingredients.

3 Drain noodles; place in casserole. Top with chicken mixture. Cover; bake 30 minutes. Stir; bake uncovered about 15 minutes longer or until liquid is absorbed.

To Make Ahead: Cover baked casserole with aluminum foil. Freeze no longer than 2 months. About 1 hour before serving, heat oven to 350°F. Bake in covered casserole 45 minutes. Uncover and bake 10 to 15 minutes longer or until hot.

66 This is a marvelous comfort food, and I ate it many times while I was on chemo. I often take this casserole to potluck dinners, and everybody loves it!"—**Lois K. Shares Her Recipe**

High in iron; good source of fiber and folic acid

1 Serving: Calories 390 (Calories from Fat 120); Total Fat 13g (Saturated Fat 3.5g, Trans Fat 0g); Cholesterol 90mg; Sodium 1460mg; Potassium 430mg; Total Carbohydrate 39g (Dietary Fiber 4g); Protein 29g **% Daily Value:** Vitamin A 25%; Vitamin C 4%; Calcium 4%; Iron 20%; Folic Acid 30%; Magnesium 15% **Exchanges:** 1 Starch, 1 ½ Other Carbohydrate, 1 Vegetable, 3 ½ Very Lean Meat, 2 Fat **Carbohydrate Choices:** 2 ½

Humor and Healing

Think back to a time when you were really uptight or worried about something. Then remember when someone made a joke—after a hearty laugh, you instantly felt much better.

This is no accident. Studies show that laughter, particularly the kind that makes your whole body shake, promotes better blood circulation and lowers blood pressure. It also releases endorphins, the chemicals in the brain that relieve pain and have a calming effect. Keeping your spirits up and having a smile on your face make it easier to deal with the stresses and strains of the world around you. Laughter has been called an inexpensive and effective wonder drug and a universal medicine.

Let your family know how important humor is to you. They may be hesitant, so you may have to take the first step and crack the first jokes. Because laughter is contagious, once people get the message, they will start to lighten up and share funny stories with you. If you have trouble getting going, try a few humor starters that have worked for others:

- Laugh at yourself. Lots of funny things occur to all of us on any given day. Choosing to laugh rather than get upset will brighten your day and make you and others less tense.

- Schedule a laughter break. Everyone who attends must bring a funny story or something humorous to share.

- Request a cartoon or humorous book as a gift. The giver will also enjoy the hunt for the humor.

- Rent videos that tickle your funny bone and have a laugh fest with friends.

- Start a humor basket. Anyone who visits adds a funny saying, a funny story or a joke contribution to the basket.

A Note from Dr. Ghosh This recipe is a great source of many essential minerals. Lack of magnesium, one of the minerals here, can become a problem if malnutrition occurs, as it can during cisplatin chemotherapy. Magnesium deficiencies can lead to weakness, lethargy, nausea and vomiting.

The Ultimate Chicken Casserole

Prep Time: 30 Minutes | **Start to Finish:** 1 Hour 15 Minutes | 8 to 10 servings

1 tablespoon vegetable oil

2 lb uncooked chicken breast tenders (not breaded)

2 boxes (9 oz each) frozen broccoli spears, thawed, drained

1 can (8 oz) sliced water chestnuts, drained

1 can (10 ¾ oz) condensed cream of chicken soup

½ cup reduced-fat mayonnaise

1 teaspoon lemon juice

½ cup milk

½ teaspoon curry powder, if desired

½ cup shredded reduced-fat Cheddar cheese (2 oz)

½ cup unseasoned dry bread crumbs

1 can (2.8 oz) French-fried onions

¼ cup slivered almonds

1 Heat oven to 350°F. In 12-inch skillet, heat oil over medium-high heat. Add chicken; cook 5 to 6 minutes, stirring occasionally, until chicken is no longer pink in center.

2 In ungreased 13x9-inch (3-quart) glass baking dish, layer broccoli spears, water chestnuts and chicken.

3 In small bowl, mix soup, mayonnaise, lemon juice, milk and curry powder; pour over chicken and broccoli. Sprinkle with cheese, bread crumbs, onions and almonds.

4 Cover tightly with foil; bake 30 minutes. Uncover; bake about 15 minutes longer or until broccoli is tender.

To Make Ahead: Cover baked casserole with aluminum foil. Freeze no longer than 2 months. About 1 hour before serving, heat oven to 350°F. Bake in covered baking dish 45 minutes. Uncover and bake 10 to 15 minutes longer or until hot.

❝When I don't feel well, I don't like fussing in the kitchen. This was such an easy recipe, I was up to preparing it even when I was very tired. It's also great for entertaining."—**Ellen T. Shares Her Recipe**

High in vitamins A and C; good source of fiber

1 Serving: Calories 360 (Calories from Fat 160); Total Fat 17g (Saturated Fat 4.5g, Trans Fat 0g); Cholesterol 60mg; Sodium 720mg; Potassium 220mg; Total Carbohydrate 21g (Dietary Fiber 3g); Protein 31g **% Daily Value:** Vitamin A 15%; Vitamin C 20%; Calcium 10%; Iron 6%; Folic Acid 10%; Magnesium 6% **Exchanges:** 1 Starch, 1 Vegetable, 3 ½ Very Lean Meat, 3 Fat **Carbohydrate Choices:** 1 ½

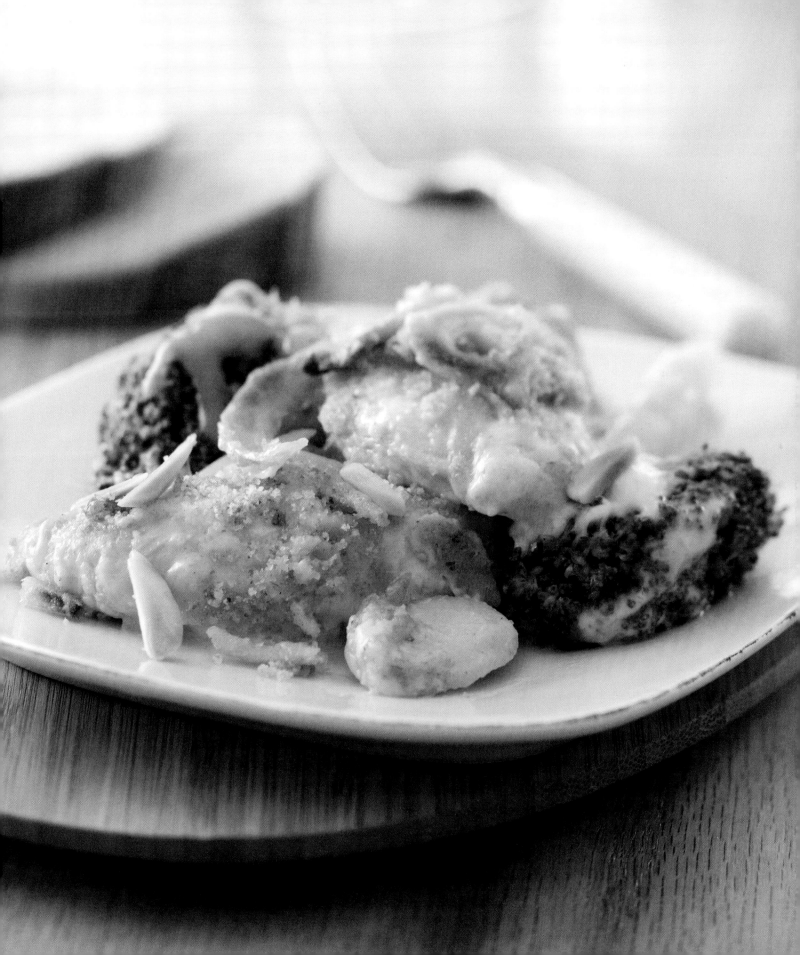

A Note from Dr. Ghosh Iron is an important mineral needed to help fight fatigue and is especially key during chemotherapy and radiation.

Chicken Soup with Homemade Noodles

Prep Time: 25 Hours | **Start to Finish:** 1 Hour 30 Minutes | 6 servings

CHICKEN

1	cut-up whole chicken (3 to 3 ½ lb)
4 ½	cups cold water
1	teaspoon salt
½	teaspoon pepper
1	medium stalk celery with leaves, cut up
1	medium onion, cut up
1	medium carrot, cut up

SOUP

4	cups water
1	teaspoon chicken bouillon granules
1	cup frozen sweet peas
2	medium stalks celery, sliced (1 cup)
1	medium onion, sliced
2	medium carrots, sliced (1 cup) or 1 bag (8 oz) ready-to-eat baby-cut carrots

NOODLES

2	eggs, beaten
¼	cup milk or water
1	cup all-purpose flour
¼	teaspoon salt
	Dash pepper

1 Remove excess fat from chicken. Place chicken in 4-quart Dutch oven. Add 4 ½ cups cold water and remaining chicken ingredients. Heat to boiling. Reduce heat; cover and simmer about 45 minutes or until juice of chicken is clear when thickest pieces are cut to bone (at least 165°F).

2 Remove chicken from broth. Cool chicken about 10 minutes or just until cool enough to handle. Skim fat from broth. Strain broth; discard vegetables. Remove skin and bones from chicken. Cut chicken into ½-inch pieces.

3 Return chicken and broth to Dutch oven. Stir in 4 cups water and the bouillon. Heat to boiling. Reduce heat; stir in peas and sliced celery, onion and carrots. Simmer uncovered 15 minutes.

4 In small bowl, mix noodle ingredients (batter will be thick). Press a few tablespoons of the batter at a time through colander (preferably one with large holes) into boiling soup. Stir soup once or twice to prevent sticking. Cook about 5 minutes or until noodles rise to surface and are tender.

To Make Ahead: Cook chicken and broth one day. Refrigerate separately. The next day, skim fat from broth, and continue with Step 2.

To freeze after preparing entire recipe, cool soup 30 minutes. Place in 2-quart airtight freezer container and label. Freeze no longer than 2 months.

66 When I was growing up, my mother always served chicken soup when I was sick. It is still a comforting food for me today, and I make it often for my family. I made this a make-ahead recipe by cooking the chicken and stock one day, then finishing the rest the next day."—**Joan K. Shares Her Recipe**

High in vitamin A; good source of fiber and iron

1 Serving: Calories 420 (Calories from Fat 120); Total Fat 13g (Saturated Fat 3.5g, Trans Fat 0g); Cholesterol 200mg; Sodium 850mg; Potassium 640mg; Total Carbohydrate 27g (Dietary Fiber 3g); Protein 48g
% Daily Value: Vitamin A 120%; Vitamin C 6%; Calcium 8%; Iron 20%; Folic Acid 20%; Magnesium 15%
Exchanges: 1 Starch, ½ Other Carbohydrate, 1 ½ Vegetable, 4 ½ Very Lean Meat, 1 ½ Lean Meat, 1 Fat
Carbohydrate Choices: 2

Food for Thought Packed with vegetables and legumes, this is a tasty vegetarian delight. MyPlate recommends a plant-based diet, loaded with fiber, vitamins and minerals, and this soup fits the bill.

Crowd-Size Minestrone

Prep Time: 25 Minutes | **Start to Finish:** 1 Hour 40 Minutes | 10 servings

1 tablespoon vegetable oil

2 cloves garlic, finely chopped

1 medium onion, chopped (½ cup)

4 cups chicken broth or water

4 cups tomato juice

1 cup dry red wine or water

1 tablespoon dried basil leaves

1 teaspoon salt

½ teaspoon dried oregano leaves

¼ teaspoon pepper

2 small zucchini, chopped (2 cups)

2 medium carrots, sliced (1 cup)

2 medium stalks celery, chopped (1 cup)

1 can (28 oz) diced tomatoes, undrained

2 cans (15 to 16 oz each) kidney, garbanzo or great northern beans, drained, rinsed

1 In 8-quart Dutch oven, heat oil over medium heat. Add garlic and onion; cook about 2 minutes, stirring occasionally, until onion is tender.

2 Stir in remaining ingredients. Heat to boiling. Reduce heat; cover and simmer 1 hour.

66 Soup is healing to the soul as well as the body. Though this recipe looks long, it serves many and keeps a long time in the freezer. Just store in individual containers and heat when ready to serve." —Judy O.

High in vitamins A and C, iron, folic acid, magnesium and potassium; excellent source of fiber

1 Serving: Calories 170 (Calories from Fat 20); Total Fat 2.5g (Saturated Fat 0g, Trans Fat 0g); Cholesterol 0mg; Sodium 1270mg; Potassium 700mg; Total Carbohydrate 27g (Dietary Fiber 6g); Protein 9g **% Daily Value:** Vitamin A 60%; Vitamin C 30%; Calcium 6%; Iron 15%; Folic Acid 30%; Magnesium 10% **Exchanges:** ½ Starch, ½ Other Carbohydrate, 2 Vegetable, ½ Very Lean Meat, ½ Fat **Carbohydrate Choices:** 2

Food for Thought Brimming with beans—navy beans, that is—this recipe is rich in fiber. Typically Americans don't eat enough fiber. Experts recommend we eat 25 to 30 grams of fiber daily for good health and to prevent constipation.

White Turkey Chili

Prep Time: 15 Minutes | **Start to Finish:** 9 Hours 30 Minutes | 8 servings

1   bag (1 lb) dried navy beans (2 cups), sorted, rinsed

8   cups water

2   tablespoons chicken bouillon granules

2   tablespoons chopped fresh cilantro or parsley

2   teaspoons ground cumin

1 ½   teaspoons dried basil leaves

¼   teaspoon ground cloves

⅛   teaspoon ground red pepper (cayenne)

1   medium onion, chopped (½ cup)

4   cloves garlic, finely chopped

2   cans (4.5 oz each) chopped green chiles, undrained

6   cups water

1   lb turkey breast tenderloins, cut into ½-inch pieces

½   cup shredded reduced-fat mozzarella or Cheddar cheese (2 oz)

1 In 4-quart Dutch oven, place beans and water. Soak at least 8 hours but no longer than 10 hours.

2 Drain beans; return beans to Dutch oven. Stir in remaining ingredients except turkey and cheese. Heat to boiling. Reduce heat; cover and simmer about 1 hour or until beans are tender.

3 Stir in turkey. Simmer uncovered about 15 minutes or until turkey is no longer pink in center. Sprinkle with cheese.

To Make Ahead: Divide chili among 3 airtight 2-quart freezer containers and label. Cool quickly and freeze no longer than 2 months. Remove lid from 1 freezer container; place upside down in 1-quart microwavable casserole. Microwave on High 5 minutes; remove container. Cover and microwave on High 20 to 25 minutes, breaking up and stirring every 5 minutes, until hot.

"This is such an easy recipe to put together. I soak the beans overnight, drain them in the morning and finish the rest of the cooking just in time for lunch. Eating my main meal of the day at lunch worked better for me; I just felt more like eating then."
—Joan K. Shares Her Recipe

High in magnesium, iron and folic acid; excellent source of fiber

1 Serving: Calories 290 (Calories from Fat 25); Total Fat 3g (Saturated Fat 1g, Trans Fat 0g); Cholesterol 40mg; Sodium 810mg; Potassium 680mg; Total Carbohydrate 39g (Dietary Fiber 14g); Protein 26g
% Daily Value: Vitamin A 4%; Vitamin C 8%; Calcium 20%; Iron 25%; Folic Acid 45%; Magnesium 25%
Exchanges: 2 Starch, 1 ½ Vegetable, 2 Very Lean Meat, ½ Lean Meat **Carbohydrate Choices:** 2 ½

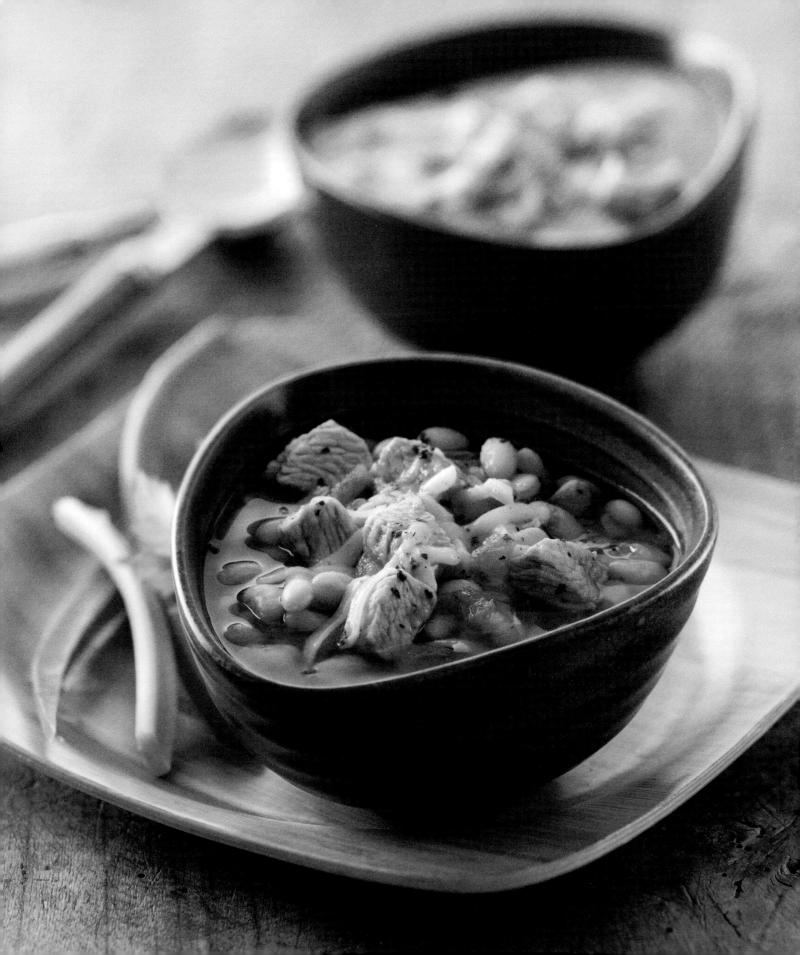

Food for Thought If your body weight is getting too low, you probably need more calories. One way to increase the calorie content of a recipe is by adding heavy cream. Cream, butter and margarine are easy high-calorie additions for soups, stews, sauces and gravies.

Beef-Vegetable Soup

Prep Time: 20 Minutes | **Start to Finish:** 3 Hours 50 Minutes | 6 servings (1 ½ cups each)

2 tablespoons vegetable oil

2 lb beef shank cross-cuts or soup bones

1 medium onion, sliced (1 cup)

6 cups cold water

1 teaspoon salt

1 dried bay leaf

1 tablespoon pickling spice

1 can (10 ½ oz) condensed beef broth

2 medium potatoes, cubed (2 cups)

2 medium carrots, sliced (1 cup)

2 medium stalks celery, sliced (1 cup)

2 cups shredded cabbage

½ cup ketchup

1 can (15 oz) sliced beets, drained, cut in half

¾ cup whipping cream

1 In 4-quart Dutch oven, heat oil over medium heat. Add beef and onion; cook until beef is brown on both sides. Add water; heat to boiling. Skim foam from broth. Stir in salt, bay leaf and pickling spice. Reduce heat; cover and simmer 3 hours.

2 Remove beef from broth. Cool beef about 10 minutes or just until cool enough to handle. Strain broth; discard vegetables and seasonings. Remove beef from bones. Cut beef into ½-inch pieces. Skim fat from broth.

3 Add enough canned broth to broth from beef to measure 5 cups. Return broth and beef to Dutch oven. Stir in potatoes, carrots, celery, cabbage, ketchup and beets. Heat to boiling. Reduce heat; cover and simmer about 30 minutes or until vegetables are tender. Cool 10 minutes. Stir in whipping cream.

To Make Ahead: Cook beef bones and water one day. Refrigerate separately. The next day, skim fat from broth, and continue with Step 2.

To freeze, cool soup 30 minutes. Place in 2-quart freezer container. Freeze no longer than 2 months. About 35 minutes before serving, remove lid from freezer container; place container upside down in 2-quart microwavable casserole. Cover and microwave on Medium (50%) 25 minutes; remove container. Break up and stir. Cover and microwave on Medium about 20 minutes longer, stirring 2 or 3 times, until hot.

❝Soups, like this one, became one of my favorite foods because it went down so easily. Other favorites: fruit cocktail, grapes, plums, watermelon, frozen pops and gelatin.❞—**MaryElaine W. Shares Her Recipe**

High in iron, potassium and vitamin A; good source of fiber

1 Serving: Calories 380 (Calories from Fat 170); Total Fat 19g (Saturated Fat 9g, Trans Fat 0.5g); Cholesterol 90mg; Sodium 1120mg; Potassium 970mg; Total Carbohydrate 27g (Dietary Fiber 4g); Protein 25g **% Daily Value:** Vitamin A 80%; Vitamin C 20%; Calcium 8%; Iron 25%; Folic Acid 15%; Magnesium 15% **Exchanges:** 1 Starch, 3 Vegetable, 2 Lean Meat, 2 ½ Fat **Carbohydrate Choices:** 2

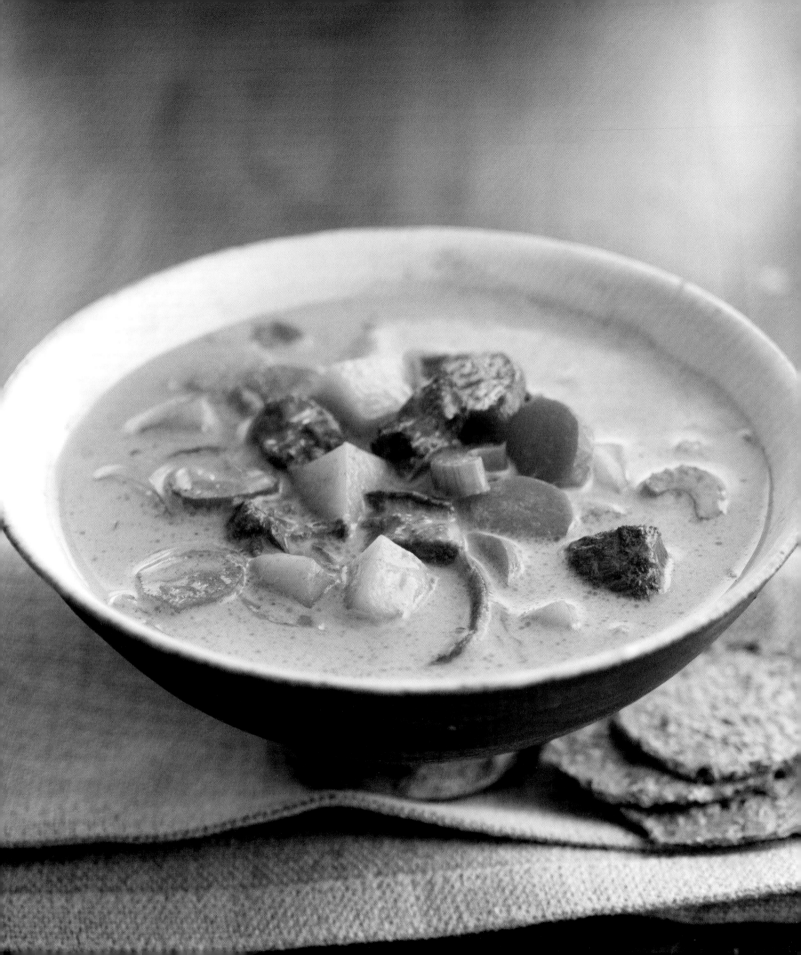

A Note from Dr. Ghosh Because of the high iron content, this recipe is a good choice for cancer patients with neutropenia, a time when white blood cell count is low and risk of infection is high. Just omit the pepper.

Layered Beef and Vegetable Dinner

Prep Time: 15 Minutes | **Start to Finish:** 1 Hour 15 Minutes | 4 servings

1 lb lean (at least 80%) ground beef

1 teaspoon salt

½ teaspoon pepper

2 medium potatoes, peeled, sliced (2 cups)

6 medium carrots (1 lb), sliced (3 cups)

1 medium onion, sliced

2 medium stalks celery, sliced (1 cup)

1 can (10 ¾ oz) condensed cream of chicken soup

1 Heat oven to 375°F. Spray 3-quart casserole with cooking spray. Crumble beef in bottom of casserole. Sprinkle with half of the salt and pepper.

2 Layer potatoes, carrots, onion and celery on beef. Sprinkle with remaining salt and pepper. Spread soup over top.

3 Cover; bake about 1 hour or until beef is brown and vegetables are tender.

To Make Ahead: Cover baked casserole with aluminum foil. Freeze no longer than 2 months. About 1 hour before serving, heat oven to 375°F. Bake in covered pan 45 minutes. Uncover and bake 15 to 20 minutes longer or until hot.

❝I found that sometimes only stubbornness and sheer will are what allow you to eat. However, the right recipes—like this easy dinner, help as well."—**Pat Y. Shares Her Recipe**

High in potassium, iron and vitamin A; excellent source of fiber

1 Serving: Calories 400 (Calories from Fat 160); Total Fat 18g (Saturated Fat 6g, Trans Fat 1g); Cholesterol 75mg; Sodium 1270mg; Potassium 940mg; Total Carbohydrate 36g (Dietary Fiber 5g); Protein 24g **% Daily Value:** Vitamin A 310%; Vitamin C 10%; Calcium 8%; Iron 15%; Folic Acid 10%; Magnesium 15% **Exchanges:** 1 Starch, ½ Other Carbohydrate, 3 Vegetable, 2 Lean Meat, 2 ½ Fat **Carbohydrate Choices:** 2 ½

Food for Thought Having beef for dinner? Beef provides a super source of the mineral zinc, which is important for growth, wound healing and your ability to taste foods.

Spaghetti and Meat Squares

Prep Time: 10 Minutes | **Start to Finish:** 25 Minutes | 6 servings

1 lb lean (at least 80%) ground beef or ground turkey

½ cup unseasoned dry bread crumbs

½ cup applesauce

1 tablespoon dried minced onion

¾ teaspoon garlic salt

¼ teaspoon pepper

6 to 7 oz uncooked spaghetti

1 jar (26 to 28 oz) tomato pasta sauce (any variety)

1 Heat oven to 400°F. In medium bowl, mix all ingredients except pasta sauce and spaghetti. Press mixture evenly in ungreased 11x7-inch pan. Cut into 1 ¼-inch squares.

2 Bake uncovered about 15 minutes or until no longer pink in center and juice is clear. Meanwhile, cook and drain spaghetti as directed on package.

3 Drain meat squares and separate. In 3-quart saucepan, mix meat squares and pasta sauce. Heat to boiling. Reduce heat; simmer uncovered about 15 minutes, stirring occasionally, until hot. Serve over spaghetti.

To Make Ahead: Cool meat squares 5 minutes. Place on cookie sheet; freeze uncovered 15 minutes. Place meat squares in airtight 1 ½-quart freezer container and label. Freeze no longer than 2 months. About 45 minutes before serving, heat meat squares and pasta sauce to boiling in 3-quart saucepan. Reduce heat; simmer uncovered about 25 minutes, stirring occasionally, until hot. Serve over spaghetti.

❝I used to make all my spaghetti sauce from scratch. Now I purchase it. That way, I have more time to rest."—Judy O.

High in iron; good source of fiber, potassium and folic acid

1 1 Serving: Calories 470 (Calories from Fat 130); Total Fat 14g (Saturated Fat 4g, Trans Fat 0.5g); Cholesterol 45mg; Sodium 1000mg; Potassium 660mg; Total Carbohydrate 64g (Dietary Fiber 4g); Protein 21g **% Daily Value:** Vitamin A 10%; Vitamin C 10%; Calcium 8%; Iron 25%; Folic Acid 25%; Magnesium 15% **Exchanges:** 3 Starch, 1 Other Carbohydrate, 1 Vegetable, 1 ½ Lean Meat, 1 ½ Fat **Carbohydrate Choices:** 4

D

A Note from Dr. Ghosh Pork is a tasty source of thiamin, or vitamin B_1. Thiamin is vitally important for energy release from foods, plus it helps keep your nervous system healthy, too.

Almond-Stuffed Pork Chops

Prep Time: 15 Minutes | **Start to Finish:** 40 Minutes | 4 servings

½ cup chicken broth

¼ cup uncooked quick-cooking brown rice

2 tablespoons finely chopped dried apricots

2 tablespoons slivered almonds, toasted*

2 teaspoons chopped fresh or ¾ teaspoon dried marjoram leaves

2 tablespoons chopped fresh parsley

4 loin pork chops, 1 inch thick (about 2 lb)

¼ cup apricot preserves

1 In 1 ½-quart saucepan, mix broth, rice, apricots, almonds and marjoram. Heat to boiling. Reduce heat to low; cover and simmer about 10 minutes or until rice is tender. Stir in parsley.

2 Cut 3-inch pocket in each pork chop, cutting from fat side almost to bone. Spoon about 2 tablespoons rice mixture into each pocket. Secure pockets with toothpicks.

3 Set oven control to broil. Place pork on rack in broiler pan. Broil with tops 5 to 6 inches from heat 10 minutes. Turn; broil 10 to 15 minutes longer until meat thermometer inserted in center reads 145°F; allow to rest for at least 3 minutes. Heat preserves; brush over pork before serving.

*To toast nuts, bake uncovered in ungreased shallow pan in 350°F oven about 10 minutes, stirring occasionally, until golden brown. Or cook in ungreased heavy skillet over medium-low heat 5 to 7 minutes, stirring frequently until browning begins, then stirring constantly until golden brown.

To Make Ahead: Place broiled pork in square baking dish, 8x8x2 inches. Wrap tightly with foil and label. Freeze no longer than 2 months. About 1 hour 15 minutes before serving, heat oven to 375°F. Bake in covered baking dish about 1 hour or until stuffing is hot in center and meat thermometer in stuffing reads 160°F. Heat preserves; brush over pork.

❝Pork with fruit and rice tastes great even on chemo. I didn't even know I liked apricots until they were one of about five fruits still left on my food list after surgery! Now I love them."—**Anne R.**

Low fiber; low residue

1 Serving: Calories 300 (Calories from Fat 90); Total Fat 10g (Saturated Fat 3g, Trans Fat 0g); Cholesterol 65mg; Sodium 180mg; Potassium 430mg; Total Carbohydrate 26g (Dietary Fiber 2g); Protein 25g
% Daily Value: Vitamin A 6%; Vitamin C 4%; Calcium 2%; Iron 8%; Folic Acid 4%; Magnesium 10%
Exchanges: ½ Starch, 1 Other Carbohydrate, 3 ½ Lean Meat **Carbohydrate Choices:** 2

Food for Thought Pasta, derived from wheat, is an easy carbohydrate source of energy. You begin breaking down carbohydrates to extract the energy they provide as soon as they enter your mouth. That's why we call carbohydrates a fast energy source.

Extra-Easy Baked Ziti

Prep Time: 20 Minutes │ **Start to Finish:** 1 Hour │ 10 to 12 servings

1 package (16 oz) ziti pasta

4 cups (¼ recipe) Italian Spaghetti Sauce (page 165)

1 ½ cups freshly shredded Parmesan cheese (6 oz)

1 Heat oven to 350°F. Cook and drain pasta as directed on package.

2 In ungreased 3-quart casserole, mix pasta, 4 cups Italian Spaghetti Sauce and ¾ cup of the cheese.

3 Cover; bake 30 minutes. Sprinkle with remaining ¾ cup cheese; bake uncovered 5 to 10 minutes longer or until cheese is melted.

To Make Ahead: Cover unbaked casserole tightly and refrigerate no longer than 24 hours. About 50 minutes before serving, heat oven to 350°F. Continue as directed in Step 4.

❝This is a great comfort food, and easy enough for my daughter to prepare when she got home from school, especially if it was ready to pop into the oven. She would add soft bread (I couldn't get hard bread down), and a salad, and our meal was complete."—**Anne R.**

High in calcium and folic acid; good source of fiber

1 Serving: Calories 410 (Calories from Fat 140); Total Fat 15g (Saturated Fat 6g, Trans Fat 0g); Cholesterol 30mg; Sodium 1230mg; Potassium 320mg; Total Carbohydrate 47g (Dietary Fiber 3g); Protein 20g **% Daily Value:** Vitamin A 10%; Vitamin C 10%; Calcium 25%; Iron 15%; Folic Acid 25%; Magnesium 10% **Exchanges:** 2 ½ Starch, ½ Other Carbohydrate, ½ Vegetable, ½ Lean Meat, 1 High-Fat Meat, 1 Fat **Carbohydrate Choices:** 3

A Note from Dr. Ghosh Ricotta, Parmesan and mozzarella cheeses are delicious sources of calcium. Vital for strong bones and teeth, calcium also helps with proper nerve and muscle function—even for the heart.

Easy Lasagna

Prep Time: 20 Minutes | **Start to Finish:** 1 Hour 35 Minutes | 12 servings

2 cups ricotta cheese

¾ cup grated Parmesan cheese

2 tablespoons chopped fresh parsley

1 tablespoon chopped fresh or 1 ½ teaspoons dried oregano leaves

8 cups (½ recipe) Italian Spaghetti Sauce (page 165)

12 uncooked lasagna noodles

2 cups shredded mozzarella cheese (8 oz)

1 Heat oven to 350°F. In medium bowl, mix ricotta cheese, ½ cup of the Parmesan cheese, the parsley and oregano.

2 In ungreased 13x9-inch (3-quart) glass baking dish, spread 2 cups of the Italian Spaghetti Sauce. Top with 4 of the noodles. Spread cheese mixture over noodles. Spread with 2 cups spaghetti sauce and top with 4 noodles; repeat with 2 cups spaghetti sauce and 4 noodles. Sprinkle with 1 ½ cups of the mozzarella cheese. Spread with remaining 2 cups spaghetti sauce. Sprinkle with remaining ¼ cup Parmesan cheese.

3 Cover with foil; bake 30 minutes. Uncover; bake about 30 minutes longer or until hot and bubbly. Sprinkle with remaining ½ cup mozzarella cheese. Let stand 15 minutes before cutting into squares.

To Make Ahead: Wrap unbaked lasagna tightly with foil and label. Freeze no longer than 2 months. About 2 hours before serving, heat oven to 350°F. Bake in covered pan 45 minutes. Uncover and bake 15 to 20 minutes longer or until hot and bubbly. Sprinkle with mozzarella cheese. Let stand 15 minutes before cutting into squares.

66 During my good week when I'm on chemo, I cook make-ahead foods and freeze them so that on the days when I have less energy and can't cook, I can just put something in the oven and still have a great meal to eat with my family. It's important to use your energy wisely when you have it because it comes and goes during treatment."—Anne R.

High in calcium and vitamins A and C; good source of fiber

1 Serving: Calories 490 (Calories from Fat 250); Total Fat 28g (Saturated Fat 13g, Trans Fat 0g); Cholesterol 65mg; Sodium 1550mg; Potassium 510mg; Total Carbohydrate 32g (Dietary Fiber 3g); Protein 27g **% Daily Value:** Vitamin A 20%; Vitamin C 20%; Calcium 35%; Iron 15%; Folic Acid 15%; Magnesium 10% **Exchanges:** 1 Starch, 1 Other Carbohydrate, 1 Vegetable, 2 ½ Medium-Fat Meat, ½ High-Fat Meat, 2 Fat **Carbohydrate Choices:** 2

A Note from Dr. Ghosh Popping with bell peppers and tomatoes, this recipe is loaded with vitamin C, a nutrient key to bolstering the immune system.

Italian Spaghetti Sauce

Prep Time: 15 Minutes | **Start to Finish:** 2 Hours 30 Minutes | 16 cups sauce

4 lb bulk Italian sausage

2 tablespoons olive or vegetable oil

6 medium onions, finely chopped (3 cups)

1 large bell pepper, finely chopped (1 ½ cups)

12 cloves garlic, finely chopped

4 cans (14.5 oz each) diced tomatoes, undrained

3 cans (15 oz each) tomato sauce

¼ cup chopped fresh or 2 tablespoons dried basil leaves

¼ cup chopped fresh or 2 tablespoons dried oregano leaves

2 tablespoons sugar

2 teaspoons salt

½ teaspoon pepper

1 cup dry red wine or beef broth

1 In 6-quart Dutch oven, cook sausage over medium-high heat about 15 minutes, stirring occasionally, until no longer pink. Remove from Dutch oven; drain.

2 In same Dutch oven, heat oil over medium heat. Add onions, bell pepper and garlic; cook, stirring occasionally, until onions are tender. Stir in sausage and remaining ingredients except wine. Heat to boiling, stirring occasionally. Reduce heat; simmer uncovered 1 hour, stirring occasionally.

3 Stir in wine. Simmer uncovered 1 hour longer, stirring occasionally.

To Make Ahead: Place sauce in 4 upright, airtight 1-quart freezer containers and label. Cool quickly and freeze no longer than 2 months. About 10 minutes before serving, place in 1 ½-quart microwavable casserole. Cover tightly and microwave on High 6 to 8 minutes, stirring after 3 minutes, until hot.

66My neighbor makes me homemade spaghetti sauce and spaghetti, that way the smells don't upset my stomach and I still get to eat some really great food. She also feels like she is really helping me out, and she is!"—**Anne R.**

High in potassium and vitamins A and C; good source of fiber

1 Cup: Calories 370 (Calories from Fat 220); Total Fat 25g (Saturated Fat 8g, Trans Fat 0g); Cholesterol 45mg; Sodium 1950mg; Potassium 620mg; Total Carbohydrate 20g (Dietary Fiber 3g); Protein 18g
% Daily Value: Vitamin A 20%; Vitamin C 30%; Calcium 6%; Iron 15%; Folic Acid 6%; Magnesium 8%
Exchanges: ½ Starch, ½ Other Carbohydrate, 1 Vegetable, 1 Medium-Fat Meat, 1 High-Fat Meat, 2 ½ Fat
Carbohydrate Choices: 1

A Note from Dr. Ghosh Green leafy vegetables such as spinach are a good source of vitamin K, essential for normal blood clotting. If taking a blood thinner such as Coumadin®, however, avoid excessive intake of dietary vitamin K because it may interfere with the medication.

Sausage, Vegetable and Cheese Strata

Prep Time: 30 Minutes | **Start to Finish:** 5 Hours 45 Minutes | 12 servings

½ lb bulk mild pork sausage

½ lb bulk hot pork sausage

1 tablespoon butter or margarine

1 box (9 oz) frozen chopped spinach, thawed, squeezed to drain, or ½ lb fresh spinach

4 small zucchini (1 lb), sliced

2 medium green bell peppers, sliced

1 medium onion, sliced

10 slices white bread

7 eggs

1 ½ cups low-fat milk

1 teaspoon ground mustard

1 teaspoon salt

½ teaspoon pepper

2 cups shredded reduced-fat Cheddar cheese (8 oz)

2 cups shredded mozzarella cheese (8 oz)

1 Spray 13x9-inch (3-quart) glass baking dish with cooking spray. In 12-inch skillet, cook sausage over medium heat 7 to 8 minutes, stirring occasionally, until no longer pink. Drain sausage in colander; set aside.

2 In same skillet, melt butter over medium-high heat. Add spinach, zucchini, bell peppers and onion; cook about 5 minutes, stirring frequently, until zucchini is crisp-tender.

3 Break each bread slice into 4 pieces. Layer sausage, vegetables and bread in baking dish. In medium bowl, beat eggs, milk, mustard, salt and pepper with hand beater or whisk until blended; pour over bread. Sprinkle cheeses over top. Cover tightly with foil; refrigerate at least 4 hours but no longer than 24 hours.

4 Heat oven to 325°F. Bake covered 30 minutes. Uncover; bake about 45 minutes longer or until top is golden brown and knife inserted in center comes out clean.

"I served this at brunch the day after my daughter Amy's wedding, and it was a real hit! It was convenient for me because the assembly is done the day before; all I had to do the day of serving was bake it."
—**Kathy S. Shares Her Recipe**

High in calcium and vitamins A and C

1 Serving: Calories 290 (Calories from Fat 140); Total Fat 15g (Saturated Fat 7g, Trans Fat 0g); Cholesterol 155mg; Sodium 830mg; Potassium 380mg; Total Carbohydrate 17g (Dietary Fiber 2g); Protein 20g **% Daily Value:** Vitamin A 45%; Vitamin C 20%; Calcium 40%; Iron 10%; Folic Acid 20%; Magnesium 10% **Exchanges:** ½ Starch, ½ Other Carbohydrate, 1 Vegetable, 1 ½ Lean Meat, 1 High-Fat Meat, ½ Fat **Carbohydrate Choices:** 1

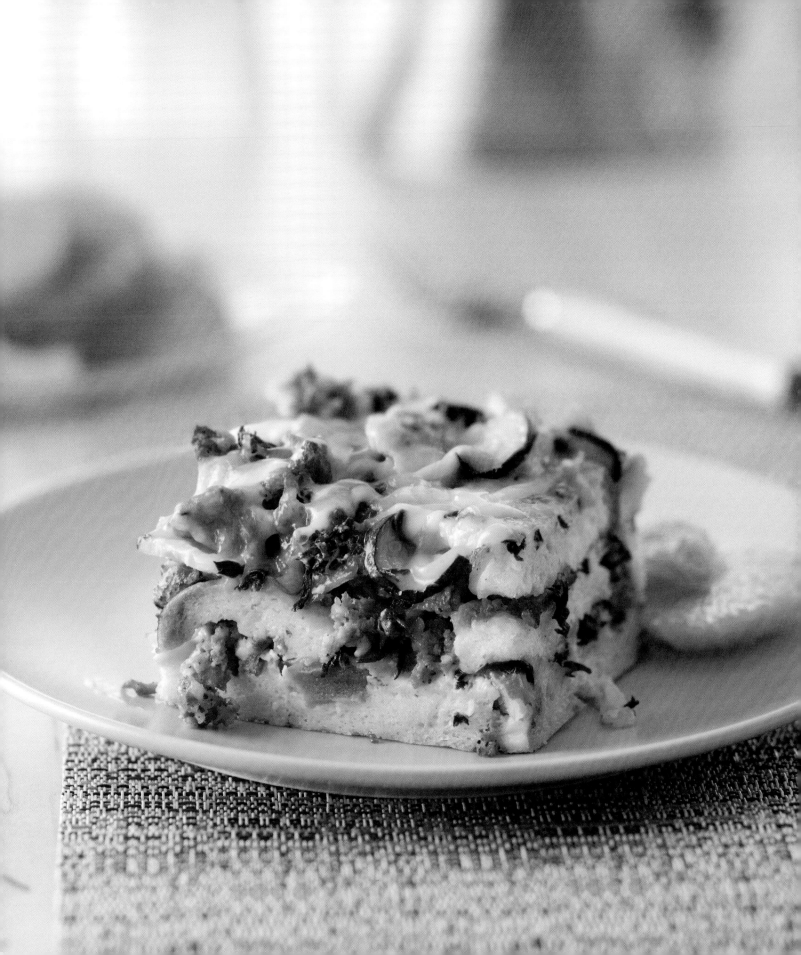

A Note from Dr. Ghosh You can reduce the residue of this recipe by omitting the almonds and using white rice instead of wild rice. (If using white rice, remember to omit the soaking step and reduce the cooking time.) Avoid high-residue diets when having intestinal problems.

Wild Rice, Sausage and Mushroom Casserole

Prep Time: 25 Minutes | **Start to Finish:** 3 Hours 45 Minutes | 6 servings (1 cup each)

1 cup uncooked wild rice

2 cups water

1 lb bulk pork sausage

1 medium onion, chopped (½ cup)

2 medium stalks celery, sliced (1 cup)

1 can (10 ¾ oz) condensed cream of mushroom soup

1 jar (6.5 oz) sliced mushrooms, drained

¼ cup slivered almonds (2 oz)

1 In 2-quart saucepan, place wild rice and water. Soak 2 hours or overnight. Do not drain; heat to boiling. Reduce heat; cover and simmer 20 minutes.

2 Meanwhile, heat oven to 350°F. Grease bottom and side of 2-quart casserole with shortening or cooking spray. In 10-inch skillet, cook sausage, onion and celery over medium heat 8 to 10 minutes, stirring occasionally, until sausage is no longer pink; drain.

3 In casserole, mix sausage mixture, soup, mushrooms and cooked wild rice. Sprinkle with almonds. Cover; bake about 1 hour or until hot and bubbly.

To Make Ahead: Cover unbaked casserole tightly and refrigerate no longer than 24 hours. About 1 hour before serving, heat oven to 350°F. Bake uncovered 45 to 50 minutes or until center is hot.

❝ Soaking the rice cuts down on the cooking time. I would make this the day before my chemo, refrigerate and bake it that evening. It helped to know that I had my family's favorite casserole in the refrigerator and all I had to do was heat it."—**Marilyn T. Shares Her Recipe**

High in calcium, folic acid and vitamins A and C; good source of fiber

1 Serving: Calories 350 (Calories from Fat 160); Total Fat 18g (Saturated Fat 4.5g, Trans Fat 0g); Cholesterol 30mg; Sodium 1090mg; Potassium 410mg; Total Carbohydrate 32g (Dietary Fiber 4g); Protein 14g **% Daily Value:** Vitamin A 0%; Vitamin C 0%; Calcium 6%; Iron 10%; Folic Acid 10%; Magnesium 20% **Exchanges:** 1 ½ Starch, ½ Other Carbohydrate, 1 Vegetable, 1 High-Fat Meat, 2 Fat **Carbohydrate Choices:** 2

A Note from Dr. Ghosh This tasty low-fiber egg dish is great for anyone who needs to restrict fiber, particularly those who have had stomach or intestinal surgery. To eat well, try adding a colorful napkin or a small centerpiece or light a candle to put yourself in an eating mood.

Crab Scramble Casserole

Prep Time: 10 Minutes | **Start to Finish:** 5 Hours | 8 servings

1   tablespoon butter or margarine, melted

12   eggs

½   cup milk

1   teaspoon salt

½   teaspoon white pepper

1 ½   teaspoons chopped fresh or ½ teaspoon dried dill weed

1   cup chopped cooked crabmeat or imitation crabmeat

1   package (8 oz) reduced-fat cream cheese (Neufchâtel), cut into ½-inch cubes

2   medium green onions, sliced (2 tablespoons)

   Paprika

1 Pour butter into 8-inch square (2-quart) glass baking dish; tilt dish to coat bottom. In large bowl, beat eggs, milk, salt, white pepper and dill weed with fork or whisk. Stir in crabmeat, cream cheese and onions. Pour into baking dish. Cover; refrigerate at least 4 hours but no longer than 24 hours.

2 Heat oven to 350°F. Sprinkle paprika over egg mixture. Bake uncovered 45 to 50 minutes or until center is set.

❝So quick to put together, refrigerate and bake later. I liked having this easy recipe for times when I needed to bring something to a potluck but didn't want to spend much time putting it together or baking it."—**Mary W.**

Good source of vitamin A; low fiber

1 Serving: Calories 230 (Calories from Fat 150); Total Fat 16g (Saturated Fat 7g, Trans Fat 0g); Cholesterol 350mg; Sodium 650mg; Potassium 200mg; Total Carbohydrate 4g (Dietary Fiber 0g); Protein 15g **% Daily Value:** Vitamin A 20%; Vitamin C 0%; Calcium 10%; Iron 6%; Folic Acid 10%; Magnesium 6% **Exchanges:** ½ Starch, 2 Medium-Fat Meat, 1 Fat **Carbohydrate Choices:** 0

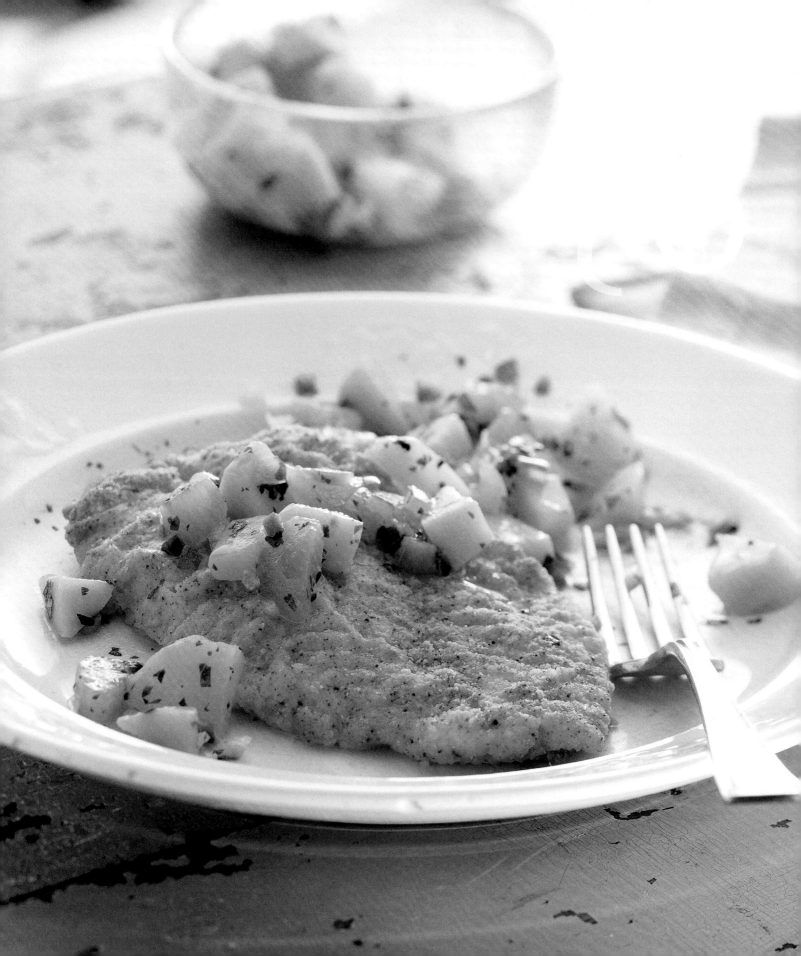

Family-Pleasing Main Dishes }

172   Creamy Corn and Garlic Risotto

173   Spaghetti and "Meatballs"

174   Ravioli with Tomato-Alfredo Sauce

176   Potato and Tomato Pizza

177   Acorn Squash and Apple Soup

178   Cheesy Vegetable Soup

179   Fresh Spinach and New Potato Frittata

180   Hash Brown Frittata

181   Salmon Burgers

182   Layered Tuna Casserole

183   Lemony Fish over Vegetables and Rice

184   Crispy Baked Fish with Tropical Salsa

186   Chicken and Vegetable Stir-Fry

187   Cheesy Chicken and Vegetable Dinner

188   Chicken and Green Beans with Rice

189   Turkey Tetrazzini

190   Turkey Club Squares

192   Old-Fashioned Beef Pot Roast

193   Cheesy Beef Enchiladas

194   Beef Fajita Bowls

196   Beef-Barley Stew

198   Beef and Bean Dinner

199   Breaded Pork Chops

200   Zesty Autumn Pork Stew

Food for Thought Though the calories in this dish are high, the amount of fat is low. This risotto also contains a very high amount of your body's favorite fuel source, carbohydrates.

Creamy Corn and Garlic Risotto

Prep Time: 45 Minutes | **Start to Finish:** 45 Minutes | 4 servings

3 ¾ cups vegetable broth

4 cloves garlic, finely chopped

1 cup uncooked Arborio or medium-grain white rice

3 cups frozen whole kernel corn

½ cup grated Parmesan cheese

⅓ cup shredded mozzarella cheese

¼ cup chopped fresh parsley

1 In 12-inch skillet or 4-quart saucepan, heat ⅓ cup of the broth to boiling. Add garlic; cook 1 minute, stirring occasionally. Stir in rice and frozen corn. Cook 1 minute, stirring occasionally.

2 Stir in remaining broth; heat to boiling. Reduce heat to medium; cook uncovered 15 to 20 minutes, stirring occasionally, until rice is tender and mixture is creamy. Remove from heat. Stir in cheeses and parsley.

❝This is a very tasty main dish, one that my whole family just loves! When my 14-year-old daughter was doing the cooking, this was one of her favorites! We used chopped garlic from a jar, which made the preparation even easier."—Anne R.

High in calcium and folic acid; good source of fiber

1 Serving: Calories 390 (Calories from Fat 60); Total Fat 7g (Saturated Fat 4g, Trans Fat 0g); Cholesterol 15mg; Sodium 1230mg; Potassium 320mg; Total Carbohydrate 68g (Dietary Fiber 4g); Protein 15g **% Daily Value:** Vitamin A 25%; Vitamin C 10%; Calcium 30%; Iron 15%; Folic Acid 30%; Magnesium 15% **Exchanges:** 3 Starch, 1 ½ Other Carbohydrate, 1 Lean Meat, ½ Fat **Carbohydrate Choices:** 4 ½

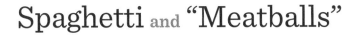

Food for Thought These "meatballs" are rolled in a small amount of wheat germ, which gives them a golden brown color and just a bit of crunch. Wheat germ has a nutty flavor and provides vitamin E, an antioxidant that helps protect cells from damaging substances.

Spaghetti and "Meatballs"

Prep Time: 25 Minutes | **Start to Finish:** 25 Minutes | 6 servings

1   package (16 oz) uncooked spaghetti

2   cups cooked brown or white rice

½   cup quick-cooking oats

1   medium onion, chopped (½ cup)

¼   cup unseasoned dry bread crumbs

¼   cup milk

1   tablespoon chopped fresh or 1 teaspoon dried basil leaves

2   teaspoons chopped fresh or ½ teaspoon dried oregano leaves

¼   teaspoon ground red pepper (cayenne), if desired

1   egg, beaten

½   cup wheat germ

1   tablespoon vegetable oil

2   cups tomato pasta sauce

Shredded Parmesan cheese, if desired

1 Cook and drain spaghetti as directed on package.

2 In large bowl, mix rice, oats, onion, bread crumbs, milk, basil, oregano, red pepper and egg. Shape into 12 balls. Roll balls in wheat germ.

3 In 10-inch skillet, heat oil over medium heat. Add rice balls; cook about 10 minutes, turning occasionally, until golden brown.

4 Heat pasta sauce until hot. Serve sauce and rice balls over spaghetti. Sprinkle with cheese.

66 This is a vegetarian spaghetti and meatballs, but my family didn't notice the difference, and they're pretty determined meat eaters. Spaghetti tastes great after chemo, and it is easy to reheat in single servings in the microwave. However, the real meatballs taste like aluminum foil and these don't, so they are a great alternative."
—**Anne R.**

High in iron, folic acid and magnesium; excellent source of fiber

1 Serving: Calories 610 (Calories from Fat 90); Total Fat 10g (Saturated Fat 2g, Trans Fat 0g); Cholesterol 35mg; Sodium 750mg; Potassium 550mg; Total Carbohydrate 108g (Dietary Fiber 9g); Protein 20g **% Daily Value:** Vitamin A 10%; Vitamin C 6%; Calcium 8%; Iron 30%; Folic Acid 50%; Magnesium 30% **Exchanges:** 6 Starch, 1 Other Carbohydrate, 1 ½ Fat **Carbohydrate Choices:** 7

Food for Thought This heavenly combo of tomato and cheese is brimming with calcium, an important healing nutrient. Calcium is key to strong bones and teeth and helps prevent osteoporosis. For women in menopause, maintaining strong bones can be a challenge, so sufficient calcium and vitamin D are necessary to prevent bone fractures. Regular health maintenance is very important during cancer treatment.

Ravioli with Tomato-Alfredo Sauce

Prep Time: 10 Minutes | **Start to Finish:** 20 Minutes | 6 servings

2   packages (9 oz each) refrigerated cheese-filled ravioli

1   package (8 oz) sliced fresh mushrooms (3 cups)

1   large onion, coarsely chopped (1 cup)

1   jar (24 to 28 oz) tomato pasta sauce

½   cup half-and-half or refrigerated nondairy creamer

¼   cup grated Parmesan cheese

¼   cup chopped fresh parsley

1   Cook and drain ravioli as directed on package; keep warm.

2   Spray same saucepan with cooking spray; heat over medium heat. Add mushrooms and onion; cook about 5 minutes, stirring frequently, until onion is crisp-tender.

3   Stir in pasta sauce and half-and-half. Heat to boiling. Reduce heat to low; stir in ravioli, cheese and parsley.

66 I love pasta because it is easy to make and then reheat in small portions. It is also so satisfying. I really feel like I've eaten good-for-me food, even if I eat only five or six ravioli squares at a serving."—**Anne R.**

High in calcium and vitamins A and C; good source of fiber and potassium

1 Serving: Calories 290 (Calories from Fat 110); Total Fat 12g (Saturated Fat 4.5g, Trans Fat 0g); Cholesterol 55mg; Sodium 1060mg; Potassium 660mg; Total Carbohydrate 36g (Dietary Fiber 3g); Protein 10g **% Daily Value:** Vitamin A 20%; Vitamin C 15%; Calcium 20%; Iron 15%; Folic Acid 10%; Magnesium 10% **Exchanges:** 1 ½ Starch, 1 Other Carbohydrate, ½ Medium-Fat Meat, 1 ½ Fat **Carbohydrate Choices:** 2 ½

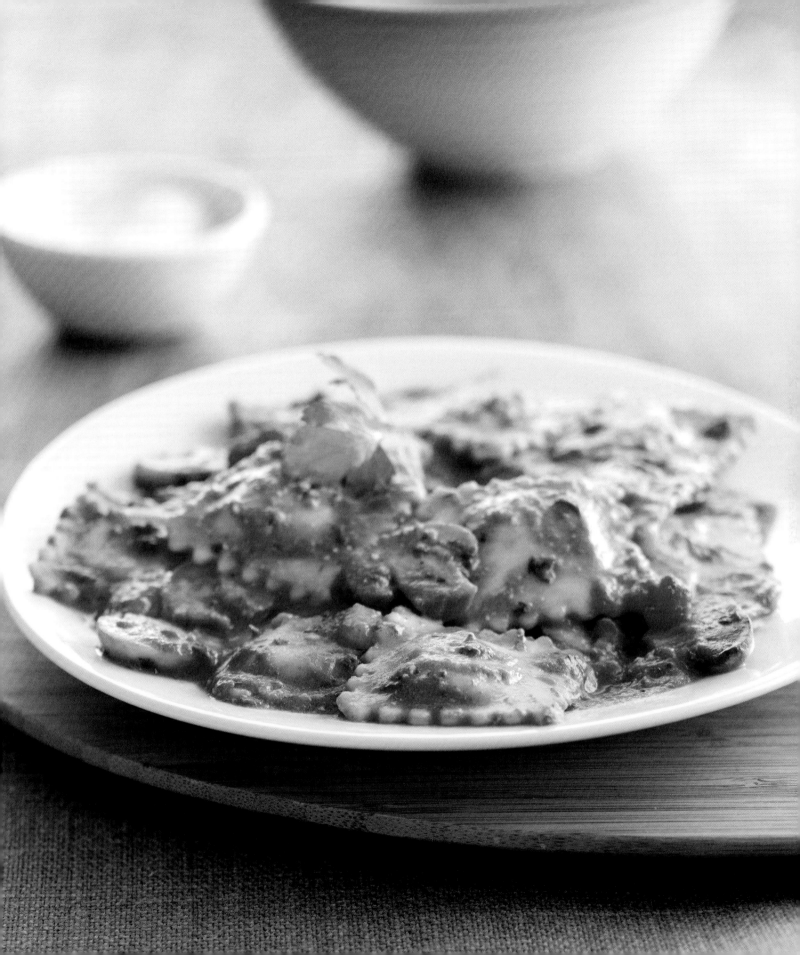

Food for Thought This is a fun twist on a traditional Italian pizza. For variety, try adding mushrooms, artichoke hearts or any leftover cooked vegetable.

Potato and Tomato Pizza

Prep Time: 15 Minutes | **Start to Finish:** 40 Minutes | 6 servings

1 can (13.8 oz) refrigerated classic pizza crust

2 cups frozen potato wedges with skins, thawed (about 32 pieces)

1 tablespoon Dijon mustard

1 medium zucchini, cut lengthwise in half, then cut crosswise into slices

3 medium plum (Roma) tomatoes, coarsely chopped (1 ½ cups)

½ teaspoon dried basil leaves

¼ teaspoon coarsely ground pepper

1 cup shredded mozzarella cheese (4 oz)

1 Heat oven to 425°F. Spray 14-inch pizza pan with cooking spray. Press pizza crust dough in pan.

2 Toss potatoes and mustard until potatoes are coated; arrange on crust. Top with zucchini, tomatoes, basil, pepper and cheese.

3 Bake 20 to 25 minutes or until cheese is melted and crust is golden brown.

❝In between treatments, I went to Italy with my daughter and the Latin Club. We couldn't believe the first time we were served 'American pizza,' which was cheese pizza covered with French fries. This recipe reminds me of that, and is a quick and easy meal for the entire family."—Anne R.

Good source of fiber and magnesium

1 Serving: Calories 280 (Calories from Fat 70); Total Fat 8g (Saturated Fat 3g, Trans Fat 0g); Cholesterol 10mg; Sodium 530mg; Potassium 240mg; Total Carbohydrate 41g (Dietary Fiber 3g); Protein 11g **% Daily Value:** Vitamin A 8%; Vitamin C 8%; Calcium 15%; Iron 15%; Folic Acid 20%; Magnesium 6% **Exchanges:** 2 ½ Starch, ½ Vegetable, 1 ½ Fat **Carbohydrate Choices:** 3

A Note from Dr. Ghosh Fruits and vegetables are important sources of fiber, vitamins and minerals. Hundreds of studies have shown there may be a protective effect against certain types of cancers when plant foods, such as fruits and vegetables, are consumed in quantity.

Acorn Squash and Apple Soup

Prep Time: 20 Minutes | **Start to Finish:** 1 Hour | 6 servings (1 cup each)

1 medium acorn or butternut squash (1 ½ to 2 lb)

2 tablespoons butter or margarine

1 medium yellow onion, sliced (½ cup)

2 medium tart cooking apples (Granny Smith, Greening or Haralson), peeled, sliced

1 teaspoon dried thyme leaves

¼ teaspoon dried basil leaves

2 cans (14 oz each) chicken broth (4 cups)

½ cup half-and-half

1 teaspoon ground nutmeg

½ teaspoon salt

¼ teaspoon white or black pepper

1 Heat oven to 350°F. Cut squash in half; remove seeds and fibers. Place cut sides up in 13x9-inch pan. Pour ¼ inch water into pan. Bake uncovered about 40 minutes or until tender. Cool; remove pulp from rind and set aside.

2 Meanwhile, in heavy 3-quart saucepan, melt butter over medium heat. Add onion; cook 2 to 3 minutes, stirring occasionally, until crisp-tender. Stir in apples, thyme and basil. Cook 2 minutes, stirring constantly. Stir in broth. Heat to boiling. Reduce heat; simmer uncovered 30 minutes.

3 Remove 1 cup apples with slotted spoon; set aside. Place one-third each of the remaining apple mixture and squash in blender or food processor. Cover; blend on medium speed about 1 minute or until smooth, then pour into bowl. Continue to blend in small batches until all soup is pureed.

4 Return blended mixture and 1 cup reserved apples to saucepan. Stir in half-and-half, nutmeg, salt and pepper; cook over low heat until thoroughly heated.

66 I found ways to make meals a time of enjoyment. Candles, music, a glass of wine and good company do wonders for the appetite. Great recipes, such as this soup, also boost my spirit."—**Mary W. Shares Her Recipe**

Good source of potassium; excellent source of fiber

1 Serving: Calories 190 (Calories from Fat 70); Total Fat 7g (Saturated Fat 4g, Trans Fat 0g); Cholesterol 20mg; Sodium 670mg; Potassium 690mg; Total Carbohydrate 26g (Dietary Fiber 6g); Protein 5g **% Daily Value:** Vitamin A 15%; Vitamin C 15%; Calcium 8%; Iron 8%; Folic Acid 6%; Magnesium 15% **Exchanges:** 1 Starch, ½ Other Carbohydrate, ½ Vegetable, 1 ½ Fat **Carbohydrate Choices:** 2

A Note from Dr. Ghosh Soothing to a sore mouth, this creamy soup can really bring comfort. If the larger pieces of veggies are difficult to swallow, try pureeing the cooked veggies in the blender or food processor to smooth out the texture of the soup.

Cheesy Vegetable Soup

Prep Time: 15 Minutes | **Start to Finish:** 15 Minutes | 4 servings

4   oz reduced-fat prepared cheese product (from 16-oz loaf), cubed

3 ½   cups fat-free (skim) milk

½   teaspoon chili powder

2   cups cooked brown or white rice

1   bag (1 lb) frozen cauliflower, carrots and snow pea pods (or other combination), thawed, drained

1   In 3-quart saucepan, heat cheese and milk over low heat, stirring occasionally, until cheese is melted.

2   Stir in chili powder. Stir in rice and vegetables; cook until hot.

66 Soup is a comfort food, and since the whole family loves it, we eat soup often at our house. This is one of my favorite recipes because I can use whatever combination of vegetables I want, and if I cook the rice ahead of time, it comes together in just a few minutes."
—Mary W.

High in calcium and vitamin A

1 Serving: Calories 280 (Calories from Fat 40); Total Fat 4.5g (Saturated Fat 2.5g, Trans Fat 0g); Cholesterol 15mg; Sodium 840mg; Potassium 650mg; Total Carbohydrate 42g (Dietary Fiber 6g); Protein 18g **% Daily Value:** Vitamin A 60%; Vitamin C 30%; Calcium 45%; Iron 6%; Folic Acid 15%; Magnesium 20% **Exchanges:** 1 ½ Starch, 1 Skim Milk, 1 Vegetable, ½ Medium-Fat Meat **Carbohydrate Choices:** 3

A Note from Dr. Ghosh Spinach is a wonderful source of so many nutrients, including folic acid. We need folic acid for all cells to operate properly and to prevent birth defects to the brain and spinal cord of developing unborn babies.

Fresh Spinach and New Potato Frittata

Prep Time: 25 Minutes | **Start to Finish:** 35 Minutes | 4 servings

6	eggs
2	tablespoons milk
¼	teaspoon dried marjoram leaves
¼	teaspoon salt
2	tablespoons butter or margarine
6	or 7 small red potatoes, thinly sliced (2 cups)
¼	teaspoon salt
1	cup firmly packed bite-size pieces spinach
¼	cup oil-packed sun-dried tomatoes, drained, sliced
3	medium green onions, cut into ¼-inch pieces
½	cup shredded Swiss cheese (2 oz)

1 In medium bowl, beat eggs, milk, marjoram and ¼ teaspoon salt; set aside.

2 In 10-inch nonstick skillet, melt butter over medium heat. Add potatoes to skillet; sprinkle with ¼ teaspoon salt. Cover; cook 8 to 10 minutes, stirring occasionally, until potatoes are tender.

3 Stir in spinach, tomatoes and onions. Cook, stirring occasionally, just until spinach is wilted; reduce heat to low.

4 Carefully pour egg mixture over potato mixture. Cover; cook 6 to 8 minutes or just until top is set. Sprinkle with cheese. Cover; cook about 1 minute or until cheese is melted.

"After surgery, I was put on a low-residue diet. All of a sudden, green beans and spinach were my only choices for green leafy vegetables. This recipe tastes great even without the onions and tomatoes, which aren't on my low-residue list. I used onion salt to get the onion flavor I like. Frittatas, easy to make and reheat in small slices, are great for grazing!"—Anne R.

High in calcium, vitamins A and C and potassium; excellent source of fiber

1 Serving: Calories 470 (Calories from Fat 170); Total Fat 19g (Saturated Fat 9g, Trans Fat 0g); Cholesterol 345mg; Sodium 510mg; Potassium 1590mg; Total Carbohydrate 56g (Dietary Fiber 6g); Protein 20g **% Daily Value:** Vitamin A 35%; Vitamin C 30%; Calcium 20%; Iron 25%; Folic Acid 30%; Magnesium 25% **Exchanges:** 3 Starch, ½ Other Carbohydrate, 1 Vegetable, 1 Medium-Fat Meat, 2 ½ Fat **Carbohydrate Choices:** 4

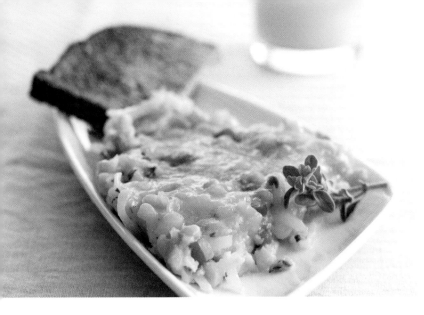

Food for Thought Offering a great source of potassium, potatoes can help maintain the body's fluid balance. Potassium is also key for proper nerve and muscle function.

Hash Brown Frittata

Prep Time: 10 Minutes | **Start to Finish:** 35 Minutes | 4 servings

2 cups refrigerated shredded hash brown potatoes

1 can (11 oz) whole kernel corn with red and green peppers, drained

1 teaspoon onion salt

2 teaspoons vegetable oil

5 eggs or 1 cup fat-free egg product

⅓ cup milk

1 ½ teaspoons chopped fresh or ½ teaspoon dried marjoram leaves

½ teaspoon red pepper sauce

⅔ cup shredded Cheddar cheese

1 In medium bowl, mix potatoes, corn and onion salt. In 10-inch nonstick skillet, heat oil over medium heat. Pack potato mixture firmly into skillet, leaving ½-inch space around edge. Reduce heat to medium-low; cook uncovered about 10 minutes or until bottom starts to brown.

2 Meanwhile, in another medium bowl, mix eggs, milk, marjoram and pepper sauce. Pour egg mixture over potato mixture. Cook uncovered over medium-low heat. As mixture begins to set on bottom and side, gently lift cooked portions with pancake turner so that thin, uncooked portion can flow to bottom; avoid constant stirring. Cook about 5 minutes or until eggs are thickened throughout but still moist.

3 Sprinkle with cheese. Reduce heat to low; cover and cook about 10 minutes or until center is set and cheese is bubbly. Loosen bottom of frittata with pancake turner. Cut frittata into 4 wedges.

❝For a couple of days after my chemotherapy treatments, I lived on refrigerated potatoes. Not only were they easy to get down and soothing to my mouth, I could keep them on hand and put them in tasty recipes like this.❞—Susan S.

High in potassium and folic acid; good source of calcium and fiber

1 Serving: Calories 480 (Calories from Fat 230); Total Fat 26g (Saturated Fat 13g, Trans Fat 0.5g); Cholesterol 310mg; Sodium 940mg; Potassium 750mg; Total Carbohydrate 43g (Dietary Fiber 4g); Protein 17g **% Daily Value:** Vitamin A 20%; Vitamin C 15%; Calcium 15%; Iron 10%; Folic Acid 20%; Magnesium 15% **Exchanges:** 2 ½ Starch, ½ Other Carbohydrate, 1 Medium-Fat Meat, 4 Fat **Carbohydrate Choices:** 3

A Note from Dr. Ghosh Salmon contains a vitamin called pantothenic acid, which we don't often hear about. Pantothenic acid helps release energy from carbohydrate-containing foods, plus it helps manufacture certain body hormones.

Salmon Burgers

Prep Time: 25 Minutes | **Start to Finish:** 25 Minutes | 5 sandwiches

CUCUMBER SAUCE

⅓ cup finely chopped seeded peeled cucumber

¼ cup plain yogurt

¼ cup mayonnaise or salad dressing

1 teaspoon chopped fresh or ¼ teaspoon dried tarragon leaves

BURGERS

1 can (14 ¾ oz) salmon, drained, flaked

½ cup crushed round buttery crackers

2 tablespoons chopped fresh parsley

½ teaspoon grated lemon peel

1 tablespoon lemon juice

2 medium green onions, sliced (2 tablespoons)

1 egg

2 tablespoons vegetable oil

5 English muffins, split, toasted

1 In small bowl, mix cucumber sauce ingredients; set aside.

2 In medium bowl, mix all burger ingredients except oil and muffins. Shape mixture into 5 patties.

3 In 10-inch skillet, heat oil over medium heat. Add patties; cook 8 to 10 minutes, turning once, until golden brown. Serve patties on muffins with cucumber sauce.

66 Salmon is great-tasting, even during chemo, and the cool taste of the cucumbers is super. Quick and easy is good! This recipe makes me think spring."—Anne R.

High in calcium and folic acid

1 Sandwich: Calories 420 (Calories from Fat 200); Total Fat 22g (Saturated Fat 4g, Trans Fat 0g); Cholesterol 110mg; Sodium 680mg; Potassium 370mg; Total Carbohydrate 32g (Dietary Fiber 2g); Protein 24g **% Daily Value:** Vitamin A 8%; Vitamin C 6%; Calcium 35%; Iron 20%; Folic Acid 10%; Magnesium 10% **Exchanges:** 1 ½ Starch, 1 ½ Vegetable, ½ Lean Meat, 1 ½ Medium-Fat Meat, 2 ½ Fat **Carbohydrate Choices:** 2

Food for Thought This recipe supplies many essential nutrients, such as niacin, that are key to the release of energy from foods. Niacin is important for healthy skin, mouth and nervous system.

Layered Tuna Casserole

Prep Time: 10 Minutes | **Start to Finish:** 45 Minutes | 4 servings (1 ½ cups each)

1   package (6 oz) chow mein noodles (3 cups)

1   can (10 ¾ oz) condensed cream of celery soup

1   can (5 oz) evaporated milk (⅔ cup)

1   can (6 oz) tuna packed in water or 1 can (5 oz) chunk chicken, drained

1   can (10 ¾ oz) condensed chicken rice soup

¼   to ½ cup unseasoned dry bread crumbs or crushed potato chips

1 Heat oven to 350°F. Spray 3-quart casserole with cooking spray. Layer all ingredients except bread crumbs in casserole in order listed. Sprinkle with bread crumbs.

2 Bake uncovered 30 to 35 minutes or until bread crumbs are brown and tuna mixture is hot and bubbly in center.

❝Stress can affect digestion, so relax and breathe deeply when you are eating. And remember, you have all the time in the world, so enjoy your food. Foods like this casserole are too good to hurry through—enjoy it."—**Pat Y. Shares Her Recipe**

High in calcium, iron and vitamin A; good source of fiber

1 Serving: Calories 430 (Calories from Fat 180); Total Fat 20g (Saturated Fat 4.5g, Trans Fat 0g); Cholesterol 25mg; Sodium 890mg; Potassium 370mg; Total Carbohydrate 43g (Dietary Fiber 2g); Protein 19g
% Daily Value: Vitamin A 15%; Vitamin C 0%; Calcium 15%; Iron 20%; Folic Acid 15%; Magnesium 15%
Exchanges: 2 ½ Starch, ½ Other Carbohydrate, 1 ½ High-Fat Meat, 1 ½ Fat **Carbohydrate Choices:** 3

Food for Thought This simple recipe is a huge help when you need to prepare dinner in a flash. If you don't like the frozen vegetable combination, select one you prefer and prepare the dish the same way.

Lemony Fish over Vegetables and Rice

Prep Time: 15 Minutes | **Start to Finish:** 30 Minutes | 4 servings

1 box (6 oz) fried rice (rice and vermicelli mix with almonds and Asian seasonings)

2 tablespoons butter or margarine

2 cups water

½ teaspoon grated lemon peel

1 bag (1 lb) frozen broccoli, corn and peppers (or other combination)

1 lb cod, haddock or other medium-firm fish fillets, about ½ inch thick, cut into 4 serving pieces

½ teaspoon lemon-pepper seasoning

1 tablespoon lemon juice

Chopped fresh parsley, if desired

1 In 12-inch nonstick skillet, cook rice and butter over medium heat about 3 minutes, stirring occasionally, until rice is golden brown. Stir in water, seasoning packet from rice mix and lemon peel. Heat to boiling. Reduce heat to low; cover and simmer 10 minutes.

2 Stir in frozen vegetables. Heat to boiling over medium-high heat, stirring occasionally. Arrange fish on rice mixture. Sprinkle fish with lemon-pepper seasoning; drizzle with lemon juice.

3 Reduce heat to low. Cover; simmer 8 to 12 minutes or until fish flakes easily with fork and vegetables are tender. Sprinkle with parsley.

❝This tastes great on the post-chemo days after a bout with diarrhea. I eat this with a large strawberry smoothie made with strawberries, frozen daiquiri mix and ice cubes in the blender. It's a great potassium booster that tastes sensational, too.❞—Anne R.

High in vitamins A and C and folic acid; good source of fiber

1 Serving: Calories 250 (Calories from Fat 70); Total Fat 8g (Saturated Fat 4g, Trans Fat 0g); Cholesterol 75mg; Sodium 620mg; Potassium 560mg; Total Carbohydrate 19g (Dietary Fiber 3g); Protein 26g **% Daily Value:** Vitamin A 25%; Vitamin C 35%; Calcium 6%; Iron 10%; Folic Acid 15%; Magnesium 20% **Exchanges:** 1 Starch, 1 Vegetable, 3 Very Lean Meat, 1 Fat **Carbohydrate Choices:** 1

A Note from Dr. Ghosh Potassium is a mineral essential for muscle function. Additional sources of potassium are needed during times of prolonged vomiting, diarrhea or diuretic use or when taking certain antibiotics.

Crispy Baked Fish with Tropical Salsa

Prep Time: 20 Minutes | **Start to Finish:** 30 Minutes | 4 servings

FISH

- 3 tablespoons butter or margarine
- ⅔ cup Original Bisquick® mix
- ¼ cup yellow cornmeal
- 1 teaspoon chili powder
- 1 ¼ teaspoons salt
- 1 lb orange roughy or other white fish fillets
- 1 egg, beaten

FRUIT SALSA

- 1 can (8 oz) pineapple chunks, drained
- 1 tablespoon finely chopped red onion
- 1 tablespoon chopped fresh cilantro
- 1 tablespoon lime juice
- 1 kiwifruit, peeled, chopped
- 1 mango or papaya, cut lengthwise in half, pitted and chopped
- 1 jalapeño chile, seeded, finely chopped

1 Heat oven to 425°F. In 13x9-inch pan, melt butter in oven.

2 In small bowl, mix Bisquick mix, cornmeal, chili powder and salt. Dip fish fillets into egg, then coat with Bisquick mixture. Place in pan.

3 Bake uncovered 10 minutes. Turn fish; bake about 15 minutes longer or until fish flakes easily with fork.

4 Meanwhile, in glass or plastic bowl, mix all fruit salsa ingredients. Serve salsa with fish.

❝Food is always more appetizing when beautifully presented. The bright colors of the fruit in the salsa make this a very pretty dish, so refreshing and healthy, too.❞—**Mary W.**

High in potassium, magnesium, folic acid and vitamins A and C; good source of fiber

1 Serving: Calories 390 (Calories from Fat 130); Total Fat 15g (Saturated Fat 7g, Trans Fat 1g); Cholesterol 140mg; Sodium 1170mg; Potassium 610mg; Total Carbohydrate 37g (Dietary Fiber 3g); Protein 27g **% Daily Value:** Vitamin A 20%; Vitamin C 35%; Calcium 6%; Iron 10%; Folic Acid 15%; Magnesium 20% **Exchanges:** ½ Starch, ½ Fruit, 1 ½ Other Carbohydrate, 3 ½ Very Lean Meat, 2 ½ Fat **Carbohydrate Choices:** 2 ½

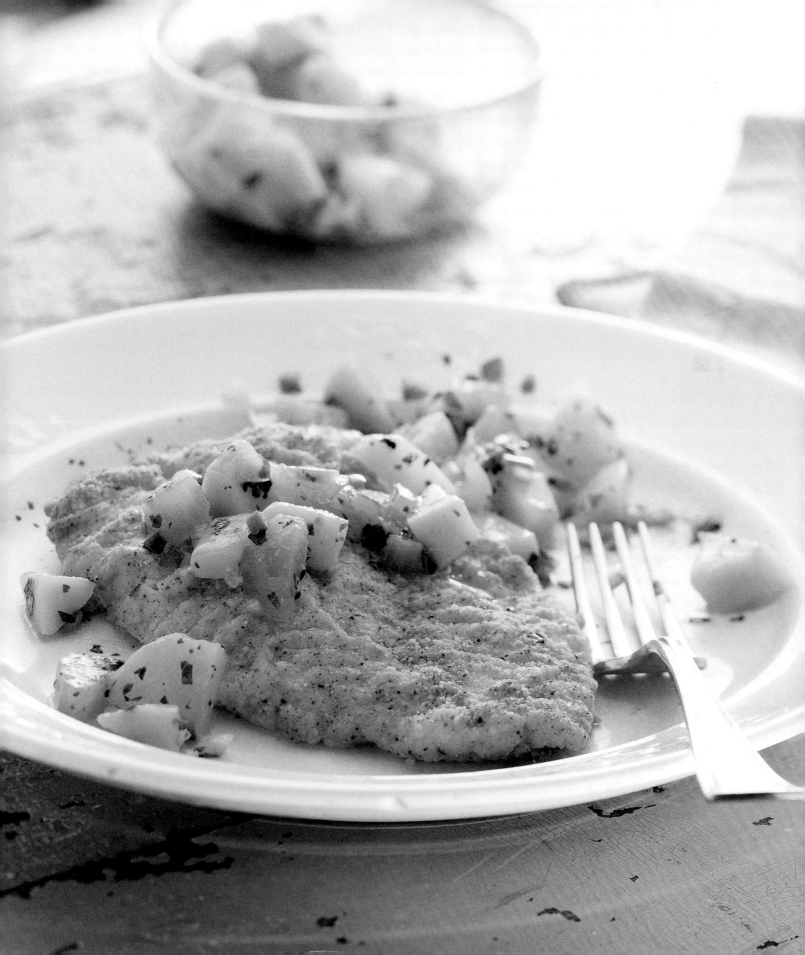

N

Food for Thought Loaded with nutrients, this chicken and veggie dish is outstanding. If you need a bit of extra flavor, add a dash or two of red pepper flakes to bring on the heat.

Chicken and Vegetable Stir-Fry

Prep Time: 25 Minutes | **Start to Finish:** 25 Minutes | 4 servings

1 cup uncooked regular long-grain rice

2 teaspoons vegetable oil

1 lb boneless skinless chicken breasts, cut into ½-inch pieces

¼ teaspoon salt

1 bag (1 lb) fresh (refrigerated) stir-fry vegetables (4 cups)

½ cup water

½ cup classic-style stir-fry sauce

1 tablespoon honey

2 cups chow mein noodles

¼ cup cashew pieces

1 Cook rice as directed on package. Meanwhile, in 12-inch nonstick skillet, heat oil over medium-high heat. Add chicken; sprinkle with salt. Stir-fry 4 to 6 minutes or until brown.

2 Add vegetables and water to skillet. Heat to boiling. Reduce heat to medium; cover and cook 5 to 7 minutes, stirring occasionally, until vegetables are crisp-tender. Stir in stir-fry sauce and honey; cook until thoroughly heated.

3 Divide rice and noodles among bowls. Top with chicken mixture. Sprinkle with cashews.

❝A satisfying meal with family and friends is a large part of a renewed emphasis on quality of life. This quick recipe, because it can easily be doubled and cooked in batches, lends itself to sharing with others."—**Mary W.**

High in potassium, iron, magnesium, folic acid and vitamins A and C; good source of fiber

1 Serving: Calories 640 (Calories from Fat 190); Total Fat 21g (Saturated Fat 5g, Trans Fat 0g); Cholesterol 80mg; Sodium 2210mg; Potassium 540mg; Total Carbohydrate 77g (Dietary Fiber 4g); Protein 34g **% Daily Value:** Vitamin A 70%; Vitamin C 15%; Calcium 6%; Iron 25%; Folic Acid 25%; Magnesium 25% **Exchanges:** 4 Starch, ½ Other Carbohydrate, 2 Vegetable, 2 ½ Lean Meat, 2 ½ Fat **Carbohydrate Choices:** 5

A Note from Dr. Ghosh Reduce the amount of cheese in this recipe if foods containing fat bother you. Sprinkling just a bit of Parmesan cheese on top of the chicken gives it a little extra zing, but not a lot of fat.

Cheesy Chicken and Vegetable Dinner

Prep Time: 20 Minutes | **Start to Finish:** 20 Minutes | 6 servings

1 teaspoon canola or vegetable oil

1 ¼ lb boneless skinless chicken breasts, cut into ¾-inch pieces

2 large carrots, cut into ⅛-inch slices (2 cups)

1 medium zucchini, cut into ⅛-inch slices (2 cups)

2 tablespoons soy sauce

8 medium green onions, sliced (½ cup)

2 cups shredded sharp reduced-fat Cheddar cheese (8 oz)

1 Heat 12-inch nonstick skillet over medium-high heat. Add oil; rotate skillet to coat bottom. Add chicken; stir-fry 4 to 5 minutes or until no longer pink in center. Remove from skillet.

2 Add carrots and zucchini to skillet; stir-fry 4 to 5 minutes or until crisp-tender. Add chicken and soy sauce; toss until chicken and vegetables are coated with soy sauce.

3 Sprinkle with onions and cheese; cover skillet until cheese is melted.

❝I do the cooking and food preparation as I feel up to it; otherwise, I let my husband take over."—**Mary W.**

High in calcium and vitamin A

1 Serving: Calories 290 (Calories from Fat 150); Total Fat 16g (Saturated Fat 9g, Trans Fat 0g); Cholesterol 100mg; Sodium 600mg; Potassium 380mg; Total Carbohydrate 4g (Dietary Fiber 1g); Protein 32g
% Daily Value: Vitamin A 30%; Vitamin C 8%; Calcium 25%; Iron 8%; Folic Acid 8%; Magnesium 10%
Exchanges: 1 Vegetable, 4 Lean Meat, 1 Fat **Carbohydrate Choices:** 0

A Note from Dr. Ghosh If you're looking for low-fiber, low-residue options after surgery, omit the celery and onion and cut the green bean amount in half for a simple casserole that can bring you comfort.

Chicken and Green Beans with Rice

Prep Time: 10 Minutes | **Start to Finish:** 1 Hour | 6 servings

2 cups cut-up cooked chicken

2 cups cooked rice

½ teaspoon salt

¼ teaspoon pepper

2 medium stalks celery, sliced (1 cup)

1 medium onion, chopped (½ cup)

1 can (14 oz) chicken broth

1 box (9 oz) frozen cut green beans, thawed

1 Heat oven to 350°F. Spray 2-quart casserole with cooking spray. Mix all ingredients in casserole.

2 Cover; bake 45 to 50 minutes or until beans are tender and mixture is hot.

❝I was told that drinking water with your meal will help settle your food, and it worked for me! Reliable recipes such as this one also helped me."—**Pat Y. Shares Her Recipe**

High in vitamin A; low fiber

1 Serving: Calories 210 (Calories from Fat 60); Total Fat 7g (Saturated Fat 2g, Trans Fat 0g); Cholesterol 40mg; Sodium 740mg; Potassium 340mg; Total Carbohydrate 20g (Dietary Fiber 2g); Protein 16g **% Daily Value:** Vitamin A 4%; Vitamin C 8%; Calcium 4%; Iron 10%; Folic Acid 10%; Magnesium 8% **Exchanges:** 1 Starch, 1 Vegetable, 1 ½ Lean Meat, ½ Fat **Carbohydrate Choices:** 1

Food for Thought Poultry, such as turkey and chicken, is a good source of zinc, a mineral needed in very small amounts. Deficiencies of zinc can lead to decreased appetite and a reduced ability to taste and smell.

Turkey Tetrazzini

Prep Time: 25 Minutes | **Start to Finish:** 55 Minutes | 5 servings (1 cup each)

1	package (7 oz) spaghetti, broken into thirds
¼	cup butter or margarine
¼	cup all-purpose flour
½	teaspoon salt
¼	teaspoon pepper
¾	cup chicken broth
1 ¼	cups milk
2	cups cubed cooked turkey or chicken
1	jar (4.5 oz) sliced mushrooms, drained
½	cup grated Parmesan cheese

1 Heat oven to 350°F. Cook spaghetti as directed on package.

2 Meanwhile, in 3-quart saucepan, melt butter over medium heat. Stir in flour, salt and pepper. Cook, stirring constantly, until mixture is bubbly; remove from heat. Stir in broth and milk. Heat to boiling, stirring constantly. Boil and stir 1 minute. Stir in turkey and mushrooms.

3 Drain spaghetti; place in ungreased 2-quart casserole. Stir in turkey mixture. Sprinkle with cheese.

4 Bake uncovered about 30 minutes or until hot and bubbly.

❝During my chemotherapy, this is the one dish everyone in my family could sit down to and enjoy. It freezes well, so it can be frozen and reheated when you need it.”—**Mary W. Shares Her Recipe**

High in calcium and folic acid; good source of fiber

1 Serving: Calories 450 (Calories from Fat 150); Total Fat 17g (Saturated Fat 9g, Trans Fat 0.5g); Cholesterol 90mg; Sodium 910mg; Potassium 360mg; Total Carbohydrate 44g (Dietary Fiber 3g); Protein 30g **% Daily Value:** Vitamin A 10%; Vitamin C 0%; Calcium 20%; Iron 15%; Folic Acid 25%; Magnesium 15% **Exchanges:** 2 ½ Starch, ½ Milk, 2 ½ Medium-Fat Meat **Carbohydrate Choices:** 3

A Note from Dr. Ghosh Low-fiber foods are good for certain kinds of cancers because they don't cause intestinal distress, especially right after surgery. To make this recipe a low-residue option, too, omit the cheese, tomato and green onions.

Turkey Club Squares

Prep Time: 20 Minutes　|　**Start to Finish:** 30 Minutes　|　6 servings

6 slices bacon

2 cups Original Bisquick® mix

⅓ cup mayonnaise or salad dressing

⅓ cup milk

2 cups cubed cooked turkey

2 medium green onions, sliced (2 tablespoons)

¼ cup mayonnaise or salad dressing

1 large tomato, chopped (1 cup)

1 cup shredded Colby-Monterey Jack cheese blend (4 oz)

1 Heat oven to 450°F. Spray cookie sheet with cooking spray. Line microwavable plate with microwavable paper towel. Place bacon on paper towel; cover with another paper towel. Microwave on High 4 to 6 minutes or until crisp. Crumble bacon; set aside.

2 Meanwhile, in medium bowl, stir Bisquick mix, ⅓ cup mayonnaise and the milk until soft dough forms. Press dough into 12x8-inch rectangle on cookie sheet. Bake 8 to 10 minutes or until crust is golden brown.

3 In medium bowl, mix turkey, onions, bacon and ¼ cup mayonnaise. Spoon over crust to within ¼ inch of edges. Sprinkle with tomato and cheese. Bake 5 to 6 minutes or until mixture is hot and cheese is melted.

❝I find that eating an early dinner allows for better digestion and sleep."—**Mary W.**

High in calcium; low fiber

1 Serving: Calories 520 (Calories from Fat 320); Total Fat 35g (Saturated Fat 10g, Trans Fat 1g); Cholesterol 75mg; Sodium 1030mg; Potassium 330mg; Total Carbohydrate 27g (Dietary Fiber 0g); Protein 24g **% Daily Value:** Vitamin A 10%; Vitamin C 4%; Calcium 25%; Iron 10%; Folic Acid 15%; Magnesium 8% **Exchanges:** 1 ½ Starch, ½ Other Carbohydrate, 2 ½ Medium-Fat Meat, 4 ½ Fat **Carbohydrate Choices:** 2

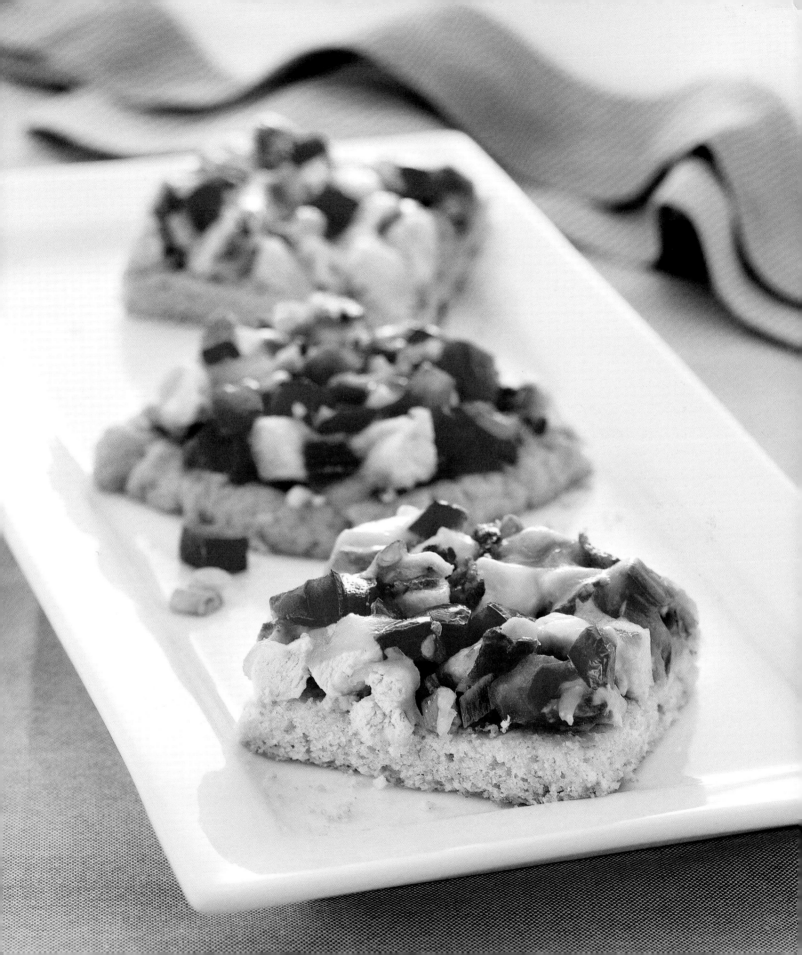

A Note from Dr. Ghosh Broiling, braising and roasting are healthy techniques to use when preparing meats. Avoid charring meats so they appear blackened, and limit consumption of processed meats because of their nitrite and nitrate content, processes that are known cancer-causing agents.

Old-Fashioned Beef Pot Roast

Prep Time: 10 Minutes | **Start to Finish:** 8 Hours 10 Minutes | 8 servings

4 medium potatoes, cut into chunks

2 lb medium carrots, cut into chunks

¼ cup water

1 can (10 ¾ oz) condensed cream of chicken soup

½ package (2-oz size) onion soup mix (1 envelope)

1 beef arm, blade or cross rib pot roast (3 lb)

1 Spray inside of 5- to 6-quart slow cooker with cooking spray. Place potatoes, carrots and water in cooker.

2 In small bowl, mix chicken soup and onion soup mix. Pour half of mixture over vegetables in cooker. Place beef on top. Pour remaining soup mixture over beef.

3 Cover; cook on Low heat setting 8 to 9 hours.

66 Simple foods that I grew up on, like pot roast, appealed to me the most."—**Marilyn T. Shares Her Recipe**

High in iron, potassium and vitamin A

1 Serving: Calories 270 (Calories from Fat 80); Total Fat 9g (Saturated Fat 3.5g, Trans Fat 0g); Cholesterol 45mg; Sodium 320mg; Potassium 790mg; Total Carbohydrate 22g (Dietary Fiber 2g); Protein 25g
% Daily Value: Vitamin A 10%; Vitamin C 10%; Calcium 2%; Iron 20%; Folic Acid 4%; Magnesium 10%
Exchanges: 1 Starch, 1 Vegetable, 1 Very Lean Meat, 1 Lean Meat, 1 Medium-Fat Meat **Carbohydrate Choices:** 1 ½

Food for Thought Try ethnic recipes; the different flavors, mix of ingredients and spices may appeal to your tastes. This Mexican-style dish is an excellent source of many important nutrients, like calcium, iron and potassium.

Cheesy Beef Enchiladas

Prep Time: 10 Minutes | **Start to Finish:** 30 Minutes | 10 servings

1 lb extra-lean (at least 90%) ground beef

½ teaspoon salt

¼ teaspoon pepper

1 medium onion, chopped (½ cup)

1 cup sour cream

1 can (11 oz) vacuum-packed super sweet yellow and white corn, drained

2 cups shredded Mexican 4-cheese blend (8 oz)

8 flour tortillas (8 inch)

1 can (10 oz) hot enchilada sauce

1 can (10 oz) mild enchilada sauce

1 Heat oven to 350°F. Sprinkle beef with salt and pepper. In 10-inch skillet, cook beef and onion over medium heat 8 to 10 minutes, stirring occasionally, until beef is brown; drain. Stir in sour cream and corn.

2 In bottom of ungreased 13x9-inch (3-quart) glass baking dish, sprinkle 1 cup of the cheese. Spoon about 2 tablespoons beef mixture onto each tortilla; top with a few drops hot enchilada sauce. Roll tortilla around filling; place seam side down on cheese in baking dish. Pour remaining hot and mild sauces over enchiladas. Sprinkle with remaining 1 cup cheese.

3 Bake uncovered about 20 minutes or until cheese is bubbly.

"You need to eat what tastes good to you. My family was very flexible. These enchiladas really hit the spot for me."—**Kathy S. Shares Her Recipe**

High in calcium, iron, potassium, folic acid and vitamin A

1 Serving: Calories 360 (Calories from Fat 160); Total Fat 18g (Saturated Fat 9g, Trans Fat 1g); Cholesterol 60mg; Sodium 950mg; Potassium 440mg; Total Carbohydrate 29g (Dietary Fiber 2g); Protein 19g **% Daily Value:** Vitamin A 10%; Vitamin C 2%; Calcium 25%; Iron 15%; Folic Acid 15%; Magnesium 10% **Exchanges:** 1 ½ Starch, 1 Vegetable, 1 ½ Very Lean Meat, ½ High-Fat Meat, 2 ½ Fat **Carbohydrate Choices:** 2

Food for Thought This beef recipe is a super source of both vitamin B$_{12}$, which is important for all body cells to function properly, and iron, a healing mineral that's vital for oxygen transfer in the blood. You cannot live without either of these vital nutrients.

Beef Fajita Bowls

Prep Time: 30 Minutes | **Start to Finish:** 30 Minutes | 4 servings

1	cup uncooked regular long-grain white rice
1	lb boneless beef sirloin steak
2	tablespoons vegetable oil
1	flour tortilla (8 inch), cut into 4x½-inch strips
1	bag (1 lb) frozen bell pepper and onion stir-fry
½	cup frozen whole kernel corn
1	cup chunky-style salsa
2	tablespoons lime juice
2	tablespoons chili sauce
½	teaspoon ground cumin
2	tablespoons chopped fresh cilantro

1 Cook rice as directed on package. Meanwhile, cut beef with grain into 2-inch strips; cut strips across grain into ⅛-inch slices. (Beef is easier to cut if partially frozen, 30 to 60 minutes.)

2 Heat 12-inch nonstick skillet over medium-high heat. Add oil; rotate skillet to coat bottom. Add tortilla strips; cook 1 to 2 minutes on each side, adding additional oil if necessary, until golden brown and crisp. Drain on paper towel.

3 Add beef to skillet; stir-fry over medium-high heat 4 to 5 minutes or until beef is brown. Remove beef from skillet. Add frozen bell pepper mixture and corn to skillet; stir-fry 1 minute. Cover; cook 2 to 3 minutes, stirring twice, until crisp-tender. Stir in beef, salsa, lime juice, chili sauce and cumin. Cook 2 to 3 minutes, stirring occasionally, until hot. Stir in cilantro.

4 Divide rice evenly among 4 bowls. Top with beef mixture and tortilla strips.

66 Stir-frying, sort of new to me, is a way of cooking that just feels healthy. I really felt like I was doing something good for myself and my family when I stir-fried meat and vegetables and ate them along with rice."—Catherine H.

High in potassium, iron, folic acid and vitamins A and C; good source of fiber

1 Serving: Calories 510 (Calories from Fat 110); Total Fat 12g (Saturated Fat 2.5g, Trans Fat 0g); Cholesterol 65mg; Sodium 1030mg; Potassium 720mg; Total Carbohydrate 66g (Dietary Fiber 4g); Protein 33g **% Daily Value:** Vitamin A 15%; Vitamin C 50%; Calcium 8%; Iron 30%; Folic Acid 35%; Magnesium 15% **Exchanges:** 3 ½ Starch, ½ Other Carbohydrate, 1 Vegetable, 3 Lean Meat **Carbohydrate Choices:** 4 ½

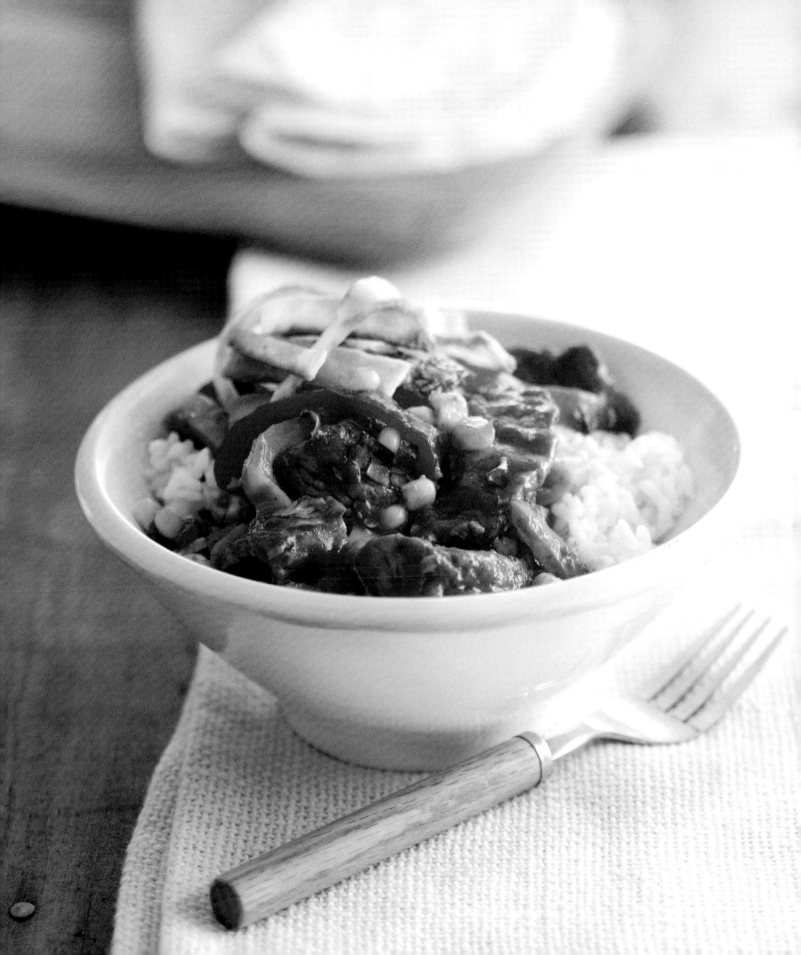

A Note from Dr. Ghosh This stew is a great meal that you can store for leftovers for when you don't feel like cooking. Remember to refrigerate all leftovers right after eating because doing so will lengthen the time that the foods can be stored.

Beef-Barley Stew

Prep Time: 15 Minutes | **Start to Finish:** 1 Hour 25 Minutes | 6 servings

1   lb extra-lean (at least 90%) ground beef

1   medium onion, chopped (½ cup)

2   cups beef broth

⅔   cup uncooked barley

2   teaspoons chopped fresh or ½ teaspoon dried oregano leaves

¼   teaspoon salt

¼   teaspoon pepper

1   can (14.5 oz) whole tomatoes, undrained

1   can (8 oz) sliced water chestnuts, undrained

2   cups frozen mixed vegetables

1 Heat oven to 350°F. In 10-inch nonstick skillet, cook beef and onion over medium heat 7 to 8 minutes, stirring occasionally, until beef is brown; drain.

2 In ungreased 3-quart casserole, mix beef mixture and remaining ingredients except frozen vegetables, breaking up tomatoes.

3 Cover; bake 30 minutes. Stir in frozen vegetables. Cover; bake 30 to 40 minutes longer or until barley is tender.

❝Good food is especially warming and nurturing to the soul. At a time when control of my life seems an issue, being able to select and prepare tasty meals gives me a sense of control over my life." —Mary W.

High in vitamins A and C and potassium; excellent source of fiber

1 Serving: Calories 280 (Calories from Fat 60); Total Fat 7g (Saturated Fat 2.5g, Trans Fat 0g); Cholesterol 45mg; Sodium 590mg; Potassium 570mg; Total Carbohydrate 34g (Dietary Fiber 8g); Protein 20g **% Daily Value:** Vitamin A 50%; Vitamin C 10%; Calcium 6%; Iron 20%; Folic Acid 8%; Magnesium 15% **Exchanges:** 1 ½ Starch, ½ Other Carbohydrate, 1 Vegetable, 2 Lean Meat **Carbohydrate Choices:** 2

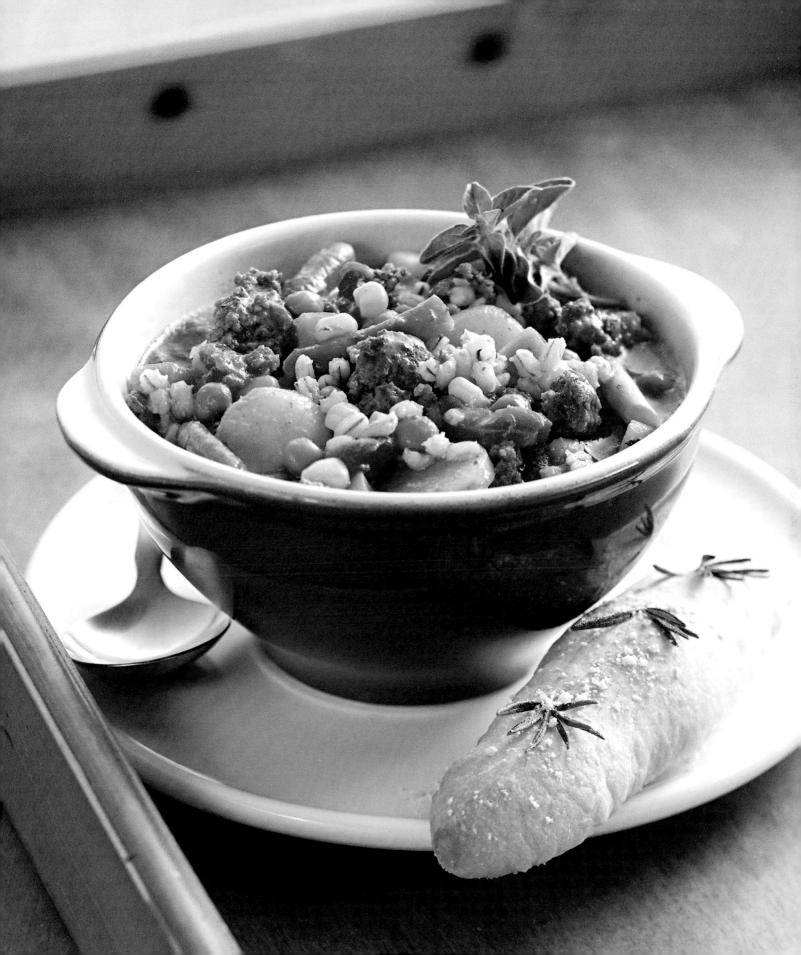

A Note from Dr. Ghosh A great source of iron, this recipe can help replenish red blood cells if you have anemia. Because maintaining iron stores during cancer treatment is very difficult, a multivitamin supplement containing iron can be used to enhance your diet.

Beef and Bean Dinner

Prep Time: 15 Minutes | **Start to Finish:** 1 Hour | 6 servings (1 ½ cups each)

1   lb lean (at least 80%) ground beef

1   medium onion, chopped (½ cup)

5   slices bacon

1   can (15 to 16 oz) lima beans, drained

1   can (15 to 16 oz) butter beans, drained

1   can (15 to 16 oz) kidney beans, drained

1   can (28 oz) baked beans

⅓   cup packed brown sugar

¼   cup ketchup

2   tablespoons Worcestershire sauce

1   Heat oven to 350°F. In 10-inch skillet, cook beef and onion over medium heat 8 to 10 minutes, stirring occasionally, until beef is brown; drain. Place beef mixture in ungreased 3-quart casserole.

2   In same skillet, cook bacon over low heat 7 to 8 minutes, turning occasionally, until crisp and brown. Drain on paper towels; cool and crumble.

3   Into beef in casserole, stir beans, brown sugar, ketchup and Worcestershire sauce. Top with bacon.

4   Cover; bake 40 to 45 minutes or until hot and bubbly.

❝I looked for foods rich in iron, and this recipe is iron-rich. An added plus is that my family thinks it tastes great, too!"—Joyce K. Shares Her Recipe

High in iron, folic acid, magnesium, potassium and vitamin A; excellent source of fiber

1 Serving: Calories 580 (Calories from Fat 110); Total Fat 12g (Saturated Fat 4.5g, Trans Fat 0.5g); Cholesterol 55mg; Sodium 1200mg; Potassium 1410mg; Total Carbohydrate 82g (Dietary Fiber 17g); Protein 36g **% Daily Value**: Vitamin A 4%; Vitamin C 4%; Calcium 10%; Iron 40%; Folic Acid 50%; Magnesium 30% **Exchanges:** 3 ½ Starch, 1 ½ Other Carbohydrate, 1 Vegetable, 3 ½ Very Lean Meat, 1 ½ Fat **Carbohydrate Choices:** 5 ½

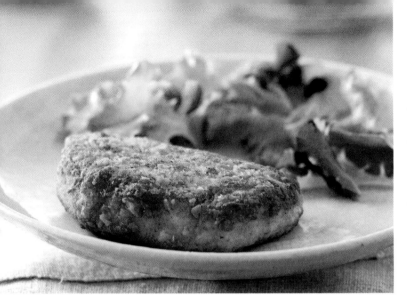

A Note from Dr. Ghosh This low-fiber, low-residue recipe is one to try when dietary restrictions apply, such as following stomach or intestinal surgery. It's so tasty, the whole family will enjoy it!

Breaded Pork Chops

Prep Time: 15 Minutes | **Start to Finish:** 15 Minutes | 8 servings

½ cup Original Bisquick® mix

12 saltine crackers, crushed (½ cup)

1 teaspoon seasoned salt

¼ teaspoon pepper

1 egg

2 tablespoons water

2 teaspoons vegetable oil

8 boneless pork loin chops, ½ inch thick (about 2 lb)

1 In shallow dish, mix Bisquick mix, cracker crumbs, seasoned salt and pepper. In another shallow dish, mix egg and water.

2 Dip pork into egg mixture, then coat with Bisquick mixture.

3 In 12-inch nonstick skillet, heat oil over medium-high heat. Add pork; cook 8 to 10 minutes, turning once, until meat thermometer inserted in center reads 145°F; allow to rest 3 minutes.

❝I found this recipe so easy, my 13-year-old son could make it all by himself. My kids enjoyed making dinner on the days I felt most ill; they really thought they were helping, and they were!"—**Anne R.**

Low fiber; low residue

1 Serving: Calories 240 (Calories from Fat 110); Total Fat 12g (Saturated Fat 3.5g, Trans Fat 0g); Cholesterol 95mg; Sodium 370mg; Potassium 330mg; Total Carbohydrate 8g (Dietary Fiber 0g); Protein 26g **% Daily Value:** Vitamin A 0%; Vitamin C 0%; Calcium 0%; Iron 8%; Folic Acid 6%; Magnesium 6% **Exchanges:** ½ Starch, 2 ½ Lean Meat, 1 Medium-Fat Meat **Carbohydrate Choices:** ½

A Note from Dr. Ghosh Most patients find comfort foods, such as stew, very satisfying. Savor hearty stews, creamy mashed potatoes or any other food that brings you comfort, and try to enjoy every moment of your meal.

Zesty Autumn Pork Stew

Prep Time: 25 Minutes | **Start to Finish:** 25 Minutes | 4 servings

1   lb pork tenderloin, cut into 1-inch cubes

2   medium dark-orange sweet potatoes, peeled, cubed (2 cups)

1   medium green bell pepper, chopped (1 cup)

2   cloves garlic, finely chopped (1 teaspoon)

1   cup coleslaw mix

1   teaspoon Cajun seasoning

1   can (14 oz) chicken broth

1   Spray 4-quart Dutch oven with cooking spray; heat over medium-high heat. Add pork; cook, stirring occasionally, until brown.

2   Stir in remaining ingredients. Heat to boiling. Reduce heat; cover and simmer about 15 minutes, stirring once, until sweet potatoes are tender.

66 Stew has always been one of my favorites. Some people have said the smell of certain foods bothered them during treatment, but it has had the opposite effect for me. Just the smell of this stew simmering on the stove made me feel more like eating."—**Mary W.**

High in potassium and vitamins A and C; good source of fiber

1 Serving: Calories 240 (Calories from Fat 45); Total Fat 5g (Saturated Fat 1.5g, Trans Fat 0g); Cholesterol 70mg; Sodium 640mg; Potassium 920mg; Total Carbohydrate 18g (Dietary Fiber 3g); Protein 30g **% Daily Value:** Vitamin A 280%; Vitamin C 40%; Calcium 4%; Iron 15%; Folic Acid 6%; Magnesium 15% **Exchanges:** 1 Starch, 4 Very Lean Meat, ½ Fat **Carbohydrate Choices:** 1

Set the Table, and Smell the Flowers

In the spirit of bringing back the joy of eating, when survivors created surroundings that were pleasant, they felt better and were able to eat more. Even little things can make a big difference.

1. Dust off the good china. Create a festive meal by setting the table with the nicest dishes you have—china or not! Use colorful pieces of dinnerware or festive disposable plates, even if they are mismatched (an eclectic mix can be fun). Try drinking your favorite warm or cold beverage from a favorite glass or mug.

2. Embrace something new. For fun, one family has a picnic in the middle of winter. They spread out a blanket on the floor and serve picnic foods like sandwiches and salads. Others create a backward dinner where dessert is served first or have a weekly pizza or pasta night.

3. Improve the mood. Light candles, use a small centerpiece, bring in unscented flowers, or unfold a colorful napkin in the middle of the table. Anything that cheers you and makes you feel better is worth a bit of extra effort.

4. Bring the outside inside. Open the window to breathe in the fresh air and gaze outside. If you do not have easy access to a window, place a picture of an outdoor scene nearby. Studies have shown that viewing an outdoor scene helps calm us and reminds us that we're part of a world that is magnificent.

5. Celebrate the small stuff. When you reach a treatment milestone or accomplish a small task, celebrate! Serve wine, sparkling water, juice or a nonalcoholic cocktail with the meal to put everyone in a festive mood. Serve a cake decorated to highlight your accomplishment.

6. Enjoy each other's company. Surround yourself with your loved ones. Take time to share with each other. If you live alone, invite a friend or family over or ask to dine at their house. If it's too much trouble to provide a meal, ask your guests to pick up a takeout meal on the way over.

7. Listen to music. Music touches your emotions. And listening to certain types of music can help you to relax and feel more like eating. Choose classical, jazz, contemporary or whatever music helps to improve the mood and soothe.

8. Walk on the wild side. Venture outdoors, even if it's just to pick up the newspaper or to walk the dog. Take a short walk when you feel up to it. Visit a nearby pond, lake or river. Nature has a wonderful way of renewing and calming us. If a walk is too much, try simply sitting outside.

Realize, too, that there may be some days when you're not up to doing any of these suggestions. One solution is to ask others to help you with these things or to do them for you. Even small efforts can be helpful. And right now, you may need all the extra encouragement you can get to relax and nourish yourself.

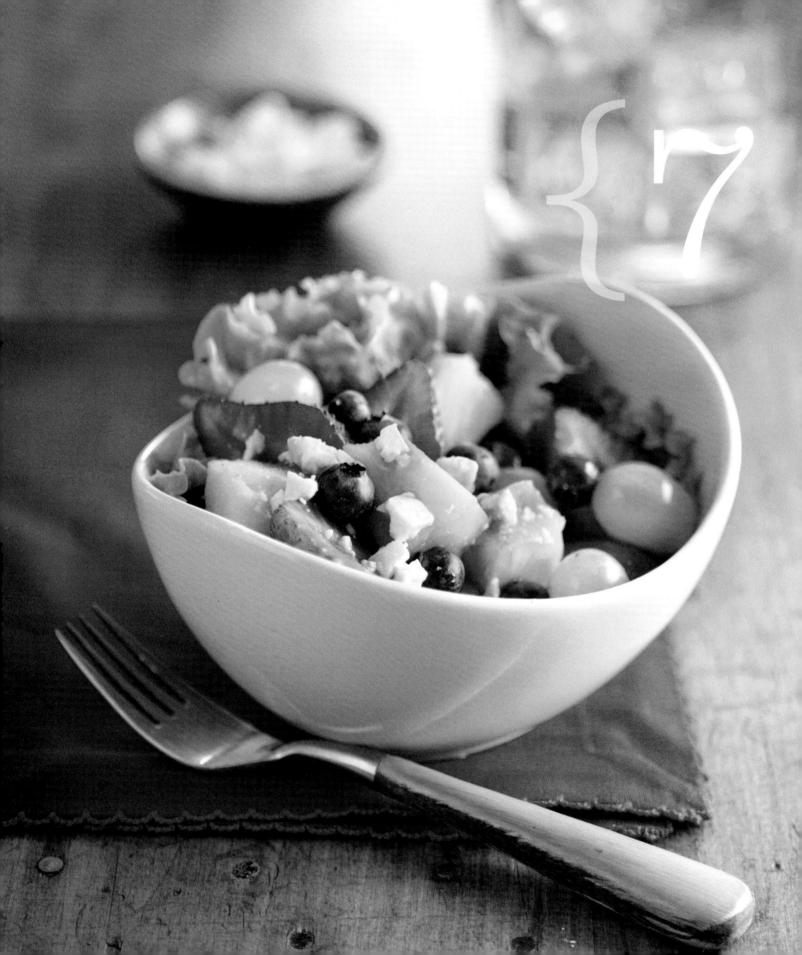

Comforting Side Dishes

}

204   Grilled Marinated Vegetables

206   Easy Creamed Vegetables

207   Stir-Fried Vegetables

208   Mashed Potatoes

209   Easy Cheesy Broccoli Bake

211   Bulgur Pilaf

212   Broccoli-Bacon Salad

214   Savory Black-Eyed Peas with Bacon

215   Wild Rice Stuffing

216   Barley and Asparagus

217   Orange-Pineapple Fruit Salad

218   Easy Fresh-Fruit Salad

A Note from Dr. Ghosh Folic acid is a nutrient needed for all cells. A diet rich in folic acid may also help to reduce heartburn and mouth sores.

Grilled Marinated Vegetables

Prep Time: 40 Minutes | **Start to Finish:** 1 Hour 15 Minutes | 8 servings (1 cup each)

ZESTY GARLIC MARINADE

½   cup water

½   cup olive or vegetable oil

1   teaspoon sesame seed

2   teaspoons white vinegar

1   teaspoon Worcestershire sauce

½   teaspoon pepper

½   teaspoon chopped fresh parsley

½   teaspoon paprika

¼   teaspoon salt

2   cloves garlic, finely chopped

GRILLED VEGETABLES

12   new potatoes

¾   lb fresh asparagus spears

2   bunches green onions

2   large portabella mushrooms, cut into ¾-inch slices

2   large red bell peppers, cut into fourths

1   large zucchini, cut into ½-inch slices

1   large yellow summer squash, cut into ½-inch slices

4   plum (Roma) tomatoes, sliced

1   In 2-gallon resealable food-storage plastic bag, place marinade ingredients. Seal bag; shake until well mixed. Set aside.

2   Cut potatoes into fourths; place on microwavable plate. Cover with microwavable plastic wrap, folding back one edge ¼ inch to vent steam. Microwave on High 5 minutes.

3   Place potatoes and remaining ingredients in bag with marinade. Seal bag; refrigerate 30 minutes.

4   Heat gas or charcoal grill. Place half of the vegetables at a time on grill over medium heat; discard marinade. Cover grill; cook 6 to 8 minutes, turning once, until vegetables are desired doneness.

66 My best friend sent me a note with the following words: Yesterday is history, tomorrow is a mystery, today is a gift. It hangs by my kitchen sink to remind me that today is indeed a gift. Another gift is good food—I love making these healthy grilled vegetables."
—Judy O. Shares Her Recipe

High in potassium, vitamins A and C and folic acid; excellent source of fiber

1 Serving: Calories 260 (Calories from Fat 130); Total Fat 14g (Saturated Fat 2g, Trans Fat 0g); Cholesterol 0mg; Sodium 105mg; Potassium 1040mg; Total Carbohydrate 27g (Dietary Fiber 6g); Protein 5g **% Daily Value:** Vitamin A 50%; Vitamin C 70%; Calcium 6%; Iron 15%; Folic Acid 30%; Magnesium 15% **Exchanges:** 1 Other Carbohydrate, 2 ½ Vegetable, 3 Fat **Carbohydrate Choices:** 2

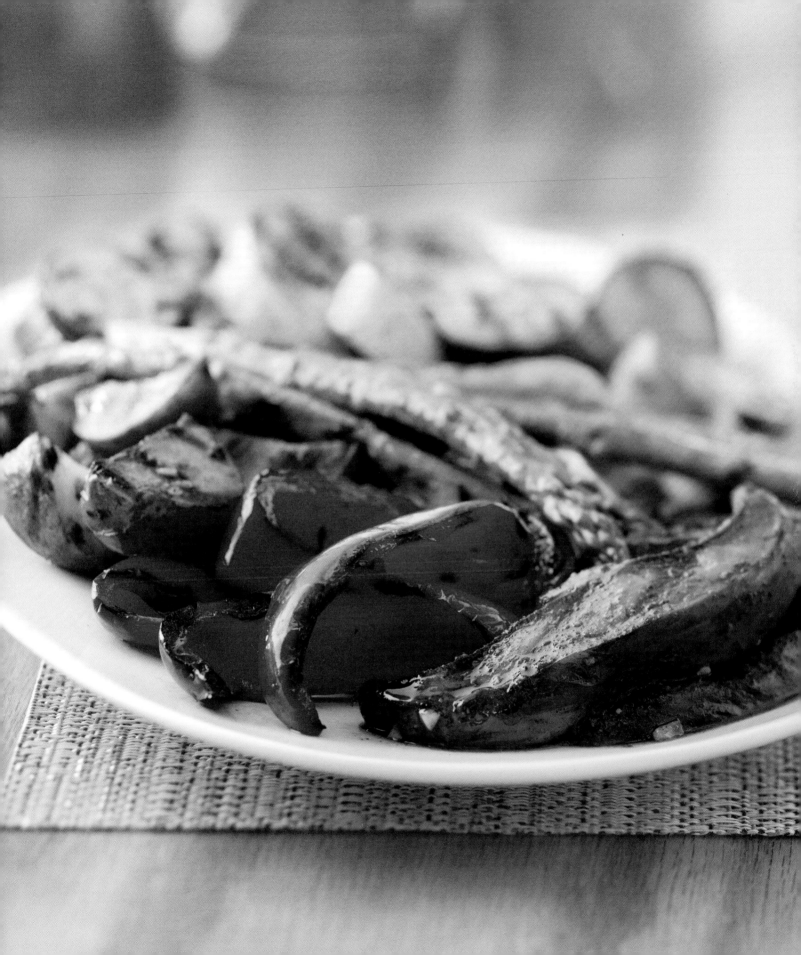

A Note from Dr. Ghosh If you decide to add meat to this dish, it is very important to chew your food well before swallowing for two reasons: (1) Your mouth has to do more of the digestion because your stomach and intestines may not be up to it right now, and (2) chewing and generating saliva can actually help prevent mouth sores and dry mouth.

Easy Creamed Vegetables

Prep Time: 15 Minutes | **Start to Finish:** 15 Minutes | 4 servings (¾ cup each)

1 can (10 ¾ oz) condensed cream of celery or cream of mushroom soup

1 bag (1 lb) frozen broccoli, cauliflower and carrots (or other combination)

1 In 2-quart saucepan, heat soup to boiling over medium heat.

2 Stir in frozen vegetables. Reduce heat to low; cover and cook about 10 minutes, stirring occasionally, until vegetables are tender.

❝When I made easy, fast foods, I didn't have to be in the kitchen all day. This recipe is delicious as a side dish or served over baked potatoes. If you add meat, it's a main dish. Either way, it was a good choice for me and my family."—**Pat Y. Shares Her Recipe**

High in vitamins A and C; good source of fiber

1 Serving: Calories 100 (Calories from Fat 40); Total Fat 4.5g (Saturated Fat 1g, Trans Fat 0g); Cholesterol 0mg; Sodium 570mg; Potassium 290mg; Total Carbohydrate 11g (Dietary Fiber 4g); Protein 3g **% Daily Value:** Vitamin A 50%; Vitamin C 30%; Calcium 8%; Iron 6%; Folic Acid 15%; Magnesium 6% **Exchanges:** 2 Vegetable, 1 Fat **Carbohydrate Choices:** 1

A Note from Dr. Ghosh Chopped fresh gingerroot, eaten raw, has been known to reduce nausea associated with chemotherapy. If the taste is too bitter for you, try sucking on crystallized ginger, which has a sweeter taste.

Stir-Fried Vegetables

Prep Time: 20 Minutes | **Start to Finish:** 20 Minutes | 6 servings (1 cup each)

1	tablespoon vegetable oil
1	tablespoon finely chopped gingerroot
1	clove garlic, finely chopped
1	medium onion, sliced
1	bag (16 oz) coleslaw mix or 3 cups shredded cabbage
2	medium stalks celery, sliced diagonally (1 cup)
2	medium red bell peppers, cut into strips
1	medium green bell pepper, cut into strips
1	tablespoon soy sauce
1	teaspoon sugar
½	teaspoon salt
¼	teaspoon pepper

1 In 10-inch skillet, heat oil over medium-high heat, rotating skillet to coat with oil. Add gingerroot, garlic and onion; stir-fry 1 minute.

2 Add coleslaw mix, celery and bell peppers; stir-fry about 5 minutes or until crisp-tender. Sprinkle with remaining ingredients.

❝Vegetable dishes without oil or cream appealed to me. These vegetables are a tasty low-fat option."—**Marie E. Shares Her Recipe**

High in vitamins A and C; good source of fiber

1 Serving: Calories 70 (Calories from Fat 20); Total Fat 2.5g (Saturated Fat 0g, Trans Fat 0g); Cholesterol 0mg; Sodium 380mg; Potassium 190mg; Total Carbohydrate 11g (Dietary Fiber 3g); Protein 2g **% Daily Value:** Vitamin A 50%; Vitamin C 80%; Calcium 6%; Iron 2%; Folic Acid 8%; Magnesium 2% **Exchanges:** ½ Other Carbohydrate, 1 Vegetable, ½ Fat **Carbohydrate Choices:** 1

Food for Thought Mashed potatoes are easy to swallow, especially when there aren't any lumps. If you would like to add a little more milk to make them more moist, try adding 1 to 2 tablespoons at a time to get just the right consistency for you.

Mashed Potatoes

Prep Time: 10 Minutes | **Start to Finish:** 40 Minutes | 4 to 6 servings

6 medium round red or white potatoes (2 lb)

⅓ to ½ cup milk

¼ cup butter or margarine, softened

½ teaspoon salt

Dash pepper

1 Place potatoes in 2-quart saucepan; add enough water just to cover potatoes. Heat to boiling. Reduce heat; cover and simmer 20 to 30 minutes or until potatoes are tender. Drain. Shake saucepan with potatoes over low heat to dry (this will help mashed potatoes be fluffier).

2 Mash potatoes in saucepan until no lumps remain. Add milk in small amounts, mashing after each addition (amount of milk needed to make potatoes smooth and fluffy depends on kind of potatoes used).

3 Add butter, salt and pepper. Mash vigorously until potatoes are light and fluffy. If desired, sprinkle with small pieces of butter or sprinkle with paprika, chopped fresh parsley or chives.

❝When the mouth sores were really bad, mashed potatoes were all I could manage to eat. I added whey powder with the butter, which made it into a meal that included a high-quality protein. It didn't change the taste, but it sure changed the nutritional benefit."
—Anne R.

High in potassium; good source of fiber; low residue if skins are removed

1 Serving: Calories 300 (Calories from Fat 110); Total Fat 12g (Saturated Fat 8g, Trans Fat 0g); Cholesterol 35mg; Sodium 400mg; Potassium 1320mg; Total Carbohydrate 42g (Dietary Fiber 5g); Protein 4g **% Daily Value:** Vitamin A 8%; Vitamin C 25%; Calcium 8%; Iron 20%; Folic Acid 4%; Magnesium 20% **Exchanges:** ½ Starch, 2 Other Carbohydrate, 1 Vegetable, 2 ½ Fat **Carbohydrate Choices:** 3

A Note from Dr. Ghosh Broccoli is a great source of folic acid, which is essential in normal body functions. Excessive folic acid intake, however, can interfere with the effectiveness of a chemotherapy called methotrexate.

Easy Cheesy Broccoli Bake

Prep Time: 10 Minutes | **Start to Finish:** 1 Hour 5 Minutes | 6 servings (1 cup each)

1 bag (1 lb) frozen broccoli cuts, thawed, drained

1 can (10 ¾ oz) condensed cream of chicken or cream of celery soup

1 jar (8 oz) process cheese sauce

1 medium onion, chopped (½ cup)

1 cup uncooked instant rice

¼ cup milk

¼ cup water

¼ teaspoon pepper

1 Heat oven to 350°F. Spray 3-quart casserole with cooking spray. Mix all ingredients in casserole.

2 Cover; bake 50 to 55 minutes or until rice is tender.

"Adding more calories was important for me, to keep up my strength. This recipe helped me to do that."—**Marilyn T. Shares Her Recipe**

High in calcium, folic acid and vitamins A and C; good source of fiber

1 Serving: Calories 260 (Calories from Fat 110); Total Fat 12g (Saturated Fat 6g, Trans Fat 0g); Cholesterol 35mg; Sodium 940mg; Potassium 280mg; Total Carbohydrate 28g (Dietary Fiber 3g); Protein 9g **% Daily Value:** Vitamin A 25%; Vitamin C 25%; Calcium 15%; Iron 10%; Folic Acid 20%; Magnesium 6% **Exchanges:** 1 ½ Starch, 1 Vegetable, 2 ½ Fat **Carbohydrate Choices:** 2

Enjoying Food during Cancer Treatment

During treatment, cancer patients often experience side effects of chemotherapy, radiation or surgery. Foods may taste metallic, patterns of hunger may be different, or, as several patients have commented, "Food just did not taste the way I remembered it before treatment."

There are ways you can bring back the joy of eating and eat well; try these suggestions.

1. Start small. Eat small quantities of food more often. You may feel full after eating only a little bit of food. Try eating a small amount, then try eating more food 30 minutes later.

2. Eat big when you can. Try eating your largest meal at a time when you are the least tired. If you are less tired in the morning or at noon, try eating your main meal then, instead of waiting until evening.

3. Have someone else cook. Food just seems to taste better when someone else cooks! Invite friends or family members to cook in your home, or pick a day when you're feeling better and try dining at their home.

4. Dine at restaurants. "If I choose good foods when eating out, it entices me to eat more because of the variety of choices," said a patient who ate many of her meals at restaurants.

5. Choose comfort foods. Everyone has a different version of comfort foods. Rice pudding, custard, mashed potatoes, oatmeal and macaroni and cheese conjure up pleasant, nostalgic thoughts, and are comforting and enjoyable for many. Use one of the many comfort food recipes in this book, or pull your favorites from your recipe collection.

6. Eat foods at room temperature. Because room-temperature foods have less aroma, this is of particular help when you are experiencing nausea.

7. Eat away from the kitchen. Avoid the smells associated with cooking by eating in a room other than the kitchen. Another environment can be quite helpful if you have nausea.

8. Eat foods that are easy to swallow. If you have mouth sores or dry mouth, this is key. "Soups, mashed potatoes and oatmeal went down easily," suggests one patient.

9. Avoid greasy or fried foods. Difficult for anyone to digest, greasy or fatty foods are particularly difficult to digest if you have an upset stomach or are feeling nauseated.

10. Eat foods that agree with you. Trial and error is the only way to know which are the best foods for your system right now. Start with small tastes of foods to see how well you tolerate them and if they taste good to you before you opt for a larger serving.

11. Enhance eating. Find simple ways to add pleasure to your dining experience. Try using colored plates, lighting candles or adding fresh flowers to improve your mood and help make you feel more like eating.

Food for Thought Bulgur is made from wheat berries that have been partially cooked and cracked. It imparts a nutty flavor with plenty of nutrients.

Bulgur Pilaf

Prep Time: 20 Minutes | **Start to Finish:** 35 Minutes | 6 servings

2 tablespoons butter or margarine

½ cup slivered almonds

1 medium onion, chopped (½ cup)

1 medium carrot, chopped (½ cup)

1 can (14 oz) chicken broth

1 cup uncooked bulgur

¼ teaspoon lemon-pepper seasoning salt or black pepper

¼ cup chopped fresh parsley

1 In 12-inch skillet, melt 1 tablespoon of the butter over medium-high heat. Add almonds; cook 2 to 3 minutes, stirring constantly, until golden brown. Remove almonds from skillet.

2 To skillet, add remaining 1 tablespoon butter, the onion and carrot. Cook about 3 minutes, stirring occasionally, until vegetables are crisp-tender.

3 Stir in broth, bulgur and lemon-pepper seasoning salt. Heat to boiling. Reduce heat; cover and simmer about 15 minutes or until bulgur is tender and liquid is absorbed. Stir in almonds and parsley.

❝A change of pace sometimes perked up my appetite. Double this recipe for tasty leftovers."—Mary W.

High in vitamin A; excellent source of fiber

1 Serving: Calories 200 (Calories from Fat 80); Total Fat 9g (Saturated Fat 3g, Trans Fat 0g); Cholesterol 10mg; Sodium 380mg; Potassium 290mg; Total Carbohydrate 23g (Dietary Fiber 6g); Protein 6g **% Daily Value:** Vitamin A 40%; Vitamin C 4%; Calcium 4%; Iron 8%; Folic Acid 6%; Magnesium 15% **Exchanges:** 1 ½ Starch, ½ Vegetable, 1 ½ Fat **Carbohydrate Choices:** 1 ½

A Note from Dr. Ghosh Tasty sunflower nuts are an excellent source of vitamin E. Working as an antioxidant, vitamin E protects body cells from damaging substances. Avoid seeds and nuts if you have an ostomy (where a portion of the intestine is brought up to the skin).

Broccoli-Bacon Salad

Prep Time: 10 Minutes | **Start to Finish:** 2 Hours 10 Minutes | 6 servings (1 cup each)

½ cup mayonnaise or salad dressing

2 tablespoons sugar

2 tablespoons white vinegar

1 lb fresh broccoli, cut into florets (5 cups)

¼ cup chopped red onion

¼ cup chopped yellow onion

¼ cup sunflower nuts

6 slices bacon, crisply cooked, crumbled

1 In large bowl, mix mayonnaise, sugar and vinegar. Stir in broccoli and onion until coated. Cover; refrigerate 2 hours to blend flavors.

2 Sprinkle with nuts and bacon before serving.

"So easy to make and so satisfying when I was tired."—**Marie E. Shares Her Recipe**

High in vitamin C

1 Serving: Calories 260 (Calories from Fat 190); Total Fat 21g (Saturated Fat 3.5g, Trans Fat 0g); Cholesterol 15mg; Sodium 310mg; Potassium 290mg; Total Carbohydrate 11g (Dietary Fiber 2g); Protein 6g
% Daily Value: Vitamin A 8%; Vitamin C 90%; Calcium 4%; Iron 6%; Folic Acid 15%; Magnesium 10%
Exchanges: ½ Starch, 1 Vegetable, ½ High-Fat Meat, 3 ½ Fat **Carbohydrate Choices:** 1

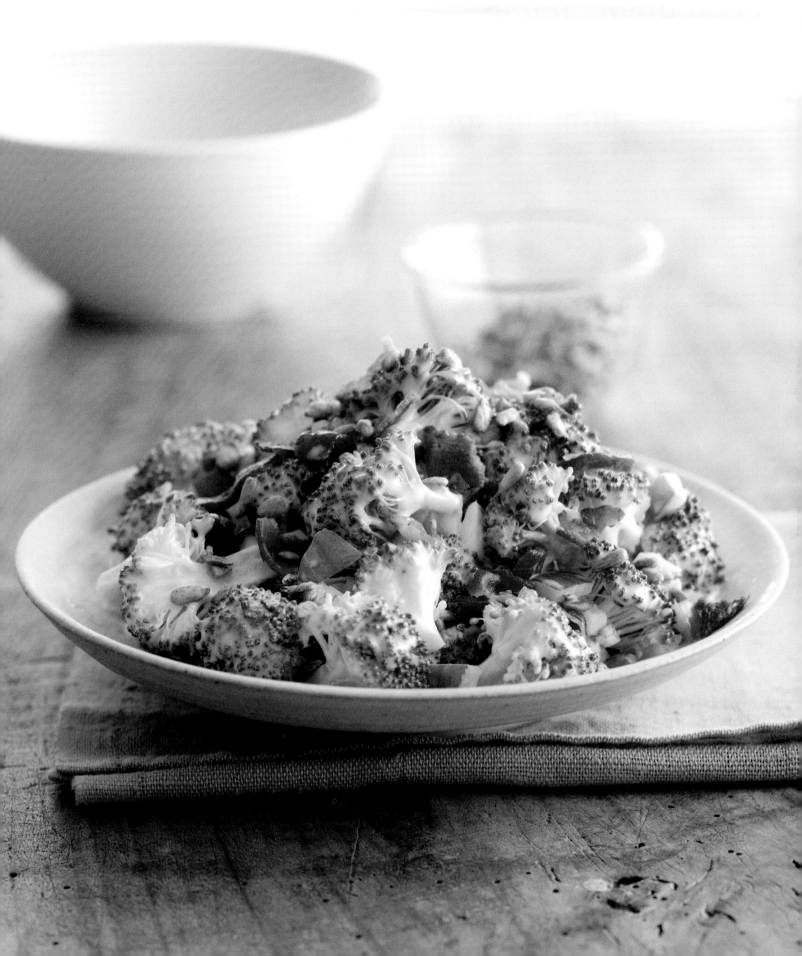

Food for Thought Be sure to include foods in your diet, such as this dish, that are nutrient-dense, meaning rich in healing nutrients—potassium, magnesium, iron, and calcium—that can aid in your recovery.

Savory Black-Eyed Peas with Bacon

Prep Time: 1 Hour 35 Minutes | **Start to Finish:** 1 Hour 35 Minutes | 4 servings (1 ½ cups each)

4 slices bacon, cut into 1-inch pieces

2 ½ cups chicken broth

1 cup dried black-eyed peas (8 oz), sorted, rinsed

2 medium stalks celery, sliced (1 cup)

1 large onion, chopped (1 cup)

1 ½ tablespoons chopped fresh or 1 ½ teaspoons dried savory leaves

1 clove garlic, finely chopped

3 medium carrots, thinly sliced (1 ½ cups)

1 large green bell pepper, cut into 1-inch pieces

½ cup shredded pepper-Jack cheese (2 oz)

1 In 10-inch skillet, cook bacon over medium heat, stirring occasionally, until crisp. Remove bacon with slotted spoon; drain. Drain fat from skillet.

2 In same skillet, heat broth, black-eyed peas, celery, onion, savory and garlic to boiling. Boil uncovered 2 minutes. Reduce heat; cover and simmer about 40 minutes, stirring occasionally, until peas are almost tender (do not boil or peas will fall apart).

3 Stir in carrots and bell pepper. Heat to simmering. Cover; simmer about 13 minutes, stirring occasionally, until vegetables are tender. Stir; sprinkle with cheese and bacon.

❝This very comforting and flavorful dish is easy to eat, even with mouth sores. Doing some of the prep work early in the day when I had more energy made dinnertime easier for me. Cooking the bacon and chopping the celery, onion, garlic and pepper are all tasks that can be done ahead of time."—**Anne R.**

High in iron, potassium, magnesium, folic acid and vitamins A and C; excellent source of fiber

1 Serving: Calories 300 (Calories from Fat 80); Total Fat 9g (Saturated Fat 4g, Trans Fat 0g); Cholesterol 20mg; Sodium 980mg; Potassium 840mg; Total Carbohydrate 36g (Dietary Fiber 10g); Protein 19g **% Daily Value:** Vitamin A 160%; Vitamin C 35%; Calcium 15%; Iron 20%; Folic Acid 70%; Magnesium 20% **Exchanges:** 1 Starch, ½ Other Carbohydrate, 2 ½ Vegetable, ½ Very Lean Meat, 1 High-Fat Meat **Carbohydrate Choices:** 2 ½

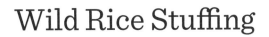

A Note from Dr. Ghosh Walnuts and peanuts are great sources of magnesium. Surgery and chemotherapy deplete the body of many essential nutrients, including magnesium, so it's important to eat foods to help replace what is lost.

Wild Rice Stuffing

Prep Time: 10 Minutes | **Start to Finish:** 1 Hour 55 Minutes | 5 servings (1 cup each)

1	cup uncooked wild rice
2 ½	cups water
⅓	cup butter or margarine, melted
1	cup orange juice
1	medium tart cooking apple, peeled, cut into 1-inch chunks
1	cup unseasoned dry bread crumbs
½	cup raisins
½	cup chopped walnuts

1 Heat oven to 325°F. In 2-quart saucepan, heat wild rice and water to boiling, stirring occasionally. Reduce heat; cover and simmer about 45 minutes or until wild rice is tender. Drain.

2 In 2-quart casserole, mix butter and orange juice. Stir in apple, wild rice, bread crumbs, raisins and walnuts. Cover; bake about 1 hour or until apple is tender.

"Eating small quantities made a big difference. Whenever I got hungry, I ate, no matter what time the clock said. This stuffing made a tasty snack."—**Kathy S. Shares Her Recipe**

High in magnesium; excellent source of fiber

1 Serving: Calories 500 (Calories from Fat 190); Total Fat 22g (Saturated Fat 9g, Trans Fat 0.5g); Cholesterol 35mg; Sodium 260mg; Potassium 460mg; Total Carbohydrate 65g (Dietary Fiber 5g); Protein 10g **% Daily Value:** Vitamin A 10%; Vitamin C 20%; Calcium 8%; Iron 15%; Folic Acid 20%; Magnesium 20% **Exchanges:** 3 ½ Starch, 1 Other Carbohydrate, 4 Fat **Carbohydrate Choices:** 4

Food for Thought Combining grains and vegetables makes an interesting and good-for-you side dish, one that's fancy enough to serve to company but easy enough to make so you don't feel exhausted. Enjoy the time you save with loved ones.

Barley and Asparagus

Prep Time: 45 Minutes | **Start to Finish:** 45 Minutes | 8 servings

3 ½   cups chicken broth

2   tablespoons vegetable oil

1   medium onion, chopped (½ cup)

1   medium carrot, chopped (½ cup)

1   cup uncooked quick-cooking barley

8   oz fresh asparagus spears (8 to 10 spears), cut into 1-inch pieces

2   tablespoons shredded Parmesan cheese

¼   teaspoon dried marjoram or thyme leaves

⅛   teaspoon pepper

1 In 2-quart saucepan, heat broth over medium heat until hot.

2 In 12-inch skillet, heat oil over medium heat. Add onion and carrot; cook 1 to 2 minutes, stirring occasionally, until crisp-tender. Stir in barley. Cook and stir 1 minute.

3 Pour 1 cup of the hot broth over barley mixture. Cook uncovered about 5 minutes, stirring occasionally, until liquid is absorbed. Stir in asparagus. Continue cooking 15 to 20 minutes, adding broth 1 cup at a time and stirring frequently, until barley is tender and liquid is absorbed.

4 Remove skillet from heat. Stir in remaining ingredients.

"If your appetite is small, make a meal of this side dish."—**Mary W.**

High in vitamin A; excellent source of fiber

1 Serving: Calories 160 (Calories from Fat 45); Total Fat 5g (Saturated Fat 1g, Trans Fat 0g); Cholesterol 0mg; Sodium 480mg; Potassium 260mg; Total Carbohydrate 23g (Dietary Fiber 5g); Protein 6g **% Daily Value:** Vitamin A 30%; Vitamin C 2%; Calcium 4%; Iron 8%; Folic Acid 6%; Magnesium 6% **Exchanges:** 1 Starch, 1 Vegetable, 1 Fat **Carbohydrate Choices:** 1 ½

A Note from Dr. Ghosh Eat this salad with a meat that's high in iron, because the vitamin C makes the iron more readily absorbed into the body. Sprinkling a little sugar over the top will add sweetness and increase the number of calories. Remember: Every calorie counts!

Orange-Pineapple Fruit Salad

Prep Time: 35 Minutes | **Start to Finish:** 2 Hours 35 Minutes | 8 servings (1 cup each)

3 medium oranges, peeled, sectioned

1 can (20 oz) pineapple chunks in juice, drained, juice reserved

¼ cup sugar

1 tablespoon lemon juice

1 tablespoon cornstarch

2 bananas, sliced

1 pint (2 cups) fresh strawberries, sliced

1 cup seedless red grapes, cut in half

2 kiwifruit, sliced or cut into chunks

1 In colander in medium bowl, place orange sections and pineapple chunks; sprinkle with sugar. Pour reserved pineapple juice over fruit, allowing juice to drain into bowl. Let stand 2 hours.

2 Pour juice from bowl into 1-quart saucepan. Stir in lemon juice and cornstarch. Heat to boiling over medium heat, stirring constantly. Boil and stir 1 minute; cool.

3 In large bowl, place oranges, pineapple, bananas, strawberries, grapes and kiwifruit. Pour sauce over fruit and gently stir. Serve immediately or chill before serving.

❝I found that fresh fruit appealed to me the most. This fruit salad was great to have on hand because I could eat it whenever I craved something sweet."—**Randie N. Shares Her Recipe**

High in vitamin C; good source of fiber

1 Serving: Calories 170 (Calories from Fat 0); Total Fat 0g (Saturated Fat 0g, Trans Fat 0g); Cholesterol 0mg; Sodium 0mg; Potassium 430mg; Total Carbohydrate 40g (Dietary Fiber 4g); Protein 1g **% Daily Value:** Vitamin A 4%; Vitamin C 130%; Calcium 4%; Iron 4%; Folic Acid 10%; Magnesium 8% **Exchanges:** ½ Starch, 1 Fruit, 1 Other Carbohydrate **Carbohydrate Choices:** 2 ½

A Note from Dr. Ghosh This salad is a great healthy snack; small meals are better tolerated during chemotherapy and radiation therapy and after surgery. Substitute process cheese for the feta cheese during times of neutropenia, when the white blood cell count is low; neutropenia usually occurs seven to fourteen days after chemotherapy.

Easy Fresh-Fruit Salad

Prep Time: 20 Minutes | **Start to Finish:** 20 Minutes | 6 servings

1 medium pineapple (2 lb), peeled, cut into 1-inch chunks (3 cups)

1 pint (2 cups) fresh strawberries, sliced

1 pint (2 cups) fresh blueberries

2 cups seedless green grapes

1 bunch leaf lettuce

½ cup raspberry vinaigrette dressing

¾ to 1 cup crumbled feta cheese (3 to 4 oz)

1 In large bowl, mix pineapple, strawberries, blueberries and grapes.

2 Line individual serving plates with lettuce. Spoon salad onto lettuce. Drizzle with dressing; sprinkle with cheese.

" This recipe was so easy. I mixed the fruit ahead of time. Then I drizzled on the dressing and added the cheese whenever I needed a little pick-me-up."—**Ellen T. Shares Her Recipe**

High in vitamin C; good source of fiber

1 Serving: Calories 260 (Calories from Fat 90); Total Fat 11g (Saturated Fat 3.5g, Trans Fat 0g); Cholesterol 15mg; Sodium 270mg; Potassium 430mg; Total Carbohydrate 36g (Dietary Fiber 4g); Protein 5g **% Daily Value:** Vitamin A 90%; Vitamin C 150%; Calcium 15%; Iron 8%; Folic Acid 15%; Magnesium 8% **Exchanges:** ½ Starch, 1 ½ Fruit, ½ Other Carbohydrate, ½ Medium-Fat Meat, 1 ½ Fat **Carbohydrate Choices:** 2 ½

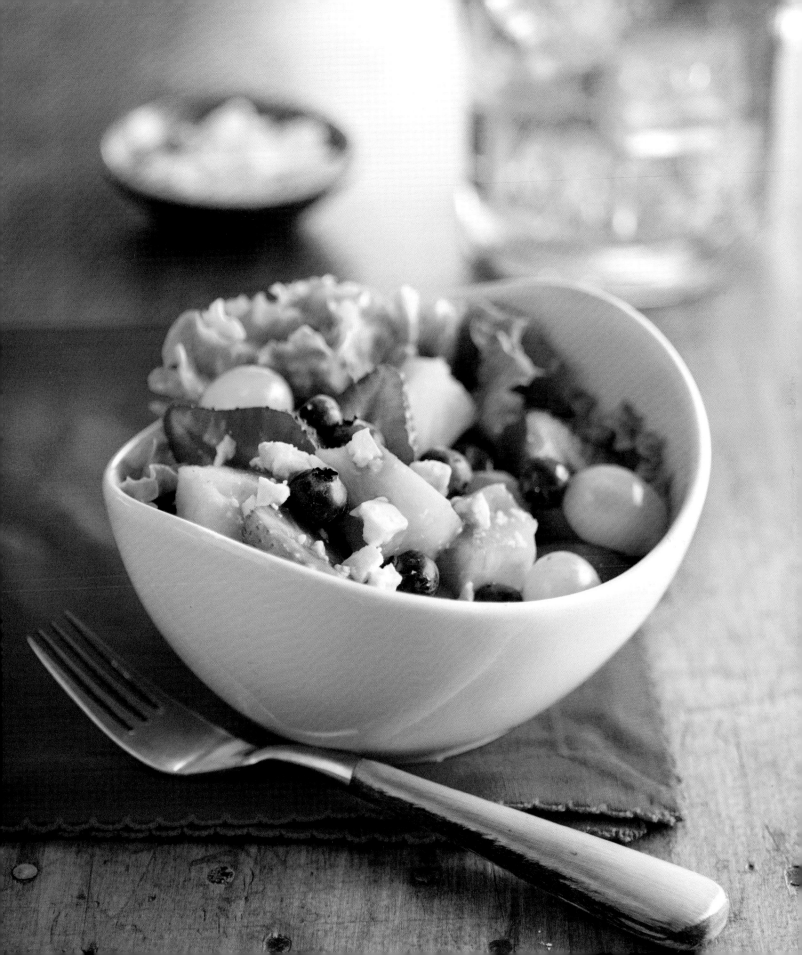

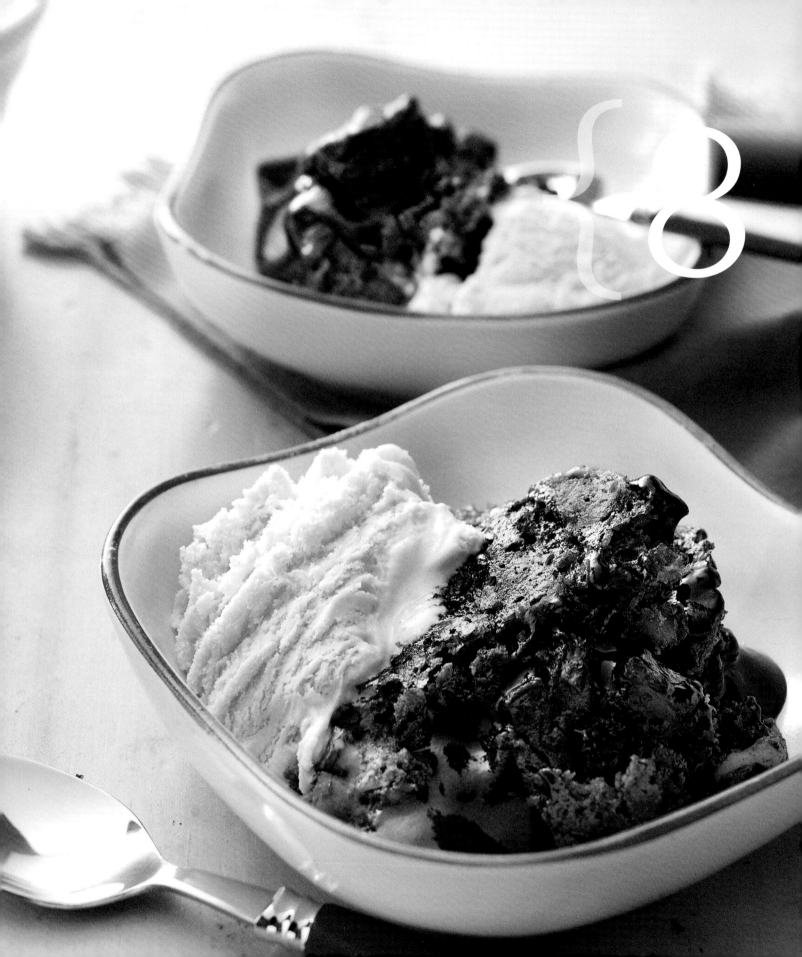

Treat-Yourself Desserts

222   Country Fruit Cobbler

224   Easy Lemon Bars

225   Pumpkin Drop Cookies

227   Rosalie's Orange Butter Cookies

228   Orange-Cream Frosty

230   Raspberry-Banana Gelatin Dessert

231   Gingerbread with Brown Sugar Meringue

232   Fudge Pudding Cake with Ice Cream

234   Baked Custard

235   Rice Pudding

A Note from Dr. Ghosh Berries are good sources of fiber and vitamin C. Adding in orange-colored fruits, such as peaches and apricots, can give you a vitamin A boost, too.

Country Fruit Cobbler

Prep Time: 10 Minutes | **Start to Finish:** 1 Hour 10 Minutes | 6 servings

¼ cup butter or margarine

1 cup all-purpose flour

1 cup sugar

2 teaspoons baking powder

¼ teaspoon salt

¾ cup milk

4 cups fresh or frozen (thawed and drained) blueberries, raspberries, sliced peaches or strawberries (or combination of fruit)

1 Heat oven to 350°F. In 1 ½-quart casserole, melt butter in oven. In medium bowl, mix flour, sugar, baking powder, salt and milk. Pour batter onto butter into casserole without mixing with butter. Spoon fruit evenly over batter.

2 Bake uncovered about 1 hour or until top is golden brown. Serve warm.

66 This was the easiest dessert to put together, and it's so good served warm with whipped cream or ice cream. Sometimes I made this with drained canned peaches if I didn't have fresh fruit on hand."
—Ellen T. Shares Her Recipe

Good source of fiber

1 Serving: Calories 360 (Calories from Fat 80); Total Fat 9g (Saturated Fat 5g, Trans Fat 0g); Cholesterol 25mg; Sodium 330mg; Potassium 150mg; Total Carbohydrate 65g (Dietary Fiber 3g); Protein 4g **% Daily Value:** Vitamin A 6%; Vitamin C 8%; Calcium 15%; Iron 8%; Folic Acid 8%; Magnesium 4% **Exchanges:** 1 ½ Starch, 1 Fruit, 2 Other Carbohydrate, 1 ½ Fat **Carbohydrate Choices:** 4

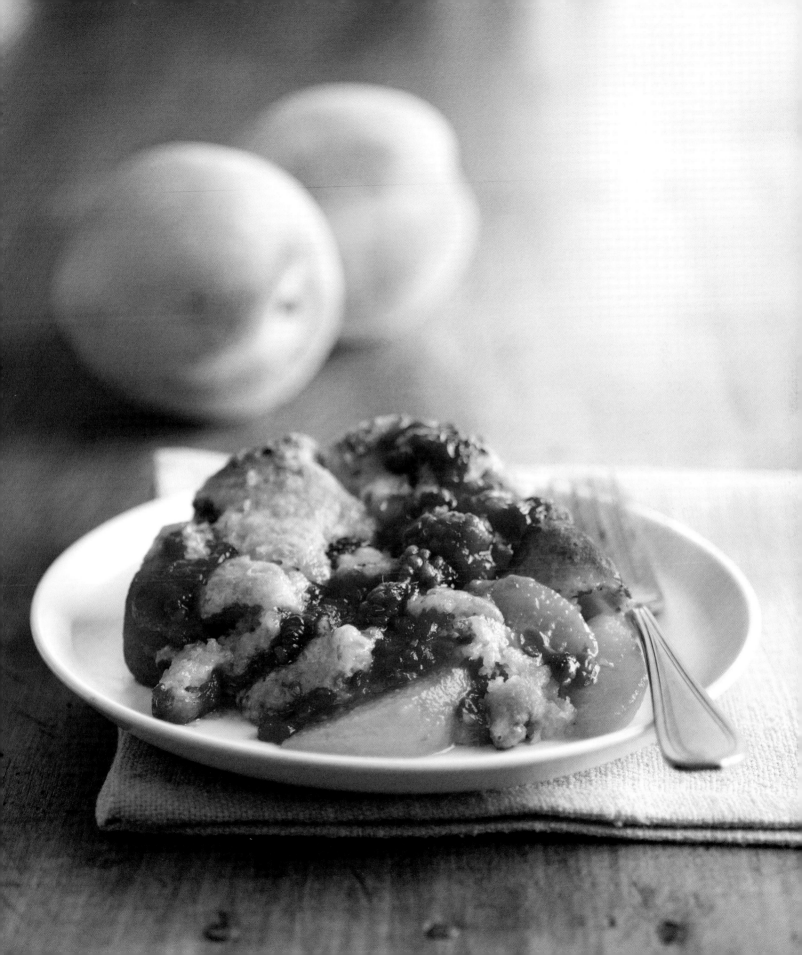

A Note from Dr. Ghosh These bars are a great snack or mini-meal when you are on the go! A daily dose of light exercise for 30 minutes can help combat your fatigue and lift your spirits.

Easy Lemon Bars

Prep Time: 25 Minutes | **Start to Finish:** 2 Hours 55 Minutes | 16 bars

1   box (1 lb 0.5 oz) lemon bar mix

Juice of 1 whole lemon (about 3 tablespoons)

½   cup vanilla-flavored protein powder

1   carton (8 oz) fat-free egg product (1 cup)

Powdered sugar, if desired

1   Heat oven to 350°F. In bottom of 8- or 9-inch square pan, press dry crust from lemon bar mix. Bake 10 minutes.

2   Meanwhile, add enough water to lemon juice to equal ½ cup. In large bowl, place filling from lemon bar mix and protein powder. Stir in egg product and lemon juice mixture with whisk until smooth.

3   Pour filling over hot crust. Bake 25 to 30 minutes or until top just begins to brown and center is set. Cool completely, about 2 hours. Sprinkle with powdered sugar. For bars, cut into 4 rows by 4 rows.

66 The best diet for me includes small meals and enough protein to help me heal and feel good during treatments. I use protein powder to boost the protein in foods that I can eat, as in these lemon bars. For a zestier lemon flavor, I add grated lemon peel to the filling."
—**Anne R. Shares Her Recipe**

Low fiber; low residue

1 Bar: Calories 140 (Calories from Fat 25); Total Fat 3g (Saturated Fat 1g, Trans Fat 1g); Cholesterol 0mg; Sodium 110mg; Potassium 50mg; Total Carbohydrate 24g (Dietary Fiber 0g); Protein 4g
% Daily Value: Vitamin A 4%; Vitamin C 0%; Calcium 0%; Iron 0%; Folic Acid 6%; Magnesium 0%
Exchanges: ½ Starch, 1 Other Carbohydrate, ½ Very Lean Meat, ½ Fat **Carbohydrate Choices:** 1 ½

A Note from Dr. Ghosh Pumpkin is rich in beta-carotene, a form of vitamin A. Studies show that vitamin A, an antioxidant vitamin, may reduce the risk of certain types of cancer.

Pumpkin Drop Cookies

Prep Time: 1 Hour | **Start to Finish:** 1 Hour | About 4 dozen cookies

½	cup butter or margarine, softened
¾	cup granulated sugar
¾	cup packed brown sugar
2	eggs
1	can (15 oz) pumpkin (not pumpkin pie mix)
2 ½	cups all-purpose flour
2 ½	teaspoons baking powder
1	teaspoon baking soda
1	teaspoon salt
1	teaspoon ground cinnamon
¼	teaspoon ground allspice
¼	teaspoon ground nutmeg
1	cup raisins

1 Heat oven to 375°F. Grease cookie sheets with shortening. In large bowl, mix butter and sugars with spoon. Beat in eggs. Stir in pumpkin. Stir in remaining ingredients except raisins. Fold in raisins.

2 Drop dough by tablespoonfuls about 2 inches apart onto cookie sheets.

3 Bake 10 to 12 minutes or until set and golden. Cool 1 to 2 minutes; remove from cookie sheets to cooling racks.

"I have always baked a lot of cookies, and my favorite recipes contained oatmeal, coconut, dried fruits or nuts, which did not fit my low-residue diet restrictions. This recipe and the following one on page 227 are low residue."—**Catherine H. Shares Her Recipe**

Low fiber; low residue

1 Cookie: Calories 80 (Calories from Fat 20); Total Fat 2g (Saturated Fat 1.5g, Trans Fat 0g); Cholesterol 15mg; Sodium 120mg; Potassium 55mg; Total Carbohydrate 15g (Dietary Fiber 0g); Protein 1g
% Daily Value: Vitamin A 30%; Vitamin C 0%; Calcium 2%; Iron 4%; Folic Acid 2%; Magnesium 0%
Exchanges: ½ Starch, ½ Other Carbohydrate, ½ Fat **Carbohydrate Choices:** 1

Great Gifts

What are the best gifts for cancer patients? Not what you might expect. Try these favorites from cancer survivors.

What to Bring

- Gift certificates—Give a gift card or certificate to a favorite restaurant or department store or for a manicure, pedicure or massage. Create a homemade certificate for a dinner you will make when the patient is home or well enough to enjoy eating, or for a household task. A certificate's underlying message that you think the patient will eventually be well brings hope.

- Books—Choose books with spiritual, uplifting messages or those with a humorous tone. Cartoons, comics and magazines are also good choices for reading when concentration may be difficult. Keep the patient's interests in mind—a mystery or the latest best-seller may be just what he or she wants for distraction.

- Balloons—Colorful get-well balloons usually last a long time and let the recipient know you are thinking of him or her. Mylar balloons make the best choice because they have no smell and stay inflated for a long time.

- Music—Cancer patients can listen at their leisure to music CDs, iPods or healing tapes to calm them or for inspiration.

- Fruit and vegetable basket—Fresh fruits and vegetables are always good choices. They contain important nutrients for healing and are easy to snack on (just rinse and enjoy). Dried fruits are a good option, too. Be wary of any produce that has a strong aroma, which might be a problem.

- Patient requests—Is there something in particular the patient wants? Funny slippers, body lotion, the latest gossip from the office? Being able to grant the patient's wish may indeed be the best gift. And sometimes, he or she may just want your company!

What Not to Bring

- Fresh flowers—Flowers with a strong odor are not the best gift for patients who often feel nauseated from cancer, medication or treatment. Ask the florist to suggest varieties (like some orchids) that offer little or no scent. Or bring a green plant to liven things up.

- Candy—Cancer patients need to eat as healthfully as possible to keep up their strength. Eating even a couple of candies may not leave an appetite for lunch or dinner. Some patients on chemotherapy have said that chocolate now just tastes sweet without the chocolate flavor.

- Anything with a strong aroma—Scented candles, bath salts and gels, lotions, powders or perfumes that are very aromatic are not the best gift choices right now. If you can find unscented versions of these gifts, the cancer patient may be more pleased.

A Note from Dr. Ghosh Pay special attention to where and at what temperature you store foods. Keep foods covered to increase storage time and to reduce odors in your kitchen. Make large quantities when you can and continue to eat, even when your appetite is down.

Rosalie's Orange Butter Cookies

Prep Time: 1 Hour | **Start to Finish:** 1 Hour 30 Minutes | About 3 ½ dozen cookies

COOKIES

⅔	cup butter or margarine, softened
¾	cup sugar
1	egg
	Grated peel of 1 large orange (about 2 tablespoons)
½	cup orange juice
2	cups all-purpose flour
½	teaspoon baking powder
½	teaspoon baking soda
½	teaspoon salt

ORANGE BUTTER FROSTING

1 ½	cups powdered sugar
2	tablespoons butter or margarine, softened
	Grated peel of 1 large orange (about 2 tablespoons)
1 ½	tablespoons orange juice

1 Heat oven to 350°F. In large bowl, mix butter, sugar and egg with spoon until creamy and well blended. Stir in orange peel and orange juice. Stir in remaining cookie ingredients.

2 Drop dough by tablespoonfuls about 2 inches apart onto ungreased cookie sheets.

3 Bake 8 to 10 minutes or until light brown around edges. Cool 1 to 2 minutes; remove from cookie sheets to cooling racks. Cool completely, about 30 minutes.

4 In medium bowl, mix frosting ingredients. Frost cooled cookies.

66 Something sweet after a meal was quite appealing. I would make up a batch of these cookies between treatments and freeze them, so it didn't take any effort to have a simple dessert or snack, even while I was on chemo."—Catherine H. Shares Her Recipe

Low fiber, low residue

1 Cookie: Calories 90 (Calories from Fat 35); Total Fat 3.5g (Saturated Fat 2g, Trans Fat 0g); Cholesterol 15mg; Sodium 75mg; Potassium 15mg; Total Carbohydrate 13g (Dietary Fiber 0g); Protein 0g
% Daily Value: Vitamin A 2%; Vitamin C 0%; Calcium 0%; Iron 0%; Folic Acid 2%; Magnesium 0%
Exchanges: ½ Starch, ½ Other Carbohydrate, ½ Fat **Carbohydrate Choices:** 1

Food for Thought The coolness of this dessert and the combination of juice and yogurt may be helpful during times when foods taste metallic or you're having difficulty swallowing.

Orange-Cream Frosty

Prep Time: 5 Minutes | **Start to Finish:** 5 Minutes | 6 servings (about 1 ½ cups each)

½ gallon (8 cups) orange, vanilla or peach frozen yogurt

1 can (6 oz) frozen (thawed) calcium-fortified orange juice concentrate

1 cup milk

1 In blender, place half each of the frozen yogurt, juice concentrate and milk. Cover; blend on medium speed about 45 seconds, stopping blender occasionally to scrape sides, until thick and smooth.

2 Pour into 3 glasses. Repeat with remaining yogurt, juice concentrate and milk.

66 This was so refreshing and went down easily when I had problems swallowing other foods. For variety, I used grape juice concentrate instead of orange juice concentrate."—**Carol N.**

High in potassium, calcium, vitamin C and folic acid; low fiber

1 Serving: Calories 430 (Calories from Fat 60); Total Fat 6g (Saturated Fat 4g, Trans Fat 0g); Cholesterol 25mg; Sodium 220mg; Potassium 910mg; Total Carbohydrate 77g (Dietary Fiber 1g); Protein 17g **% Daily Value:** Vitamin A 8%; Vitamin C 70%; Calcium 70%; Iron 2%; Folic Acid 20%; Magnesium 15% **Exchanges:** ½ Fruit, 3 Other Carbohydrate, 1 Skim Milk, 1 Low-Fat Milk **Carbohydrate Choices:** 5

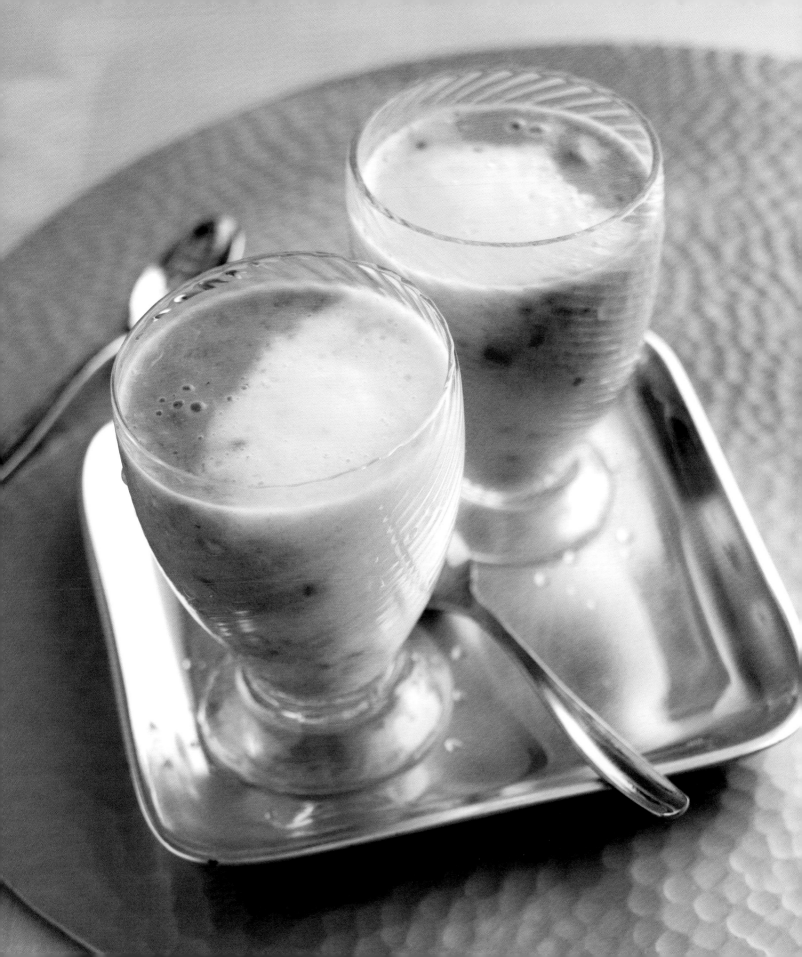

A Note from Dr. Ghosh During times of nausea, gelatin can help settle the stomach. To lessen the nausea, avoid acidic, sweet and high-fat foods. Crackers and dry toast can help combat nausea in the morning. Drinking plenty of fluids can also be a big help.

Raspberry-Banana Gelatin Dessert

Prep Time: 10 Minutes | **Start to Finish:** 3 Hours 40 Minutes | 8 servings (1 cup each)

1 box (8-serving size) raspberry-flavored gelatin

2 cups boiling water

1 pint (2 cups) vanilla ice cream

1 can (20 oz) crushed pineapple in juice, drained

2 medium bananas, thinly sliced

1 Place gelatin in medium bowl. Add boiling water; stir until gelatin is dissolved. Stir in ice cream. Refrigerate about 30 minutes or until partially set.

2 Spray 2-quart mold with cooking spray. Stir pineapple and bananas into gelatin. Spoon into mold. Cover; refrigerate at least 3 hours until firm. Unmold gelatin onto serving plate.

"I made gelatin recipes often—they helped my nausea. This one is cool and comforting."—**Randie N. Shares Her Recipe**

Low fiber

1 Serving: Calories 210 (Calories from Fat 35); Total Fat 3.5g (Saturated Fat 2g, Trans Fat 0g); Cholesterol 15mg; Sodium 130mg; Potassium 240mg; Total Carbohydrate 42g (Dietary Fiber 1g); Protein 3g **% Daily Value:** Vitamin A 4%; Vitamin C 15%; Calcium 6%; Iron 0%; Folic Acid 2%; Magnesium 6% **Exchanges:** 1 Starch, ½ Fruit, 1 ½ Other Carbohydrate, ½ Fat **Carbohydrate Choices:** 3

A Note from Dr. Ghosh Molasses is a great source of iron and magnesium, plus gingerbread offers big taste from the spices. If you're not up to preparing the meringue, serve it with applesauce for an afternoon snack.

Gingerbread with Brown Sugar Meringue

Prep Time: 20 Minutes | **Start to Finish:** 1 Hour 10 Minutes | 9 servings

GINGERBREAD

2 ⅓ cups all-purpose flour

½ cup butter or margarine

⅓ cup sugar

1 cup full-flavor or mild-flavor molasses

¾ cup hot water

1 teaspoon baking soda

1 teaspoon ground ginger

1 teaspoon ground cinnamon

¾ teaspoon salt

1 egg

BROWN SUGAR MERINGUE

2 egg whites

¼ teaspoon cream of tartar

½ cup packed brown sugar

1 Heat oven to 325°F. Grease bottom and side of 9-inch springform pan or 9-inch square pan with shortening; lightly flour. In large bowl, beat gingerbread ingredients with electric mixer on low speed 30 seconds, scraping bowl constantly. Beat on medium speed 3 minutes, scraping bowl occasionally. Pour into pan.

2 Bake about 50 minutes or until toothpick inserted in center comes out clean.

3 Meanwhile, in medium bowl, beat egg whites and cream of tartar with electric mixer on high speed until foamy. Beat in brown sugar, 1 tablespoon at a time; continue beating until stiff peaks form and mixture is glossy. Do not underbeat.

4 Increase oven temperature to 400°F. Spread meringue over hot gingerbread. Bake 8 to 10 minutes longer or until meringue is light brown. Serve warm. Store covered in refrigerator.

"Gingerbread. Ginger cookies. Ginger ale. Who knew they could lessen nausea so much? My mom makes me ginger cookies every time I have chemo. My neighbor brings over gingerbread. These foods sure hit the spot now."—**Anne R.**

High in iron, magnesium and potassium; low fiber

1 Serving: Calories 410 (Calories from Fat 100); Total Fat 11g (Saturated Fat 7g, Trans Fat 0g); Cholesterol 50mg; Sodium 450mg; Potassium 640mg; Total Carbohydrate 73g (Dietary Fiber 1g); Protein 5g **% Daily Value:** Vitamin A 6%; Vitamin C 0%; Calcium 10%; Iron 20%; Folic Acid 10%; Magnesium 25% **Exchanges:** 1 ½ Starch, 3 ½ Other Carbohydrate, 2 Fat **Carbohydrate Choices:** 5

A Note from Dr. Ghosh Dessert can be an important part of a meal because it often provides plenty of calories per bite. If you are too full to eat dessert after a meal, try eating it as a snack between meals. Enjoy!

Fudge Pudding Cake with Ice Cream

Prep Time: 15 Minutes | **Start to Finish:** 1 Hour 10 Minutes | 9 servings

1	cup all-purpose flour
¾	cup granulated sugar
2	tablespoons unsweetened baking cocoa
2	teaspoons baking powder
¼	teaspoon salt
½	cup milk
2	tablespoons vegetable oil
1	teaspoon vanilla
1	cup chopped nuts
1	cup packed brown sugar
¼	cup baking cocoa
1 ¾	cups boiling water
4 ½	cups vanilla ice cream

1 Heat oven to 350°F. In ungreased 9-inch square pan, mix flour, granulated sugar, 2 tablespoons cocoa, the baking powder, and salt. Stir in milk, oil and vanilla with fork until smooth. Stir in nuts. Spread evenly in pan.

2 In small bowl, mix brown sugar and ¼ cup cocoa; sprinkle over batter. Pour boiling water over batter.

3 Bake 40 minutes. Let stand 15 minutes. Spoon cake and sauce into individual dishes. Top each with ice cream.

Microwave Directions: In 2-quart microwavable casserole, mix flour, granulated sugar, 2 tablespoons cocoa, the baking powder and salt. Stir in milk, oil and vanilla. Stir in nuts. Spread evenly in casserole. In small bowl, mix brown sugar and ¼ cup cocoa; sprinkle over batter. Pour boiling water over batter. Microwave uncovered on Medium (50%) 9 minutes. Rotate casserole ½ turn; microwave uncovered on High 5 to 7 minutes longer or until top is almost dry.

❝After surgery, when I was shown the list of foods not on the low-residue/low-fiber diet, I was devastated. Then I noticed chocolate. I said to my doctor, 'As long as I can eat chocolate, I'll be okay!' I can't live without my dose of chocolate every day."—**Anne R.**

Good source of calcium and fiber

1 Serving: Calories 490 (Calories from Fat 180); Total Fat 20g (Saturated Fat 6g, Trans Fat 0g); Cholesterol 30mg; Sodium 240mg; Potassium 310mg; Total Carbohydrate 71g (Dietary Fiber 3g); Protein 7g **% Daily Value:** Vitamin A 6%; Vitamin C 0%; Calcium 20%; Iron 10%; Folic Acid 8%; Magnesium 15% **Exchanges:** 2 Starch, 2 ½ Other Carbohydrate, 4 Fat **Carbohydrate Choices:** 5

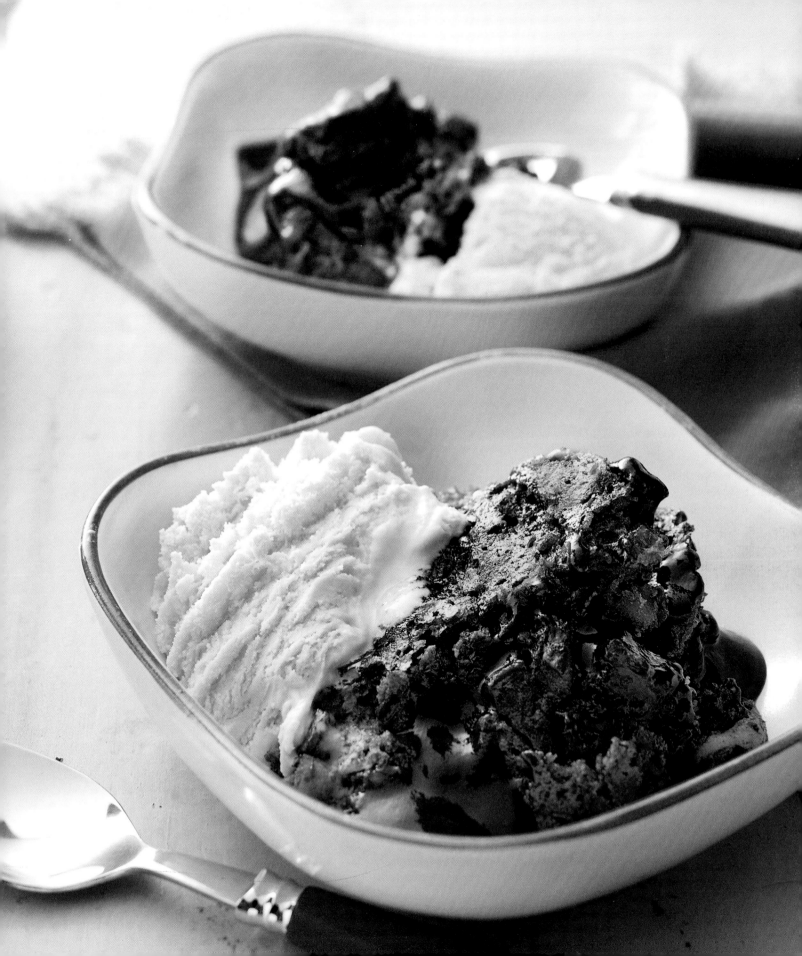

A Note from Dr. Ghosh Custard is easy to swallow when other foods just won't go down or when you're suffering from mouth sores. The smooth and soothing texture may be just what you're looking for in a dessert or snack.

Baked Custard

Prep Time: 15 Minutes | **Start to Finish:** 1 Hour 30 Minutes | 6 servings

3 large eggs, slightly beaten

⅓ cup sugar

1 teaspoon vanilla

Dash salt

2 ½ cups very warm milk (120°F to 130°F)

Ground nutmeg

1 Heat oven to 350°F. In medium bowl, beat eggs, sugar, vanilla and salt with whisk or fork. Gradually stir in milk. Pour into 6 (6-oz) custard cups. Sprinkle with nutmeg. Place cups in 13x9-inch pan.

2 Place pan on oven rack in oven. Pour very hot water into pan to within ½ inch of tops of cups.

3 Bake about 45 minutes or until knife inserted halfway between center and edge comes out clean. Remove cups from water. Cool about 30 minutes. Unmold and serve warm, or refrigerate and unmold before serving. Store covered in refrigerator.

66 This is so good, so smooth and creamy and so nutritious with all those eggs. I love this pudding when my mouth is sore. Sometimes I have a banana with it. Reminds of Grandma's banana cream pie. Mmm, good."—**Anne R.**

Low fiber

1 Serving: Calories 130 (Calories from Fat 40); Total Fat 4.5g (Saturated Fat 2g, Trans Fat 0g); Cholesterol 115mg; Sodium 95mg; Potassium 190mg; Total Carbohydrate 16g (Dietary Fiber 0g); Protein 7g **% Daily Value:** Vitamin A 6%; Vitamin C 0%; Calcium 15%; Iron 0%; Folic Acid 4%; Magnesium 4% **Exchanges:** ½ Other Carbohydrate, ½ Low-Fat Milk, ½ Very Lean Meat, ½ Fat **Carbohydrate Choices:** 1

A Note from Dr. Ghosh Puddings, custards and shakes are great comfort foods to include during cancer treatment. If you need extra protein, 2 tablespoons of protein powder can be stirred in with the cornstarch to boost the protein level of this pudding.

Rice Pudding

Prep Time: 15 Minutes | **Start to Finish:** 20 Minutes | 7 servings (½ cup each)

1	cup uncooked regular long-grain white rice
2	cups water
⅔	cup sugar
1	tablespoon cornstarch
½	teaspoon salt
2	cups milk
2	eggs, beaten
1	teaspoon vanilla
	Ground cinnamon or nutmeg
	Slivered almonds, if desired

1 Heat rice and water to boiling in 2-quart saucepan, stirring once or twice; reduce heat to low. Cover and simmer 14 to 15 minutes (do not lift cover or stir). All water should be absorbed.

2 Mix sugar, cornstarch and salt in 3-quart saucepan; gradually stir in milk. Cook over medium heat, stirring constantly, until mixture thickens and boils. Boil and stir 1 minute. Gradually stir at least half of the hot mixture into eggs, then stir back into hot mixture in saucepan. Boil and stir 1 minute; remove from heat. Stir in rice and vanilla.

3 Serve warm sprinkled with cinnamon and almonds, or cover and refrigerate about 3 hours until chilled. Store covered in refrigerator.

❝I've returned to eating many of the foods I ate as a child. It's funny, my granddaughter and I are now eating the same foods."—**Kathy S. Shares Her Recipe**

Low fiber

1 Serving: Calories 240 (Calories from Fat 30); Total Fat 3g (Saturated Fat 1.5g, Trans Fat 0g); Cholesterol 65mg; Sodium 220mg; Potassium 150mg; Total Carbohydrate 47g (Dietary Fiber 0g); Protein 6g **% Daily Value:** Vitamin A 4%; Vitamin C 0%; Calcium 10%; Iron 6%; Folic Acid 8%; Magnesium 4% **Exchanges:** 2 Starch, 1 Other Carbohydrate, ½ Fat **Carbohydrate Choices:** 3

Easy Menus During Treatment

Meal and menu planning can be difficult and time consuming, especially when you aren't feeling well. In the following pages, you'll find ideas for healthy, quick meals and snacks that meet a cancer patient's needs, all based on eating smaller meals six times a day.

The seven-day menus list meal and daily nutrient totals and include foods that are rich in the following healing nutrients: calcium, iron, magnesium and potassium. For maximum healing, it's important to consume more than 1,000 milligrams of calcium, more than 18 milligrams of iron, more than 500 milligrams of magnesium and more than 1,000 milligrams of potassium per day. In addition, a fiber intake of 25 to 35 grams each day is suggested. We've also included the meal and daily calorie levels. Instead of focusing on calories during treatment, focus on getting the minerals your body needs at this time.

You can mix and match meals and snacks from different days to add variety to your eating and to adjust for foods you may not like or may not be able to eat right now.

The menus listed are intended to be a guide for you. On days when you are not feeling well, you may look at the menus and realize you can't eat that much. That's okay, just do your best to eat whatever you can. And on the days you are feeling better, try to eat as often as you feel up to it. Remember, during treatment, your survival is linked to your ability to eat and replenish lost nutrients.

In addition to the seven days of menus, we've provided a two-day menu for each of the four most common side effects: constipation, diarrhea, mouth sores and nausea. And because finding food sources that provide enough iron can be difficult, we've included high-iron food choices in a neutropenia menu. Read on to learn about your eating options.

Menu 1

Breakfast
- 1 serving Cinnamon-Raisin Morning Mix (page 59)
- 1 serving Citrus-Peach Smoothie (page 103)

Calories	Calcium (mg)	Iron (mg)	Magnesium (mg)	Potassium (mg)
295	212	8.5	43	482

Snack
- ½ bagel with 1 tablespoon cream cheese

Calories	Calcium (mg)	Iron (mg)	Magnesium (mg)	Potassium (mg)
129	33	1	9	46

Lunch
- 1 serving Hot Turkey Sandwiches (page 90)
- 10 baby-cut carrots with 2 tablespoons Roasted Vegetable Dip (page 80)
- 1 cup fat-free (skim) milk

Calories	Calcium (mg)	Iron (mg)	Magnesium (mg)	Potassium (mg)
484	401	3	105	1237

Snack
- 2 Rosalie's Orange Butter Cookies (page 227)
- 1 cup fat-free (skim) milk

Calories	Calcium (mg)	Iron (mg)	Magnesium (mg)	Potassium (mg)
259	321	1	32	441

Dinner
- 1 baked pork chop
- 1 serving Wild Rice Stuffing (page 215)
- ½ cup spinach salad with 2 tablespoons ranch dressing

Calories	Calcium (mg)	Iron (mg)	Magnesium (mg)	Potassium (mg)
831	143	4	116	875

Snack
- 6 ounces fruited low-fat yogurt
- 1 cup apple-cranberry juice

Calories	Calcium (mg)	Iron (mg)	Magnesium (mg)	Potassium (mg)
337	276	0.3	30	397

Daily Total

Calories	Calcium (mg)	Iron (mg)	Magnesium (mg)	Potassium (mg)
2337	1386	18	336	3478

Menu 2

Breakfast

- Milk and Rice "Soup" (page 39)
- ½ cup berries
- 1 cup fat-free (skim) milk

Calories	Calcium (mg)	Iron (mg)	Magnesium (mg)	Potassium (mg)
411	519	2	87	1062

Snack

- Crunchy Fruit Snack Mix (page 43)
- 1 cup Chai Tea (page 108)

Calories	Calcium (mg)	Iron (mg)	Magnesium (mg)	Potassium (mg)
246	280	6	53	532

Lunch

- 1 serving Orange-Pineapple Fruit Salad (page 217)
- 1 roast beef sandwich with 2 slices whole wheat bread and 2 teaspoons mayonnaise and/or mustard
- 1 cup raw broccoli flowerets and cauliflowerets
- 1 cup hot tea or coffee

Calories	Calcium (mg)	Iron (mg)	Magnesium (mg)	Potassium (mg)
532	133	5	127	1186

Snack

- 1 serving String Cheese Sticks (page 86)
- 1 cup fat-free (skim) milk

Calories	Calcium (mg)	Iron (mg)	Magnesium (mg)	Potassium (mg)
389	604	1.5	51	598

Dinner

- 1 serving Turkey Tetrazzini (page 189)
- 1 serving Corn and Black Bean Salad (page 142)
- 1 serving Raspberry-Banana Gelatin Dessert (page 230)

Calories	Calcium (mg)	Iron (mg)	Magnesium (mg)	Potassium (mg)
774	356	6	132	1047

Snack

- 1 cup red or green seedless grapes

Calories	Calcium (mg)	Iron (mg)	Magnesium (mg)	Potassium (mg)
114	18	0.4	10	296

Daily Total

Calories	Calcium (mg)	Iron (mg)	Magnesium (mg)	Potassium (mg)
2466	1910	21	460	4721

Menu 3

Breakfast

- 1 serving Home-Style Oatmeal with Raisins (page 57) sprinkled with 2 tablespoons brown sugar
- 1 cup fat-free (skim) milk

Calories	Calcium (mg)	Iron (mg)	Magnesium (mg)	Potassium (mg)
539	588	3	118	1266

Snack

- Hot Fruit Compote (page 37)
- 1 cup hot herbal tea

Calories	Calcium (mg)	Iron (mg)	Magnesium (mg)	Potassium (mg)
223	32	1.5	28	436

Lunch

- 1 serving Cream of Broccoli Soup (page 136)
- 1 serving Onion and Rosemary Focaccia Wedges (page 84) with 1 to 2 teaspoons butter or margarine
- 1 medium pear

Calories	Calcium (mg)	Iron (mg)	Magnesium (mg)	Potassium (mg)
488	285	3.5	63	856

Snack

- ½ cup cottage cheese
- 2 tablespoons sunflower nuts

Calories	Calcium (mg)	Iron (mg)	Magnesium (mg)	Potassium (mg)
200	82	1	62	199

Dinner

- 1 serving Potato-Tomato-Tofu Dinner (page 132)
- 1 slice whole wheat or white bread
- Romaine salad with 2 tablespoons French dressing
- 1 cup fat-free (skim) milk

Calories	Calcium (mg)	Iron (mg)	Magnesium (mg)	Potassium (mg)
447	455	4	104	1097

Snack

- 1 serving Orange-Cream Frosty (page 228)

Calories	Calcium (mg)	Iron (mg)	Magnesium (mg)	Potassium (mg)
362	448	0.4	49	604

Daily Total

Calories	Calcium (mg)	Iron (mg)	Magnesium (mg)	Potassium (mg)
2259	1888	13	423	4457

Menu 4

Breakfast
- 1 serving Baked French Toast with Strawberry-Rhubarb Sauce (page 74)
- 1 cup calcium-fortified orange juice

Calories	Calcium (mg)	Iron (mg)	Magnesium (mg)	Potassium (mg)
534	596	5	76	865

Snack
- 1 or 2 slices Banana Bread (page 62) or Easy Brown Bread (page 64)
- 1 cup Sugar 'n Spice Green Tea (page 107)

Calories	Calcium (mg)	Iron (mg)	Magnesium (mg)	Potassium (mg)
194	24	1	19	228

Lunch
- 1 serving Zesty Autumn Pork Stew (page 200)
- 1 kiwifruit
- 1 cup fat-free (skim) milk

Calories	Calcium (mg)	Iron (mg)	Magnesium (mg)	Potassium (mg)
388	368	2.5	99	1599

Snack
- 1 serving Tomato Bruschetta (page 85)

Calories	Calcium (mg)	Iron (mg)	Magnesium (mg)	Potassium (mg)
229	96	1.7	17	107

Dinner
- 1 serving Extra-Easy Baked Ziti (page 163)
- Mixed-greens salad with 2 tablespoons Caesar dressing
- 1 serving Easy Fresh-Fruit Salad (page 218)

Calories	Calcium (mg)	Iron (mg)	Magnesium (mg)	Potassium (mg)
522	348	4	79	805

Snack
- 1 serving Easy Salmon Spread with crackers (page 102)

Calories	Calcium (mg)	Iron (mg)	Magnesium (mg)	Potassium (mg)
237	138	1	23	229

Daily Total

Calories	Calcium (mg)	Iron (mg)	Magnesium (mg)	Potassium (mg)
2104	1570	15	313	383

Menu 5

Breakfast
- 1 serving Poached Eggs in Milk (page 56)
- ¼ cup raisins or dates
- 1 cup fat-free (skim) milk

Calories	Calcium (mg)	Iron (mg)	Magnesium (mg)	Potassium (mg)
632	650	4	88	1167

Snack
- 1 serving Creamy Caramel Dip with Fruit (page 100)
- 1 cup calcium-fortified orange juice

Calories	Calcium (mg)	Iron (mg)	Magnesium (mg)	Potassium (mg)
357	451	2	49	770

Lunch
- 1 serving Cantaloupe and Chicken Salad (page 121)
- 1 whole wheat dinner roll with 2 teaspoons butter or margarine

Calories	Calcium (mg)	Iron (mg)	Magnesium (mg)	Potassium (mg)
597	90	3.5	73	500

Snack
- 2 Pumpkin Drop Cookies (page 225)
- 1 cup fat-free (skim) milk

Calories	Calcium (mg)	Iron (mg)	Magnesium (mg)	Potassium (mg)
249	350	1	40	538

Dinner
- 1 serving Layered Tuna Casserole (page 182)
- 1 cup steamed green beans
- ½ cup melon cubes
- 1 serving Easy Lemon Bars (page 224)

Calories	Calcium (mg)	Iron (mg)	Magnesium (mg)	Potassium (mg)
562	293	6.5	116	798

Snack
- ½ English muffin with 1 teaspoon peanut butter
- ½ cup apple juice

Calories	Calcium (mg)	Iron (mg)	Magnesium (mg)	Potassium (mg)
157	60	1.3	18	221

Daily Total

Calories	Calcium (mg)	Iron (mg)	Magnesium (mg)	Potassium (mg)
2554	1894	18	385	3994

Menu 6

Breakfast

- 1 serving Rise 'n Shine Muffins with Creamy Orange Glaze (page 65)
- 1 cup calcium-fortified orange juice

Calories	Calcium (mg)	Iron (mg)	Magnesium (mg)	Potassium (mg)
298	86	3	68	572

Snack

- 1 serving Quick Quesadillas (page 93)
- ¼ cup Fresh Salsa (page 98)

Calories	Calcium (mg)	Iron (mg)	Magnesium (mg)	Potassium (mg)
290	263	2	26	227

Lunch

- 1 serving Broccoli-Bacon Salad (page 212)
- 1 dinner roll with 2 teaspoons butter or margarine
- 1 serving Rice Pudding (page 235)
- 1 cup fat-free (skim) milk

Calories	Calcium (mg)	Iron (mg)	Magnesium (mg)	Potassium (mg)
738	485	3.5	93	870

Snack

- 1 soft breadstick with 2 teaspoons butter or margarine
- 1 cup tomato juice

Calories	Calcium (mg)	Iron (mg)	Magnesium (mg)	Potassium (mg)
196	50	2	36	574

Dinner

- 1 serving Hash Brown Frittata (page 180)
- 1 serving Easy Creamed Vegetables (page 206)
- ½ cup mixed fresh fruit

Calories	Calcium (mg)	Iron (mg)	Magnesium (mg)	Potassium (mg)
540	366	9	97	1188

Snack

- 1 serving Baked Custard (page 234)
- 1 cup hot herbal tea

Calories	Calcium (mg)	Iron (mg)	Magnesium (mg)	Potassium (mg)
161	168	0.6	22	248

Daily Total

Calories	Calcium (mg)	Iron (mg)	Magnesium (mg)	Potassium (mg)
2222	1417	20	342	3678

Menu 7

Breakfast

- 1 serving Blueberry Brunch Cake (page 67)
- 1 cup raspberries or 1 pear
- 1 cup fat-free (skim) milk

Calories	Calcium (mg)	Iron (mg)	Magnesium (mg)	Potassium (mg)
425	400	2	58	668

Snack

- 1 medium banana
- 1 cup fat-free (skim) milk or hot or iced tea

Calories	Calcium (mg)	Iron (mg)	Magnesium (mg)	Potassium (mg)
194	309	0.5	62	873

Lunch

- 1 serving Beef and Bean Dinner (page 198)
- 1 orange, tangerine or clementine
- 1 cup hot herbal tea or coffee

Calories	Calcium (mg)	Iron (mg)	Magnesium (mg)	Potassium (mg)
618	190	10	164	1676

Snack

- 1 cup cranberry juice
- 1 cup pretzels
- ¼ cup raisins

Calories	Calcium (mg)	Iron (mg)	Magnesium (mg)	Potassium (mg)
413	55	3	49	643

Dinner

- 1 serving Crispy Baked Fish with Tropical Salsa (page 184)
- 1 baked potato with 2 tablespoons sour cream or butter
- 1 whole-grain or white dinner roll with 2 teaspoons butter or margarine
- 1 cup fat-free (skim) milk or water

Calories	Calcium (mg)	Iron (mg)	Magnesium (mg)	Potassium (mg)
853	474	5	191	1917

Snack

- 2 graham crackers with 1 tablespoon peanut butter
- 1 cup fat-free (skim) or low-fat milk

Calories	Calcium (mg)	Iron (mg)	Magnesium (mg)	Potassium (mg)
291	315	1	62	561

Daily Total

Calories	Calcium (mg)	Iron (mg)	Magnesium (mg)	Potassium (mg)
2794	1743	22	568	6339

A Two-Day Suggested Eating Plan for Constipation

Eating high-fiber foods and drinking plenty of liquids, at least eight glasses of water daily, is important. Drink a hot beverage about half an hour before your usual time for a bowel movement. See page 36 for other tips on handling constipation. Here's a sampling of foods to assist you when you're feeling constipated:

Day 1

Breakfast
- Rise 'n Shine Muffins with Creamy Orange Glaze (page 65)
- 1 cup hot herbal tea

Snack
- Hot Fruit Compote (page 37)
- 1 cup water

Lunch
- Spaghetti and "Meatballs" (page 173)
- ½ cup fat-free (skim) milk

Snack
- ¼ cup dried apricots or raisins
- 2 or 3 tablespoons toasted soybeans
- 1 cup water

Dinner
- Corn and Black Bean Salad (page 142)
- 1 slice whole-grain bread
- 1 cup fruit juice

Snack
- Easy Fresh-Fruit Salad (page 218)
- 1 cup mineral water

Day 2

Breakfast
- Potato Pancakes with Cinnamon Apples (page 72)
- ½ cup prune juice

Snack
- 1 kiwifruit
- 1 cup water

Lunch
- Barley and Asparagus (page 216)
- Stir-Fried Vegetables (page 207)
- 1 cup hot tea

Snack
- ⅓ to ½ cup high-fiber cereal with milk
- 1 cup water

Dinner
- White Turkey Chili (page 156)
- Whole-grain breadsticks or bread
- 1 cup fat-free (skim) milk

Snack
- Creamy Caramel Dip with Fruit (page 100)
- 1 cup fruit juice

A Two-Day Suggested Eating Plan for Diarrhea

Replenishing lost fluids is of great importance when you have diarrhea. One way to ensure fluid replacement is to drink plenty of water and other liquids throughout the day, at least eight glasses. If you can, consume foods and beverages that contain extra potassium and sodium, because these nutrients are lost during bouts of diarrhea. See page 38 for hints on helping to calm diarrhea. Below is a sampling of foods that may help soothe diarrhea:

Day 1

Breakfast
- Milk and Rice "Soup" (page 39)
- 1 cup water

Snack
- 1 or 2 slices Banana Bread (page 62)
- ½ cup apple juice

Lunch
- 1 baked potato with sour cream or butter
- 1 scrambled egg
- 1 slice white bread, toasted
- 1 cup fat-free (skim) milk

Snack
- 1 container (6 ounces) fruited yogurt
- ½ cup sports drink

Dinner
- Salmon Burgers (page 181)
- ½ cup Orange-Pineapple Fruit Salad (page 217), canned mandarin orange segments or pineapple chunks
- 1 cup orange juice

Snack
- Saltine crackers with creamy peanut butter
- 1 cup fat-free (skim) milk

Day 2

Breakfast
- Home-Style Oatmeal with Raisins (page 57)
- 1 cup fat-free (skim) milk

Snack
- 1 banana
- 1 cup grape juice

Lunch
- Cantaloupe and Chicken Salad (page 121)
- 1 slice French bread
- 1 cup tomato juice

Snack
- Citrus-Peach Smoothie (page 103)
- 1 cup water

Dinner
- Old-Fashioned Beef Pot Roast (page 192)
- 1 slice white bread
- 1 cup water

Snack
- Rice Pudding (page 235)
- 1 cup hot herbal tea

A Two-Day Suggested Eating Plan for Mouth Sores

See page 40 for hints to help you soothe your mouth sores. Here's a sampling of foods that may also be of help:

Day 1

Breakfast
- Poached Eggs in Milk (page 56)
- ½ cup applesauce
- ½ cup apple juice

Snack
- Watermelon-Kiwi-Banana Smoothie (page 104)
- 1 cup water

Lunch
- Cream of Broccoli Soup (page 136)
- Crackers moistened with soup
- 1 cup fat-free (skim) milk

Snack
- 1 banana
- 1 frozen ice pop
- 1 cup water

Dinner
- Loaded Potatoes (puree if necessary) (page 134)
- 1 cup fat-free (skim) milk

Snack
- Baked Custard (page 234)
- 1 cup hot herbal tea

Day 2

Breakfast
- Home-Style Oatmeal with Raisins (page 57)
- 1 cup fat-free skim milk

Snack
- ½ cup cottage cheese
- 1 cup peach or apricot nectar

Lunch
- Easy Salmon Spread (page 102)
- Soft crackers
- ½ cup watermelon

Snack
- Creamy Caramel Dip with Fruit (page 100) with canned peaches or pears as dippers
- 1 cup water

Dinner
- Acorn Squash and Apple Soup (page 177)
- 1 or 2 soft breadsticks
- ½ cup mashed or pureed vegetables, such as peas or carrots

Snack
- Raspberry-Banana Gelatin Dessert (page 230)
- 1 cup water

A Two-Day Suggested Eating Plan For Nausea

Though you may not feel like eating when you have nausea, it's important to keep eating. Eating will actually help you regain your strength and your appetite as well. If your doctor has prescribed antinausea medicine, be sure to take it, and drink plenty of clear liquids. See pages 32 and 77 for specific hints on easing nausea. Listed below is a sampling of foods that you may eat for two days when nausea strikes:

Day 1

Breakfast
- Fruit Parfaits (page 60)
- 1 cup water

Snack
- 1 or 2 slices toast dry, or with a small amount of butter or margarine
- ½ cup fat-free (skim) milk

Lunch
- Chicken Soup with Homemade Noodles (page 154)
- Oyster crackers
- ½ cup fat-free (skim) milk

Snack
- 1 container (6 ounces) low-fat fruited yogurt
- ½ glass sparkling water or soda

Dinner
- Dijon Chicken (page 148)
- Mashed Potatoes (page 208)
- ½ cup canned green beans, corn or peas
- ½ cup fat-free (skim) milk

Snack
- ½ cup frozen sherbet
- 1 cup sparkling water or soda

Day 2

Breakfast
- Home-Style Oatmeal with Raisins (page 57)
- ½ cup fat-free (skim) milk

Snack
- Pretzels
- ½ cup apple-cranberry juice

Lunch
- Macaroni Pasta "Soup" (page 135)
- Rice Pudding (page 235)

Snack
- Canned peaches, pears or other canned bland fruit
- ½ glass sparkling water

Dinner
- 3 ounces baked or boiled chicken, without skin
- Baking Powder Biscuits (page 68)
- Easy Creamed Vegetables (page 206)
- 1 cup water

Snack
- Orange-Cream Frosty (page 228)
- ½ cup apple juice

A Two-Day Suggested Eating Plan For Neutropenia

Approximately seven to fourteen days after receiving chemotherapy, developing an abnormally low white blood cell count is common; this is called neutropenia. When your blood cell counts drop, you need to get plenty of iron from the foods you eat. In addition, your doctor may suggest you take iron supplements to be certain you're getting enough iron. A sampling of some high-iron foods to eat during neutropenia is listed below:

Day 1

Breakfast
- Cinnamon-Raisin Snack Mix (page 59)
- Berry-Banana Smoothie (page 29)

Snack
- Roasted Vegetable Dip (page 80) with broccoli flowerets and cauliflowerets

Lunch
- Chicken and Vegetable Stir-Fry (page 186)
- 1 cup tomato juice

Snack
- Savory Black-Eyed Peas with Bacon (page 214)
- ½ cup cooked spinach
- 1 cup fat-free (skim) milk

Dinner
- Beef and Bean Dinner (page 198)
- 1 cup fat-free (skim) milk

Snack
- Gingerbread with Brown Sugar Meringue (page 231)
- 1 cup orange juice

Day 2

Breakfast
- Tropical Pancakes (page 70)
- ½ cup strawberries
- 1 cup fat-free (skim) milk

Snack
- ⅓ cup raisins
- ½ cup pretzels
- 1 cup sparkling water

Lunch
- Philly Beef Sandwiches (page 92)
- Canned mandarin orange segments

Snack
- Streusel-Topped Fruit Brunch Cake (page 66)
- 1 cup fat-free (skim) milk

Dinner
- Crowd-Size Minestrone (page 155)
- Soft breadsticks
- 1 cup water

Snack
- 2 graham crackers with peanut butter
- 1 cup apple juice

Recipes to Use After Treatment

The ABCs for a Healthy Lifestyle after cancer treatment are discussed on pages 24–25. The three steps include Be Active Daily, Eat Plant Foods and Make Sensible Choices. Many of the recipes in this cookbook fit these guidelines and can be useful even after treatment. (And they also taste great!) Following is a list of recipes that offer many nutrients:

Chapter 1

- Berry-Banana Smoothie (page 29)
- Hot Fruit Compote (page 37)
- Milk and Rice "Soup" (page 39)
- Creamy Seafood Risotto (page 41)
- Crunchy Fruit Snack Mix (page 43)
- Lentil-Rice Casserole (page 45)
- Roasted Garlic Mashed Potatoes (page 47)

Chapter 2

- Country Eggs in Tortilla Cups (page 52)
- Cheesy Ham and Asparagus Bake (page 54)
- Poached Eggs in Milk (page 56)
- Home-Style Oatmeal with Raisins (page 57)
- Cinnamon-Raisin Morning Mix (page 59)
- Fruit Parfaits (page 60)
- Tropical Pancakes (page 70)
- Cheesy Pear Oven Pancake (page 71)
- Baked French Toast with Strawberry-Rhubarb Sauce (page 74)
- Make-Ahead Waffles with Peanut Butter Spread (page 76)

Chapter 3

- Roasted Vegetable Dip (page 80)
- Easy Chicken Nuggets (page 91)
- Philly Beef Sandwiches (page 92)
- Chicken Salad in Pitas (page 94)
- Mozzarella and Tomatoes (page 97)
- Creamy Caramel Dip with Fruit (page 100)
- Spinach Dip in Bread Bowl (page 101)
- Citrus-Peach Smoothie (page 103)
- Watermelon-Kiwi-Banana Smoothie (page 104)
- Orange-Pineapple Smoothie (page 106)

Chapter 4

- Fettuccine with Asparagus and Mushrooms (page 112)
- Angel Hair Pasta with Avocado and Tomatoes (page 114)
- Creamy Quinoa Primavera (page 116)
- Mediterranean Couscous and Beans (page 118)
- Honey-Mustard Turkey with Snap Peas (page 120)
- Cantaloupe and Chicken Salad (page 121)
- Caribbean Chicken Salad (page 122)
- Spinach-Shrimp Salad with Hot Bacon Dressing (page 124)
- Chutney-Salmon Salad (page 125)
- Savory Scallops and Shrimp (page 126)
- Chopped Vegetable and Crabmeat Salad (page 128)
- Fiesta Taco Salad (page 131)
- Loaded Potatoes (page 134)
- Cream of Broccoli Soup (page 136)
- Easy Beef Stroganoff (page 138)
- Caramelized Pork Slices (page 139)

Chapter 5

- Corn and Black Bean Salad (page 142)
- Layered Chicken Salad (page 145)
- Southwestern Pork Salad (page 146)
- The Ultimate Chicken Casserole (page 152)
- Crowd-Size Minestrone (page 155)
- White Turkey Chili (page 156)
- Beef-Vegetable Soup (page 158)
- Layered Beef and Vegetable Dinner (page 160)
- Spaghetti and Meat Squares (page 161)
- Sausage, Vegetable and Cheese Strata (page 166)

Chapter 6

- Spaghetti and "Meatballs" (page 173)
- Ravioli with Tomato-Alfredo Sauce (page 174)
- Fresh Spinach and New Potato Frittata (page 179)
- Hash Brown Frittata (page 180)
- Layered Tuna Casserole (page 182)
- Lemony Fish over Vegetables and Rice (page 183)
- Crispy Baked Fish with Tropical Fruit Salsa (page 184)
- Chicken and Vegetable Stir-Fry (page 186)
- Old-fashioned Beef Pot Roast (page 192)
- Cheesy Beef Enchiladas (page 193)
- Beef Fajita Bowls (page 194)
- Beef-Barley Stew (page 196)
- Beef and Bean Dinner (page 198)
- Zesty Autumn Pork Stew (page 200)

Chapter 7

- Grilled Marinated Vegetables (page 204)
- Easy Cheesy Broccoli Bake (page 206)
- Stir-Fried Vegetables (page 207)
- Bulgur Pilaf (page 211)
- Savory Black-Eyed Peas with Bacon (page 214)
- Wild Rice Stuffing (page 215)
- Barley and Asparagus (page 216)
- Orange-Pineapple Fruit Salad (page 217)
- Easy Fresh-Fruit Salad (page 218)

Chapter 8

- Country Fruit Cobbler (page 222)
- Pumpkin Drop Cookies (page 225)
- Orange-Cream Frosty (page 228)
- Gingerbread with Brown Sugar Meringue (page 231)

Nutrition and Medical Glossary

Medical and nutrition terms can sometimes be confusing, so we have gathered definitions of the nutrition and medical terms used in this cookbook.

Acupuncture—The insertion of needles into specific points on the body to help the body heal.

Alternative therapies—Treatment options that include thoughts and emotions as an integral part of healing. These may be used in combination with conventional forms of treatment.

Antioxidant—A substance that inhibits oxidation in plant and animal cells. Scientists believe that having a diet high in antioxidants may contribute to reducing disease.

Aromatherapy—The use of essential oils to increase relaxation, improve mood, and enhance circulation.

Ayurveda—An ancient medical practice that originated in India, based on the concept that energy keeps the mind and body alive.

Body Mass Index (BMI)—A measure used to compare the height and weight of adult men and women to their risk of disease.

Bodywork—A catchall term for a variety of techniques that treat ailments and promote relaxation through proper movement, posture, exercise or massage.

Calcium—A mineral in dairy foods that is important for maintaining strong bones and teeth and nerve and muscle function. Calcium aids recovery.

Cancer—The abnormal growth of any cells in the body.

Carbohydrates—Providing quick energy, they are the body's favorite fuel source. The carbohydrate content of each recipe in this book is listed under the recipe.

Chemotherapy—Systemic drugs that target and kill rapidly dividing cells, including cancer cells.

Chi—The flow of energy; based on the belief that energy flows between body organs along channels. Healing occurs when the flow of energy in the entire body is balanced.

Cholesterol—Fatlike substance, found primarily in animal foods, that is important for cell structures, hormones and nerve coverings. It is also manufactured in our bodies.

Complementary therapies—See "Alternative therapies."

Coronary Heart Disease (CHD)—A buildup of fatty, cholesterol-filled deposits in the arteries that block the normal flow of blood and can ultimately cause a heart attack.

Cruciferous—Vegetables from the cabbage family, including broccoli, cabbage, cauliflower and Brussels sprouts, which are thought to be somewhat protective against certain types of cancer when eaten as part of a low-fat, healthy diet.

Diet Exchanges—Developed by the American Dietetic Association and the American Diabetes Association, Diet Exchanges categorize foods based on their nutritional content.

Dietary Guidelines for Americans—Developed in 2010 by the U.S. Departments of Agriculture and Health and Human Services, these guidelines help people to develop a healthy lifestyle including healthy eating and daily activity.

Fat—A necessary nutrient, fat helps build new cells, shuttles vitamins through the body and makes certain hormones that regulate blood pressure.

Fiber—The type of carbohydrate that is not broken down before passing through to the stool.

Herbs—Specific plants or parts of plants that impart flavor and have medicine-like qualities.

High blood pressure (hypertension)—A condition that occurs when blood pressure is equal to or greater than 140/90 millimeters of mercury.

Iron—A mineral that carries much-needed oxygen to body cells, is vital for life and aids recovery. Iron is found in meats, spinach and fortified cereal.

Liquid diet—A clear liquid diet is mainly comprised of liquids and provides only about 500 calories per day. It should be used for only short lengths of time.

Low-residue diet—A diet made up of foods that, when eaten, leave little material in the colon after digestion. Cancer patients who have had stomach or colon surgery may need to eat a low-residue diet.

Magnesium—A nutrient (mineral) that helps release carbohydrate energy from foods and aids recovery. Magnesium is found in nuts and spinach.

Massage—The manipulation of soft tissue to relieve sore muscles and promote relaxation.

Meditation—Quiet forms of contemplation and mindfulness used to establish a sense of peace, inner calm and relaxation.

Minerals—Organic compounds, needed in very small amounts, that help the body with many functions. Minerals beneficial to cancer treatment are calcium, iron, magnesium and potassium.

MyPlate—A nutrition education resource that helps people learn how to eat a healthy balance of different foods.

MyPyramid—A nutrition education guide developed to help people learn how to eat a healthy balance of a variety of foods and include daily exercise.

Naturopathy—With an emphasis on preventive care, it takes advantage of the body's natural healing powers.

Neuropathy—Tingling and numbness in the fingers and toes that can develop in cancer patients when undergoing chemotherapy.

Neutropenia—A condition that occurs when white blood cell counts fall below 500 cells per cubic millimeter of blood; often occurs seven to ten days after beginning chemotherapy treatment.

Nutrient—Catchall term that describes substances necessary for life that build, repair and maintain body cells. Protein, carbohydrates, fats, water, vitamins and minerals are all examples of nutrients.

% Daily Value—A standard for nutrition labeling of foods that is based on a 2,000-calorie daily diet. It applies to healthy people of various ages and represents the highest recommended level of each nutrient. It replaces the former U.S. Recommended Daily Allowance (RDA).

Phytochemicals—Umbrella term used to describe many naturally occurring substances found in plant foods that may have disease-fighting properties.

Potassium—A nutrient (mineral) that helps maintain the body's fluid balance and aids recovery. Potassium is found in fruits, vegetables and dairy foods.

Protein—This nutrient helps build new cells, makes hormones and enzymes that keep the body functioning and generates antibodies to fight off infection. During cancer treatment, the body has an increased need for protein.

Radiation (radiotherapy)—The use of concentrated energy to target and kill cancer cells.

Residue—The material left in the colon after digestion, including intestinal cells and breakdown products such as fiber from the foods you eat.

Saturated fat—Solid at room temperature, these fats tend to elevate blood cholesterol levels and usually come from animal sources, such as beef, pork, poultry, eggs and dairy foods including cheese, whole milk and butter. Also included are palm oil and coconut oil, even though they are liquids.

Shiatsu—A form of Japanese acupressure that uses finger pressure on specific body sites to increase circulation and improve energy flow.

Unsaturated fat—Liquid at room temperature, these fats do not tend to elevate blood cholesterol levels. They usually come from plant sources such as olive oil, sunflower oil, corn oil, nuts and avocados.

Vitamins—A group of vital nutrients, found in small amounts in a variety of foods, that are key to developing cells, control- ling body functions and helping release energy from fuel sources. Vitamins are different from minerals in that they contain the element carbon; minerals do not.

Yoga—An ancient practice and philosophy first developed and practiced in India, yoga is based on stretching and strengthening exercises, ethical beliefs and dietary restrictions to balance the mind, body and spirit.

Additional Resources

Books and Publications

Cancer Talk: Voices of Hope and Endurance from "The Group Room," the World's Largest Cancer Support Group. Schimmel, Selma R., with Barry Fox, Ph.D. New York: Broadway Books, 1999.

Eating Hints for Cancer Patients. National Institutes of Health, U.S. Public Health Service, 2006.

Fighting Cancer with Knowledge and Hope: A Guide for Patients, Families, and Health Care Providers. Richard C. Frank, MD and Gale V. Parsons. New Haven, CT: Yale University Press, 2009.

Help Me Live: 20 Things People with Cancer Want You to Know. Lori Hope. Berkeley, CA: Celestial Arts, 2005.

It All Begins with Hope: Patients, Caregivers, and the Bereaved Speak Out. Jevne, Ronna Fay. Philadelphia, PA: Innisfree Press, 1991.

Cancer Resources Web Sites

American Cancer Society of Clinical Oncology: www.cancer.net/portal/site/patient

American Institute for Cancer Research: www.aicr.org

National Cancer Institute: www.cancer.gov

Women's Cancer Network: www.wcn.org

Nutrition Resources Web Sites

American Dietetic Association: www.eatright.org/public

Dietary Guidelines: www.cnpp.usda.gov/dietaryguidelines.htm

MyPlate: www.choosemyplate.gov

MyPyramid: www.mypyramid.gov

Metric Conversion Guide

Volume

U.S. Units	Canadian Metric	Australian Metric
¼ teaspoon	1 mL	1 ml
½ teaspoon	2 mL	2 ml
1 teaspoon	5 mL	5 ml
1 tablespoon	15 mL	20 ml
¼ cup	50 mL	60 ml
⅓ cup	75 mL	80 ml
½ cup	125 mL	125 ml
⅔ cup	150 mL	170 ml
¾ cup	175 mL	190 ml
1 cup	250 mL	250 ml
1 quart	1 liter	1 liter
1 ½ quarts	1.5 liters	1.5 liters
2 quarts	2 liters	2 liters
2 ½ quarts	2.5 liters	2.5 liters
3 quarts	3 liters	3 liters
4 quarts	4 liters	4 liters

Weight

U.S. Units	Canadian Metric	Australian Metric
1 ounce	30 grams	30 grams
2 ounces	55 grams	60 grams
3 ounces	85 grams	90 grams
4 ounces (¼ pound)	115 grams	125 grams
8 ounces (½ pound)	225 grams	225 grams
16 ounces (1 pound)	455 grams	500 grams
1 pound	455 grams	½ kilogram

Note: The recipes in this cookbook have not been developed or tested using metric measures. When converting recipes to metric, some variations in quality may be noted.

Measurements

Inches	Centimeters
1	2.5
2	5.0
3	7.5
4	10.0
5	12.5
6	15.0
7	17.5
8	20.5
9	23.0
10	25.5
11	28.0
12	30.5
13	33.0

Temperatures

Fahrenheit	Celsius
32°	0°
212°	100°
250°	120°
275°	140°
300°	150°
325°	160°
350°	180°
375°	190°
400°	200°
425°	220°
450°	230°
475°	240°
500°	260°

Recipe Testing and Calculating Nutrition Information

Recipe Testing:

- Large eggs and 2% milk were used unless otherwise indicated.
- Fat-free, low-fat, low-sodium or lite products were not used unless indicated.
- No nonstick cookware and bakeware were used unless otherwise indicated. No dark-colored, black or insulated bakeware was used.
- When a pan is specified, a metal pan was used; a baking dish or pie plate means ovenproof glass was used.
- An electric hand mixer was used for mixing only when mixer speeds are specified.

Calculating Nutrition:

- The first ingredient was used wherever a choice is given, such as $\frac{1}{3}$ cup sour cream or plain yogurt.
- The first amount was used wherever a range is given, such as 3- to 3 $\frac{1}{2}$-pound whole chicken.
- The first serving number was used wherever a range is given, such as 4 to 6 servings.
- "If desired" ingredients were not included.
- Only the amount of a marinade or frying oil that is absorbed was included.

Index

Note: *Italicized* page references indicate photographs.

A

Acorn Squash and Apple Soup, 177

Acupuncture, 22

Alfredo, tomato-, sauce, ravioli with, 174, 175

Almond-Stuffed Pork Chops, 162

Angel Hair Pasta with Avocado and Tomatoes, 114, 115

Appetite, lack of, easing, 42

Apple(s)

  acorn squash and, soup, 177

  cinnamon, 73

    potato pancakes with, 72, 73

Aromatherapy, 22

Asparagus

  barley and, 216

  fettuccine with mushrooms and, 112, 113

  ham and, bake, cheesy, 54

Attitude, good, tips for, 201

Ayurveda, 22

B

Bacon

  broccoli-, salad, 209

  dressing, hot, spinach-shrimp salad with, 124

Baked Custard, 234

Baked French Toast with Strawberry-Rhubarb Sauce, 50, 74, 75

Baking Powder Biscuits, 68, 69

Banana(s)

  berry-, smoothie, 29

Bread, 62, 63

  in Milk and Rice "Soup," 39

  raspberry-, gelatin dessert, 228, 229

  watermelon, and kiwi smoothie, 104, 105

Barley, beef-, stew, 196, 197

Barley and Asparagus, 216

Beans

  beef and, dinner, 198

  black, corn and, salad, 142, 143

  couscous and, 118

  green, chicken and, with rice, 188

Beef

  -Barley Stew, 196, 197

  and Bean Dinner, 198

  enchiladas, cheesy, 193

  Fajita Bowls, 194

  pot roast, old-fashioned, 192

  in Spaghetti and Meat Squares, 161

  stroganoff, easy, 138

  Philly sandwiches, 92

  and vegetable dinner, layered, 160

  -Vegetable Soup, 158, 159

Berry-Banana Smoothie, 29

Beverages. *See* Drink; Smoothie; Tea

Biscuits, baking powder, 68, 69

Blueberry Breakfast Bake, 55

Blueberry Brunch Cake, 67

Body Mass Index (BMI), 24

Bodywork, 22

Bone marrow transplant, 20

Bread

  banana, 62, 63

  bowl, spinach dip in, 101

  brown, easy, 64

Breaded Pork Chops, 199

Broccoli

  -Bacon Salad, 212, 213

  bake, cheesy, easy, 209

  soup, cream of, 136, 137

Bruschetta, tomato, 85

Bulgur Pilaf, 210

Burgers, salmon, 180

C

Cake

  blueberry brunch, 67

  fudge pudding, 220, 232, 233

  streusel-topped fruit brunch, 66

Calcium, foods rich in, 13–14

Cancer. *See also* specific treatments

  coping with, 8–24

  mind-body-spirit healing connection, 21–23

  nutritional needs, 13–21, 24–25

Cantaloupe and Chicken Salad, 121

Caramel dip, creamy, with fruit, 100

Caramelized Pork Slices, 139

Carbohydrates, 13

Caribbean Chicken Salad, 110, 122, 123

Carrot-Tuna Salad, 130

Casserole. *See also* Strata

  chicken, ultimate, 152, 153

  chicken noodle, 150

  crab scramble, 169

  lentil-rice, 45

  tuna, layered, 182

  wild rice, sausage and mushroom, 168

Chai Tea, 108

Cheese. *See also* Cheesy; Mozzarella

  Grits, 58

  sandwiches, grilled, 87

  sausage, and vegetable strata, 166, 167

  string, sticks, 86

  veggies and, mini-pizzas, 88, 89

Cheesy Beef Enchiladas, 193

Cheesy Chicken and Vegetable Dinner, 187

Cheesy Ham and Asparagus Bake, 54

Cheesy Pear Oven Pancake, 71

Cheesy Vegetable Soup, 178

Chemotherapy, about, 8, 10, 14, 17, 21

  enjoying food during treatment, 210

  neutropenic diet for, 20

Chicken

  Dijon, 148

  casserole, ultimate, 152, 153

  in chili sauce, pasta with, 119

  and Green Beans with Rice, 188

  Noodle Casserole, 150

  nuggets, easy, 91

  rolls, Italian, 149

  salad

    cantaloupe and, 121

    Caribbean, 110, 122, 123

layered, 145

in pitas, 94, 95

Soup with Homemade Noodles, 154

spicy citrus, 31

and vegetable dinner, cheesy, 187

and Vegetable Stir-Fry, 186

Chili, white turkey, 140, 156, 157

Chili sauce, pasta with chicken in, 119

Chopped Vegetable and Crabmeat Salad, 128, 129

Chutney-Salmon Salad, 125

Cinnamon

apples. *See* Apples

-Raisin Snack Mix, 59

Citrus-Peach Smoothie, 103

Club, turkey, squares, 190, 191

Cobbler, fruit, country, 222, 223

Complementary therapies, 21–23

Compote, hot fruit, 37

Constipation, about

coping with, 36, 49

eating plan for, 240

Constipation, recipes to ease

Baked French Toast with Strawberry-Rhubarb Sauce, 50, 74, 75

Barley and Asparagus, 216

Beef and Bean Dinner, 198

Beef Fajita Bowls, 194, 195

Beef-Barley Stew, 196, 197

Berry-Banana Smoothie, 29

Bulgur Pilaf, 211

Chicken Noodle Casserole, 150

Chicken Salad in Pitas, 94, 95

Chopped Vegetable and Crabmeat Salad, 128, 129

Corn and Black Bean Salad, 142, 143

Country Eggs in Tortilla Cups, 52, 53

Creamy Quinoa Primavera, 116, 117

Crispy Baked Fish with Tropical Fruit Salsa, 170, 184, 185

Crowd-Size Minestrone, 155

Fettuccine with Asparagus and Mushrooms, 112, 113

Fiesta Taco Salad, 131

Grilled Marinated Vegetables, 204, 205

Home-Style Oatmeal with Raisins, 57

Hot Fruit Compote, 37

Layered Beef and Vegetable Dinner, 160

Lentil-Rice Casserole, 45

Loaded Potatoes, 134

Mediterranean Couscous and Beans, 118

Old-Fashioned Beef Pot Roast, 192

Potato Pancakes with Cinnamon Apples, 72, 73

Rise 'n Shine Muffins with Creamy Orange Glaze, 65

Roasted Garlic Mashed Potatoes, 47

Sausage, Vegetable and Cheese Strata, 166, 167

Savory Black-Eyed Peas with Bacon, 214

Southwestern Pork Salad, 146, 147

Spaghetti and "Meatballs," 173

White Turkey Chili, 140, 156, 157

Cookies

drop, pumpkin, 225

Rosalie's orange butter, 227

Corn and Black Bean Salad, 142, 143

Corn and garlic risotto, creamy, 172

Country Eggs in Tortilla Cups, 52, 53

Country Fruit Cobbler, 222, 223

Couscous and beans, Mediterranean, 118

Crabmeat, chopped vegetable and, salad, 128, 129

Crab Scramble Casserole, 169

Cranberry–Herbal Tea Granita, 26, 35

Cream of Broccoli Soup, 136, 137

Creamy Caramel Dip with Fruit, 100

Creamy Corn and Garlic Risotto, 172

Creamy Quinoa Primavera, 116, 117

Creamy Seafood Risotto, 41

Crispy Baked Fish with Tropical Fruit Salsa, 170, 184, 185

Crowd-Size Minestrone, 155

Crunchy Fruit Snack Mix, 43

Cucumber sauce, 181

Custard, baked, 234

D

Diarrhea, about

coping with, 38, 49

eating plan for, 241

Diarrhea, recipes to ease

Almond-Stuffed Pork Chops, 162

Baking Powder Biscuits, 68, 69

Banana Bread, 62, 63

Blueberry Brunch Cake, 67

Caramelized Pork Slices, 139

Chai Tea, 108

Chicken and Green Beans with Rice, 188

Cinnamon Apples, 73

Country Eggs in Tortilla Cups, 52, 53

Country Fruit Cobbler, 222, 223

Crab Scramble Casserole, 169

Cream of Broccoli Soup, 136, 137

Creamy Caramel Dip with Fruit, 100

Dijon Chicken with Orzo Rice, 148

Easy Brown Bread, 64

Easy Salmon Spread, 102

Gingerbread with Brown Sugar Meringue, 231

Hot Fruit Compote, 37

Hot Turkey Sandwiches, 90

Italian Chicken Rolls, 149

Lemony Fish over Vegetables and Rice, 183

Macaroni Pasta "Soup," 135

Make-Ahead Waffles with Peanut Butter Spread, 76

Milk and Rice "Soup," 39

Orange-Pineapple Smoothie, 106

Pasta with Chicken in Chili Sauce, 119

Pumpkin Drop Cookies, 225

Raspberry-Banana Gelatin Dessert, 230

Rice Pudding, 235

Rosalie's Orange Butter Cookies, 227

Sausage, Vegetable and Cheese Strata, 166, 167

Spaghetti and Meat Squares, 161

Tropical Pancakes, 70

Wild Rice Stuffing, 215

Diets. *See also* Nutrition

liquid, 20

neutropenic, 20–21

special, 19–21

Dijon Chicken with Orzo Rice, 148

Dip. *See also* Salsa

creamy caramel, with fruit, 100

roasted vegetable, 80, 81

spinach, in bread bowl, 101

Dressing

hot bacon, spinach-shrimp salad with, 124

lime, 128

lime, creamy, 146

Drink, lemon-lime, 33

Dry mouth, coping with, 30, 34

E

Easy Beef Stroganoff, 138

Easy Brown Bread, 64

Easy Cheesy Broccoli Bake, 209

Easy Chicken Nuggets, 91

Easy Creamed Vegetables, 206

Easy Fresh-Fruit Salad, 202, 218, 219

Easy Lasagna, 164

Easy Lemon Bars, 224

Easy Salmon Spread, 102

Eggs. *See also* Frittata

in Crab Scramble Casserole, 169

poached, in milk, 56

in tortilla cups, country, 52, 53

Enchiladas, cheesy beef, 193

Exercise, 12, 23, 24

Extra-Easy Baked Ziti, 163

F

Fajita, beef, bowls, 194, 195

Fat, about, 13, 14, 16, 25

Fat calories, 25

Fatigue, coping with, 28

Fettuccine with Asparagus and Mushrooms, 112, 114

Fiber, diets low and high in, 19, 20

Fiesta Taco Salad, 131

Fish

crispy baked, with tropical fruit salsa, 170, 184, 185

lemony, over vegetables and rice, 183

Flavor booster tips, 127

Focaccia wedges, onion and rosemary, 84

French toast, with strawberry-rhubarb sauce, 50, 74, 75

Fresh Salsa, 78, 98, 99

Frittata

hash brown, 180

spinach and new potato, 179

Frosting, orange butter, 227

Frosty, orange-cream, 228

Fruit. *See also* specific names

brunch cake, 67

caramel dip with, 100

cobbler, country, 222, 223

compote, hot, 37

Parfaits, 60, 61

salad, easy fresh-, 218, 219

salad, orange-pineapple, 217

tropical, salsa, crispy baked fish with, 170, 184, 185

Fudge Pudding Cake with Ice Cream, 220, 232, 233

G

Gelatin, raspberry-banana, dessert, 230

Gift suggestions, 226

Gingerbread with Brown Sugar Meringue, 231

Glaze, creamy orange, 65

Granita, cranberry–herbal tea, 26, 35

Grilled Marinated Vegetables, 204, 205

Grits, cheese, 58

Grocery shopping, 15, 17

H

Ham and asparagus bake, cheesy, 54

Hash Brown Frittata, 180

Heartburn, coping with, 44

Herbal medicine, 23

Herbal tea granita, cranberry–, 26, 35

High-fiber diet, 20

High-residue diet, 20

Home-Style Oatmeal with Raisins, 57

Honey-Mustard Turkey with Snap Peas, 120

Hot Fruit Compote, 37

Hot Turkey Sandwiches, 90

I

Ice cream, fudge pudding cake with, 220, 232, 233

Iron, foods rich in, 13–15

Italian Chicken Rolls, 149

Italian Spaghetti Sauce, 165

K

Kiwi, watermelon, and banana smoothie, 104, 105

L

Lasagna, easy, 164

Laughter, healing and, 11, 151

Layered Beef and Vegetable Dinner, 160

Layered Chicken Salad, 145

Layered Tuna Casserole, 182

Lemon bars, easy, 224

Lemon-lime drink, refreshing, 33

Lemony Fish over Vegetables and Rice, 183

Lentil-Rice Casserole, 45

Lime, lemon-, drink, 33

Lime dressing, 128, 146

Liquid diet, 20

Loaded Potatoes, 134

Low-fiber diet, 20

Low-residue diet, 19

M

Macaroni Pasta "Soup," 135

Magnesium, foods rich in, 13

Make-Ahead Waffles with Peanut Butter Spread, 76

Mashed potatoes. *See* Potatoes

Massage, 12, 22, 23

Meals

eating out, 17–18

"Meatballs," spaghetti and, 173

Meat squares, spaghetti and, 161

Meditation, 11, 12, 23

Mediterranean Couscous and Beans, 118

Meringue, brown sugar, gingerbread with, 231

Metallic taste in food, coping with, 30

Milk and Rice "Soup," 39

Mind-body-spirit connection to healing, 21–23

Minerals, about, 13, 14

Minestrone, crowd-size, 155

Mix

cinnamon-raisin snack, 59

snack, crunchy fruit, 43

Mouth sores, about

coping with, 34, 40, 48

eating plan for, 242

Mouth sores, recipes to ease

Acorn Squash and Apple Soup, 177

Angel Hair Pasta with Avocado and Tomatoes, 114, 115

Baked Custard, 234

Barley and Asparagus, 216

Beef-Vegetable Soup, 158

Berry-Banana Smoothie, 29

Blueberry Breakfast Bake, 55

Bulgur Pilaf, 211

Chai Tea, 108

Cheese Grits, 58

Cheesy Vegetable Soup, 178

Chicken and Green Beans with Rice, 188

Chicken Soup with Homemade Noodles, 154

Cinnamon Apples, 73

Country Eggs in Tortilla Cups, 52, 53

Cranberry–Herbal Tea Granita, 26, 35

Cream of Broccoli Soup, 136, 137

Creamy Corn and Garlic Risotto, 172

Creamy Seafood Risotto, 41

Easy Creamed Vegetables, 206

Easy Lemon Bars, 224

Easy Salmon Spread, 102

Fresh Spinach and New Potato Frittata, 179

Fruit Parfaits, 60, 61

Fudge Pudding Cake with Ice Cream, 220, 232, 233

Gingerbread with Brown Sugar Meringue, 231

Grilled Marinated Vegetables, 204, 205

Hash Brown Frittata, 180

Layered Beef and Vegetable Dinner, 160

Loaded Potatoes, 134

Macaroni Pasta "Soup," 135

Mashed Potatoes, 208

Milk and Rice "Soup," 39

Orange-Cream Frosty, 228

Poached Eggs in Milk, 56

Potato-Tomato-Tofu Dinner, 132, 133

Raspberry-Banana Gelatin Dessert, 230

Rice Pudding, 235

Roasted Garlic Mashed Potatoes, 47

Sausage, Vegetable and Cheese Strata, 166, 167

Savory Black-Eyed Peas with Bacon, 214

Stir-Fried Vegetables, 207

Sugar 'n Spice Green Tea, 107

Watermelon-Kiwi-Banana Smoothie, 4, 104, 105

Mozzarella and Tomatoes, 97

Muffins with creamy orange glaze, 65

Mushroom(s)

    fettuccine with asparagus and, 112, 113

    wild rice, and sausage casserole, 168

Mustard. See Dijon; Honey-mustard

MyPlate dietary guidelines, 16

N

Naturopathy, 23

Nausea, about

    coping with, 32, 48, 77

    eating plan for, 243

Nausea, recipes to ease

    Acorn Squash and Apple Soup, 177

    Angel Hair Pasta with Avocado and Tomatoes, 114, 115

    Baked Custard, 234

    Baking Powder Biscuits, 68

    Banana Bread, 62, 63

    Beef and Bean Dinner, 198

    Beef Fajita Bowls, 194, 195

    Beef-Vegetable Soup, 158, 159

    Berry-Banana Smoothie, 29

    Blueberry Brunch Cake, 67

    Breaded Pork Chops, 199

    Bulgur Pilaf, 211

    Cantaloupe and Chicken Salad, 121

    Caramelized Pork Slices, 139

    Caribbean Chicken Salad, 110, 122, 123

    Cheesy Chicken and Vegetable Dinner, 187

    Cheesy Pear Oven Pancake, 71

    Cheesy Vegetable Soup, 178

    Chicken and Green Beans with Rice, 188

Chicken and Vegetable Stir-Fry, 186

Chicken Salad in Pitas, 94, 95

Chicken Soup with Homemade Noodles, 154

Chopped Vegetable and Crabmeat Salad, 128, 129

Chutney-Salmon Salad, 125

Cinnamon-Raisin Morning Mix, 59

Citrus-Peach Smoothie, 103

Corn and Black Bean Salad, 142, 143

Country Eggs in Tortilla Cups, 52, 53

Country Fruit Cobbler, 222, 223

Cranberry–Herbal Tea Granita, 26, 35

Creamy Caramel Dip with Fruit, 100

Crispy Baked Fish with Tropical Fruit Salsa, 170, 184, 185

Crowd-Size Minestrone, 155

Easy Brown Bread, 64

Easy Cheesy Broccoli Bake, 209

Easy Creamed Vegetables, 206

Easy Fresh Fruit Salad, 202, 218, 219

Easy Lasagna, 164

Easy Lemon Bars, 224

Easy Salmon Spread, 102

Extra-Easy Baked Ziti, 163

Fresh Salsa, 78, 98, 99

Fresh Spinach and New Potato Frittata, 179

Fruit Parfaits, 60, 61

Fudge Pudding Cake with Ice Cream, 220, 232, 233

Gingerbread with Brown Sugar Meringue, 231

Grilled Marinated Vegetables, 204, 205

Hash Brown Frittata, 180

Home-Style Oatmeal with Raisins, 57

Honey-Mustard Turkey with Snap Peas, 120

Hot Turkey Sandwiches, 90

Layered Chicken Salad, 145

Lemony Fish over Vegetables and Rice, 183

Loaded Potatoes, 134

Macaroni Pasta "Soup," 135

Old-Fashioned Beef Pot Roast, 192

Onion and Rosemary Focaccia Wedges, 84

Orange-Cream Frosty, 228

Orange-Pineapple Fruit Salad, 217

Orange-Pineapple Smoothie, 106

Oven-Fried Potato Wedges, 83

Pasta with Chicken in Chili Sauce, 119

Poached Eggs in Milk, 56

Potato and Tomato Pizza, 176

Potato-Tomato-Tofu Dinner, 132, 133

Pumpkin Drop Cookies, 225

Raspberry-Banana Gelatin Dessert, 230

Ravioli with Tomato-Alfredo Sauce, 174, 175

Refreshing Lemon-Lime Drink, 33

Rice Pudding, 235

Roasted Vegetable Dip, 80, 81

Rosalie's Orange Butter Cookies, 227

Salmon Burgers, 181

Sausage, Vegetable and Cheese Strata, 166, 167

Savory Scallops and Shrimp, 126

Spaghetti and "Meatballs," 173

Stir-Fried Vegetables, 207

Sugar 'n Spice Green Tea, 107

Tropical Pancakes, 70

Turkey Club Squares, 190, 191

Turkey Tetrazzini, 189

Watermelon-Kiwi-Banana Smoothie, 4, 104, 105

Wild Rice Stuffing, 215

Neutropenia
diet for, 20, 21
two-day eating plan for, 244

Noodle(s)
chicken, casserole, 150
homemade, chicken soup with, 154

Nutrition, sound
foods rich in essential nutrients, 13
importance of, 13–14, 24–25
special diets, 19–20

O

Oatmeal with raisins, home-style, 57

Old-Fashioned Beef Pot Roast, 192

Onion and Rosemary Focaccia Wedges, 84

Orange Butter Frosting, 227

Orange-Cream Frosty, 228. 229

Orange-Pineapple Fruit Salad, 217

Orange-Pineapple Smoothie, 106

Oven-Fried Potato Wedges, 83

P

Pancake(s)
cheesy pear oven, 71
potato, with cinnamon apples, 72, 73
tropical, 70

Pantry, stocking, 17

Parfaits, fruit, 60, 61

Pasta. See also specific names
salad, seven-layer, 144
with Chicken in Chili Sauce, 119

Peach, citrus-, smoothie, 103

Peanut butter spread, waffles with, 76

Pear oven pancake, cheesy, 71

Peas
black-eyed, with bacon, 214
snap, honey-mustard turkey with, 120

Philly Beef Sandwiches, 92

Pilaf, bulgur, 211

Pineapple. See Orange- pineapple

Pitas, chicken salad in, 94, 95

Pizza(s)
mini-, veggies and cheese, 88, 89
potato and tomato, 176

Poached Eggs in Milk, 56

Pork. See also Ham
chops, almond-stuffed, 162
chops, breaded, 199
salad, southwestern, 146, 147
slices, caramelized, 139
stew, zesty autumn, 200

Positive attitude, 11

Potassium, foods rich in, 13–14

Potato(es)
Hash Brown Frittata, 180
loaded, 134
mashed, 208
mashed, roasted garlic, 47
Pancakes with Cinnamon Apples, 72, 73
spinach and, frittata, 179
wedges, oven-fried, 83
and Tomato Pizza, 176
-Tomato-Tofu Dinner, 132, 133

Pot roast, beef, 192

Prayer, 11

Primavera, creamy quinoa, 116, 117

Protein, about, 14, 16

Pudding
fudge, cake, 220, 232, 233
rice, 235

Pumpkin Drop Cookies, 225

Q

Quesadillas, quick, 93

Quinoa primavera, creamy, 116, 117

R

Radiation (radiotherapy), 8, 14, 210
remedies, 14
enjoying food during treatment, 210

Raisin(s)
cinnamon-, snack mix, 59
oatmeal with, 57

Raspberry-Banana Gelatin Dessert, 230

Ravioli with Tomato-Alfredo Sauce, 174, 175

Refreshing Lemon-Lime Drink, 33

Relaxation techniques, 11, 12, 22–23

Residue, foods for low- and high-residue diets, 19–20

Rhubarb, strawberry-, sauce, 74

Rice
chicken and green beans with, 188
lemony fish over, 183
lentil-, casserole, 45
milk and, "soup," 39
pudding, 235
wild, sausage and mushroom casserole, 168
wild, stuffing, 215

Rise 'n Shine Muffins with Creamy Orange Glaze, 65

Risotto, creamy
corn and garlic, 172
seafood, 41

Roasted Garlic Mashed Potatoes, 47

Roasted Vegetable Dip, 80, 81

Rosalie's Orange Butter Cookies, 227

S

Salad
broccoli-bacon, 212, 213
carrot-tuna, 130
chicken. See Chicken salad
chopped vegetable and crabmeat, 128, 129
chutney-salmon, 125
corn and black bean, 142, 143
fiesta taco, 131
fruit. See Fruit salad
orange-pineapple fruit, 217
pasta, seven-layer, 144
pork, southwestern, 146, 147
spinach-shrimp, 124

Salmon
Burgers, 181
chutney-, salad, 125
spread, easy, 102

Salsa
fresh, 78, 98, 99
tropical fruit, crispy baked fish with, 170, 184, 185

Sandwiches
grilled cheese, 87
Philly beef, 92
turkey, hot, 90

Sauce
chili, pasta with chicken in, 119
cucumber, 181
spaghetti, Italian, 165
strawberry-rhubarb, French toast with, 50, 74, 75

Sausage
Vegetable and Cheese Strata, 166, 167
wild rice, and mushroom casserole, 168

Scallops and shrimp, savory, 126

Seafood. See specific names

Seven-Layer Pasta Salad, 144

Shiatsu, 22

Shrimp
  in Creamy Seafood Risotto, 41
  scallops and, savory, 126
  spinach-, salad, 124
Side effects. *See also* specific
    names
  common, key to, 48–49
  coping with, 27–49
Smoothie
  berry-banana, 29
  citrus-peach, 103
  orange-pineapple, 106
  watermelon-kiwi-banana, 104, 105
Snacks, tips for, 109
Snappy Stuffed Tomatoes, 96
Soup. *See also* "Soup"; Stew
  acorn squash and apple, 177
  beef-vegetable, 158, 159
  cheesy vegetable, 178
  chicken, with homemade
    noodles, 154
  cream of broccoli, 136, 137
  minestrone, crowd-size, 155
"Soup," macaroni pasta, 135
"Soup," milk and rice, 39
Southwestern Pork Salad, 146, 147
Spaghetti
  and "Meatballs," 173
  and Meat Squares, 161
  sauce, Italian, 165
Spicy Citrus Chicken, 31
Spinach
  Dip in Bread Bowl, 101
  and potato frittata, 179
  -Shrimp Salad with Hot Bacon
    Dressing, 124
Spread
  peanut butter, 76
  salmon, easy, 102

Squash, acorn, and apple soup, 177
Stew. *See also* Chili
  beef-barley, 196, 197
  pork, zesty autumn, 200
Stir-fry(ied)
  chicken and vegetable, 186
  vegetables, 207
Strata, sausage, vegetable and
    cheese, 166, 167
Strawberry-rhubarb sauce, French
    toast with, 50, 74, 75
Streusel-Topped Fruit Brunch
    Cake, 66
String Cheese Sticks, 86
Stuffing, wild rice, 215, 216
Sugar, brown, meringue, 231
Sugar 'n Spice Green Tea, 107
Surgery, 8, 14, 18, 20, 210
  enjoying food during treatment,
    210
  post-, suggestions, 18
Swallowing difficulties, coping
    with, 46

T

Table-setting tips, 201
Taco salad, fiesta, 131
Tea
  Chai, 108
  cranberry–herbal, granita, 26, 35
  green, sugar 'n spice, 107
Tetrazzini, turkey, 189
Tofu, potato, and tomato dinner,
    132, 133
Tomato(es)
  -Alfredo sauce, ravioli with, 174,
    175
  Bruschetta, 85

mozzarella and, 97
potato, and tofu dinner, 132, 133
and potato pizza, 176
snappy stuffed, 96
Tortilla cups, eggs in, 52, 53
Treatment. *See also* specific names
  complementary therapy, 21–23
  easy menus during and after,
    236–44
  enjoying food during, 210
Tropical fruit salsa, 170, 184, 185
Tropical Pancakes, 70
Tuna, carrot-, salad, 130
Tuna casserole, layered, 182
Turkey
  chili, white, 140, 156, 157
  Club Squares, 190
  ground, in Spaghetti and Meat
    Squares, 161
  honey-mustard, with snap peas,
    120
  sandwiches, hot, 90
  Tetrazzini, 189

U

Ultimate Chicken Casserole, The,
    152, 153

V

Vegetable(s). *See also* specific
    names
  beef and, dinner, layered, 160
  beef-, soup, 158, 159
  and Cheese Mini-Pizzas, 88, 89
  chicken and, dinner, cheesy, 187
  chicken and, stir-fry, 186
  dip, roasted, 80, 81

easy creamed, 206
grilled marinated, 204, 205
sausage, and cheese strata, 166,
  167
soup, cheesy, 178
stir-fried, 207
Vitamins, about, 13–18, 24
Vomiting, coping with, 32. *See also*
  Nausea

W

Waffles, with peanut butter spread,
  76
Watermelon-Kiwi-Banana
  Smoothie, 104, 105
White Turkey Chili, 156, 157
Wild rice. *See* Rice

Y

Yoga, 12, 23

Z

Zesty Autumn Pork Stew, 200
Ziti, baked, extra-easy, 163
Zucchini Bites, 82